THE ESSEN

MW01673523

Bella

AIR FRYER

Cookbook

500 SIMPLE, EASY AND DELICIOUS BELLA AIR FRYER RECIPES THAT ANYONE CAN COOK

RUDOLPH BRANDON

CONTENTS

Vegetarians Recipes 41

Appetizers And Snacks 62

INTRODUCTION

How Does the Bella Air Fryer Work

Air fryers heat food by convection air is heated to 320-400 degrees Fahrenheit and passed around your food at high speed to heat it and give it a crispy exterior. It browns food by a process known as the Maillard reaction, a chemical reaction that occurs between amino acids and reducing sugars. With air fryers, your food is not submerged in oil. All you need is to coat whatever it is you're trying to heat with a thin layer of oil, place it in the air fryer's basket, set the timer and temperature regulator, and you're good to go.

The Advantages of Your Bella Air Fryer

1. Remove Fat from Food

Air fryers use very little oil to cook. Even air fryers can cook food without oil. Foods cooked in other cooking methods contain high fat. As a result, food cooked in all these ways is not healthy. Many manufacturers claim that their air fryer removes up to 95% fat from fried foods.

Moreover, the air fryer cooks using very little oil compared to the traditional frying method. While many recipes require 3 cups of oil to cook in the traditional frying method, only 1 teaspoon of oil is required to cook the same recipe in an air fryer. However, the taste of food does not change much.

Air fryers use a special type of technology to remove excess fat from food that traps fat from food and stores it under the air fryer basket. Various experiments have shown that air fryers can cook delicious fried foods like the traditional frying method with very little oil. Which makes the food delicious and healthy at the same time.

2. To Lose Weight

Traditional fried foods not only contain extra fat but also extra calories. Excess calories will increase your weight. So if you want to lose weight, you should avoid fried foods. However, food cooked through an air fryer is extra calorie-free. Because air fryers use very little oil to cook fried food. With an air fryer, you can lose weight without avoiding fried foods.

3. Easy to Use and Clean

Air fryers are much easier to use. Most air fryers have a touch control system. Through which the temperature and time of the air fryer can be set very easily. However, many affordable air fryers have a knob control system. Air fryers can also be easily controlled through these. Air fryers are not only easy to use, but they are also very easy to clean. Because most air fryer baskets, trays, pans are dishwasher safe. As a result, they can be easily cleaned using soap and hot water. These must be thoroughly dried before re-using the air fryer.

Moreover, cooking in an air fryer does not require much oil. This makes it less messy and makes the cleaning process easier. Cooking in a drip fryer requires more oil so they are more dirty. An air fryer is much easier to clean than a drip fryer.

4. Safe to Use

Air fryers are much safer to use than other cooking utensils. The air fryer keeps the user safe from hot elements and hot oil. Sprinkling oil while cooking in a drip fryer is a regular occurrence. This can lead to accidents such as burning hands while cooking in a drip fryer. But there is no possibility of such an accident in an air fryer.

Moreover, most air fryers have cool-touch handles. Which will keep your hands safe from heated material. This allows you to cook safely in an air fryer. Modern air fryers have an automatic shut-off system. This automatically shuts off the air fryer when the cooking time is over. So there is no fear of burning food.

5. Use Little to No Oil to Cook Food

Cooking in traditional deep fryers often takes up to a gallon of oil. But it takes just one tablespoon of oil to cook any recipe in an air fryer. Moreover, many recipes can be cooked without oil.

There are several benefits to cooking in low oil. First of all, you need a little oil to cook in the air fryer so you don't have to spend extra money to buy cooking oil. Second, foods cooked with less oil are healthier. This is because foods cooked in low oil do not contain extra calories and fat. Third, the air fryer can be cooked with less oil so its baskets are not oily. Which makes it much easier to clean. Deep fryers on the other hand require a lot of oil to cook so it is very oily. Which makes the deep fryer very difficult to clean.

6. Take Little Space

Air fryers are usually small in size. As a result, they do not require much space in the kitchen. These are much smaller than other kitchen appliances. Air fryers are usually slightly larger than a coffee maker and smaller than a toaster oven. However, air fryers of different sizes are available in the market. You can buy small-size air fryers for small families and big-size air fryers for big families. All types of air fryers, small or large, do not require much space to be placed on the countertop.

Tips and Tricks on Using Your Bella Air Fryer

1. Preheat Your Bella Air Fryer

For a proper, it a normal practice that any cooking item should be preheated. Most air fryers recommend that the air fryer should be preheated to ensure even cooking. Often I do it, sometimes I don't do it, and my meal is still good. And in case your air fryer is without preheat feature, simply turn it to the desired temperature and allow it to run for about 3 minutes before bringing adding the food.

2. Use Oil For Food COOKED in the Bella Air Fryer

I like using oil for certain food to make them crisp, but some foods don't always need it. If your diet has some fat on it (dark meat chicken, ground beef, fatty cuts of meat, etc.) so you really don't need oil. I use vegetable oil (like my Breakfast Air Fried Potatoes) and any dried seafood, Like the Crispy Air Fryer Fish).

3. Grease Your Bella Air Fryer

Container Even if your food does not need oil, do take a moment to at least grease your air fryer container. I grease mine by rubbing or brushing a little bit of oil on the bottom of the grates. This will make sure the diet isn't going to stay on it.

4. Never Use Aerosol Spray Cans in Your Bella Air Fryer

The Aerosol spray cans (such as Pam and related brands) are known to cause chipping in many Air Fryer containers. The aerosol cans contain toxic chemicals that don't match with the covering on most of the containers.

5. Don't Overload the Basket

If you want your fried food to turn out to be fresh, you'll want to make sure you don't congest the refrigerator. Placing too much food in the bowl will keep the food from stretching and browning. Cook your food in containers or invest in a larger air fryer to make sure this doesn't happen.

6. Shake the Basket During Frying Wings and Other Food

When frying small items such as chicken wings and French fries, shake the basket every few minutes to ensure uniform cooking, sometimes, instead of throwing, use a pair of silicone kitchen pins to flip over larger items

When you open the basket to shake, the air fryer will stop for a while, but it will continue frying the food at the same temperature when you return to the container.

Hints on Cleaning Baked on Grease from the Bella Air Fryer

1) The most stubborn and irritating thing that can get stuck in an air fryer is the baked-on grease. The best way to ensure that the grease doesn't accumulate too much is to clean it after every use, if you do that, cleaning your air fryer should be quick and easy. Here's how to go about cleaning the grease out of your air fryer.

2) Unplug the air fryer and let it cool - Make sure the air fryer is off, unplugged and cool before beginning to clean it. These all sound obvious but taking a second to be sure that its ready will help you avoid hurting yourself or damaging the device.

3) Clean the basket and pans - In many air fryers, the removable baskets and pans are dishwasher safe. If this is the case, simply put the basket and pans into the dishwasher and let the dishwasher clean them for you. If not, you can simply soak the basket and pans in hot, soapy water for 10-15 minutes then gently scrub any food particles off with a non-abrasive sponge or towel. Finally, give the basket and pans a quick rinse and dry with a towel before putting them back in the air fryer. Check the manufacturer's instructions to see if the removable parts are dishwasher safe.

4) Clean the heating element - To clean the heating element, turn the air fryer upside down and wipe it down with a towel or non-abrasive sponge.

5) Clean the inside of the air fryer - Use a soft cloth or paper towels to wipe out any visible grease or food debris from the inside of the air fryer. Next, use a soft cloth, a non-abrasive sponge or a soft-bristled brush soaked in hot water with dish soap to gently scrub the bottom and sides of the inside of the air fryer.

6) Wipe down the outside of the air fryer - Grease does not just build up on the inside of the air fryer, it can also accumulate on the outside. After every use, wipe the outside of the air fryer down with a soft towel soaked in hot, soapy dishwater.

Poultry Recipes

Italian Roasted Chicken Thighs

Servings: 6

Cooking Time: 14 Minutes

Ingredients:

- 6 boneless chicken thighs
- ½ teaspoon dried oregano
- ½ teaspoon garlic powder
- ½ teaspoon sea salt
- ½ teaspoon black pepper
- ¼ teaspoon crushed red pepper flakes

Directions:

1. Pat the chicken thighs with paper towel.
2. In a small bowl, mix the oregano, garlic powder, salt, pepper, and crushed red pepper flakes. Rub the spice mixture onto the chicken thighs.
3. Preheat the air fryer to 400°F.
4. Place the chicken thighs in the air fryer basket and spray with cooking spray. Cook for 10 minutes, turn over, and cook another 4 minutes. When cooking completes, the internal temperature should read 165°F.

Buffalo Egg Rolls

Servings: 8

Cooking Time: 9 Minutes Per Batch

Ingredients:

- 1 teaspoon water
- 1 tablespoon cornstarch
- 1 egg
- 2½ cups cooked chicken, diced or shredded (see opposite page)
- ⅓ cup chopped green onion
- ⅓ cup diced celery
- ⅓ cup buffalo wing sauce
- 8 egg roll wraps
- oil for misting or cooking spray
- Blue Cheese Dip
- 3 ounces cream cheese, softened
- ⅓ cup blue cheese, crumbled
- 1 teaspoon Worcestershire sauce
- ¼ teaspoon garlic powder
- ¼ cup buttermilk (or sour cream)

Directions:

1. Mix water and cornstarch in a small bowl until dissolved. Add egg, beat well, and set aside.
2. In a medium size bowl, mix together chicken, green onion, celery, and buffalo wing sauce.
3. Divide chicken mixture evenly among 8 egg roll wraps, spooning ½ inch from one edge.
4. Moisten all edges of each wrap with beaten egg wash.
5. Fold the short ends over filling, then roll up tightly and press to seal edges.
6. Brush outside of wraps with egg wash, then spritz with oil or cooking spray.
7. Place 4 egg rolls in air fryer basket.
8. Cook at 390°F for 9minutes or until outside is brown and crispy.
9. While the rolls are cooking, prepare the Blue Cheese Dip. With a fork, mash together cream cheese and blue cheese.
10. Stir in remaining ingredients.
11. Dip should be just thick enough to slightly cling to egg rolls. If too thick, stir in buttermilk or milk 1 tablespoon at a time until you reach the desired consistency.
12. Cook remaining 4 egg rolls as in steps 7 and 8.
13. Serve while hot with Blue Cheese Dip, more buffalo wing sauce, or both.

Coconut Chicken With Apricot-ginger Sauce

Servings: 4

Cooking Time: 8 Minutes Per Batch

Ingredients:

- 1½ pounds boneless, skinless chicken tenders, cut in large chunks (about 1¼ inches)
- salt and pepper
- ½ cup cornstarch
- 2 eggs
- 1 tablespoon milk
- 3 cups shredded coconut (see below)
- oil for misting or cooking spray

- Apricot-Ginger Sauce
- ½ cup apricot preserves
- 2 tablespoons white vinegar
- ¼ teaspoon ground ginger
- ¼ teaspoon low-sodium soy sauce
- 2 teaspoons white or yellow onion, grated or finely minced

Directions:

1. Mix all ingredients for the Apricot-Ginger Sauce well and let sit for flavors to blend while you cook the chicken.
2. Season chicken chunks with salt and pepper to taste.
3. Place cornstarch in a shallow dish.
4. In another shallow dish, beat together eggs and milk.
5. Place coconut in a third shallow dish. (If also using panko breadcrumbs, as suggested below, stir them to mix well.)
6. Spray air fryer basket with oil or cooking spray.
7. Dip each chicken chunk into cornstarch, shake off excess, and dip in egg mixture.
8. Shake off excess egg mixture and roll lightly in coconut or coconut mixture. Spray with oil.
9. Place coated chicken chunks in air fryer basket in a single layer, close together but without sides touching.
10. Cook at 360°F for 4minutes, stop, and turn chunks over.
11. Cook an additional 4 minutes or until chicken is done inside and coating is crispy brown.
12. Repeat steps 9 through 11 to cook remaining chicken chunks.

Chicken Cordon Bleu

Servings: 2

Cooking Time: 16 Minutes

Ingredients:

- 2 boneless, skinless chicken breasts
- ¼ teaspoon salt
- 2 teaspoons Dijon mustard
- 2 ounces deli ham
- 2 ounces Swiss, fontina, or Gruyère cheese
- ⅓ cup all-purpose flour
- 1 egg
- ½ cup breadcrumbs

Directions:

1. Pat the chicken breasts with a paper towel. Season the chicken with the salt. Pound the chicken breasts to 1½ inches thick. Create a pouch by slicing the side of each chicken breast. Spread 1 teaspoon Dijon mustard inside the pouch of each chicken breast. Wrap a 1-ounce slice of ham around a 1-ounce slice of cheese and place into the pouch. Repeat with the remaining ham and cheese.
2. In a medium bowl, place the flour.
3. In a second bowl, whisk the egg.
4. In a third bowl, place the breadcrumbs.
5. Dredge the chicken in the flour and shake off the excess. Next, dip the chicken into the egg and then in the breadcrumbs. Set the chicken on a plate and repeat with the remaining chicken piece.
6. Preheat the air fryer to 360°F.
7. Place the chicken in the air fryer basket and spray liberally with cooking spray. Cook for 8 minutes, turn the chicken breasts over, and liberally spray with cooking spray again; cook another 6 minutes. Once golden brown, check for an internal temperature of 165°F.

Sweet-and-sour Chicken

Servings: 6

Cooking Time: 10 Minutes

Ingredients:

- 1 cup pineapple juice
- 1 cup plus 3 tablespoons cornstarch, divided
- ¼ cup sugar
- ¼ cup ketchup
- ¼ cup apple cider vinegar
- 2 tablespoons soy sauce or tamari
- 1 teaspoon garlic powder, divided
- ¼ cup flour
- 1 tablespoon sesame seeds
- ½ teaspoon salt
- ¼ teaspoon ground black pepper
- 2 large eggs
- 2 pounds chicken breasts, cut into 1-inch cubes
- 1 red bell pepper, cut into 1-inch pieces
- 1 carrot, sliced into ¼-inch-thick rounds

Directions:

1. In a medium saucepan, whisk together the pineapple juice, 3 tablespoons of the cornstarch, the sugar, the ketchup, the apple cider vinegar, the soy sauce or tamari, and ½ teaspoon of the garlic powder. Cook over medium-low heat, whisking occasionally as the sauce thickens, about 6 minutes. Stir and set aside while preparing the chicken.
2. Preheat the air fryer to 370°F.
3. In a medium bowl, place the remaining 1 cup of cornstarch, the flour, the sesame seeds, the salt, the remaining ½ teaspoon of garlic powder, and the pepper.
4. In a second medium bowl, whisk the eggs.
5. Working in batches, place the cubed chicken in the cornstarch mixture to lightly coat; then dip it into the egg mixture, and return it to the cornstarch mixture. Shake off the excess and place the coated chicken in the air fryer basket. Spray with cooking spray and cook for 5 minutes, shake the basket, and spray with more cooking spray. Cook an additional 3 to 5 minutes, or until completely cooked and golden brown.
6. On the last batch of chicken, add the bell pepper and carrot to the basket and cook with the chicken.
7. Place the cooked chicken and vegetables into a serving bowl and toss with the sweet-and-sour sauce to serve.

Chicken Parmesan

Servings: 4
Cooking Time: 11 Minutes

Ingredients:

- 4 chicken tenders
- Italian seasoning
- salt
- ¼ cup cornstarch
- ½ cup Italian salad dressing
- ¼ cup panko breadcrumbs
- ¼ cup grated Parmesan cheese, plus more for serving
- oil for misting or cooking spray
- 8 ounces spaghetti, cooked
- 1 24-ounce jar marinara sauce

Directions:

1. Pound chicken tenders with meat mallet or rolling pin until about ¼-inch thick.
2. Sprinkle both sides with Italian seasoning and salt to taste.
3. Place cornstarch and salad dressing in 2 separate shallow dishes.
4. In a third shallow dish, mix together the panko crumbs and Parmesan cheese.
5. Dip flattened chicken in cornstarch, then salad dressing. Dip in the panko mixture, pressing into the chicken so the coating sticks well.
6. Spray both sides with oil or cooking spray. Place in air fryer basket in single layer.
7. Cook at 390°F for 5minutes. Spray with oil again, turning chicken to coat both sides. See tip about turning.
8. Cook for an additional 6 minutes or until chicken juices run clear and outside is browned.
9. While chicken is cooking, heat marinara sauce and stir into cooked spaghetti.
10. To serve, divide spaghetti with sauce among 4 dinner plates, and top each with a fried chicken tender. Pass additional Parmesan at the table for those who want extra cheese.

Chicken Tikka

Servings: 4
Cooking Time: 15 Minutes

Ingredients:

- ¼ cup plain Greek yogurt
- 1 clove garlic, minced
- 1 tablespoon ketchup
- 1 tablespoon extra-virgin olive oil
- 1 tablespoon lemon juice
- ½ teaspoon salt
- ½ teaspoon ground cumin
- ½ teaspoon paprika
- ¼ teaspoon ground cinnamon
- ½ teaspoon ground black pepper
- ½ teaspoon cayenne pepper
- 1 pound boneless, skinless chicken thighs

Directions:

1. In a large bowl, stir together the yogurt, garlic, ketchup, olive oil, lemon juice, salt, cumin, paprika, cinnamon, black pepper, and cayenne pepper until combined.

2. Add the chicken thighs to the bow and fold the yogurt-spice mixture over the chicken thighs until they're covered with the marinade. Cover with plastic wrap and place in the refrigerator for 30 minutes.
3. When ready to cook the chicken, remove from the refrigerator and preheat the air fryer to 370°F.
4. Liberally spray the air fryer basket with olive oil mist. Place the chicken thighs into the air fryer basket, leaving space between the thighs to turn.
5. Cook for 10 minutes, turn the chicken thighs, and cook another 5 minutes (or until the internal temperature reaches 165°F).
6. Remove the chicken from the air fryer and serve warm with desired sides.

Chicken Wellington

Servings: 2
Cooking Time: 31 Minutes

Ingredients:

- 2 (5-ounce) boneless, skinless chicken breasts
- ½ cup White Worcestershire sauce
- 3 tablespoons butter
- ½ cup finely diced onion (about ½ onion)
- 8 ounces button mushrooms, finely chopped
- ¼ cup chicken stock
- 2 tablespoons White Worcestershire sauce (or white wine)
- salt and freshly ground black pepper
- 1 tablespoon chopped fresh tarragon
- 2 sheets puff pastry, thawed
- 1 egg, beaten
- vegetable oil

Directions:

1. Place the chicken breasts in a shallow dish. Pour the White Worcestershire sauce over the chicken coating both sides and marinate for 30 minutes.
2. While the chicken is marinating, melt the butter in a large skillet over medium-high heat on the stovetop. Add the onion and sauté for a few minutes, until it starts to soften. Add the mushrooms and sauté for 5 minutes until the vegetables are brown and soft. Deglaze the skillet with the chicken stock, scraping up any bits from the bottom of the pan. Add the White Worcestershire sauce and simmer for 3 minutes until the mixture reduces and starts to thicken. Season with salt and freshly ground black pepper. Remove the mushroom mixture from the heat and stir in the fresh tarragon. Let the mushroom mixture cool.
3. Preheat the air fryer to 360°F.
4. Remove the chicken from the marinade and transfer it to the air fryer basket. Tuck the small end of the chicken breast under the thicker part to shape it into a circle rather than an oval. Pour the marinade over the chicken and air-fry for 10 minutes.
5. Roll out the puff pastry and cut out two 6-inch squares. Brush the perimeter of each square with the egg wash. Place half of the mushroom mixture in the center of each puff pastry square. Place the chicken breasts, top side down on the mushroom mixture. Starting with one corner of puff pastry and working in one direction, pull the pastry up over the chicken to enclose it and press the ends of the pastry together in the middle. Brush the pastry with the egg wash to seal the edges. Turn the Wellingtons over and set aside.
6. To make a decorative design with the remaining puff pastry, cut out four 10-inch strips. For each Wellington, twist two of the strips together, place them over the chicken breast wrapped in puff pastry, and tuck the ends underneath to seal it. Brush the entire top and sides of the Wellingtons with the egg wash.
7. Preheat the air fryer to 350°F.
8. Spray or brush the air fryer basket with vegetable oil. Air-fry the chicken Wellingtons for 13 minutes. Carefully turn the Wellingtons over. Air-fry for another 8 minutes. Transfer to serving plates, light a candle and enjoy!

Poblano Bake

Servings: 4
Cooking Time: 11 Minutes Per Batch

Ingredients:

- 2 large poblano peppers (approx. 5½ inches long excluding stem)
- ¾ pound ground turkey, raw
- ¾ cup cooked brown rice
- 1 teaspoon chile powder

- ½ teaspoon ground cumin
- ½ teaspoon garlic powder
- 4 ounces sharp Cheddar cheese, grated
- 1 8-ounce jar salsa, warmed

Directions:

1. Slice each pepper in half lengthwise so that you have four wide, flat pepper halves.
2. Remove seeds and membrane and discard. Rinse inside and out.
3. In a large bowl, combine turkey, rice, chile powder, cumin, and garlic powder. Mix well.
4. Divide turkey filling into 4 portions and stuff one into each of the 4 pepper halves. Press lightly to pack down.
5. Place 2 pepper halves in air fryer basket and cook at 390°F for 10minutes or until turkey is well done.
6. Top each pepper half with ¼ of the grated cheese. Cook 1 more minute or just until cheese melts.
7. Repeat steps 5 and 6 to cook remaining pepper halves.
8. To serve, place each pepper half on a plate and top with ¼ cup warm salsa.

Chicken Souvlaki Gyros

Servings: 4

Cooking Time: 18 Minutes

Ingredients:

- ¼ cup extra-virgin olive oil
- 1 clove garlic, crushed
- 1 tablespoon Italian seasoning
- ½ teaspoon paprika
- ½ lemon, sliced
- ¼ teaspoon salt
- 1 pound boneless, skinless chicken breasts
- 4 whole-grain pita breads
- 1 cup shredded lettuce
- ½ cup chopped tomatoes
- ¼ cup chopped red onion
- ¼ cup cucumber yogurt sauce

Directions:

1. In a large resealable plastic bag, combine the olive oil, garlic, Italian seasoning, paprika, lemon, and salt. Add the chicken to the bag and secure shut. Vigorously shake until all the ingredients are combined. Set in the fridge for 2 hours to marinate.
2. When ready to cook, preheat the air fryer to 360°F.
3. Liberally spray the air fryer basket with olive oil mist. Remove the chicken from the bag and discard the leftover marinade. Place the chicken into the air fryer basket, allowing enough room between the chicken breasts to flip.
4. Cook for 10 minutes, flip, and cook another 8 minutes.
5. Remove the chicken from the air fryer basket when it has cooked (or the internal temperature of the chicken reaches 165°F). Let rest 5 minutes. Then thinly slice the chicken into strips.
6. Assemble the gyros by placing the pita bread on a flat surface and topping with chicken, lettuce, tomatoes, onion, and a drizzle of yogurt sauce.
7. Serve warm.

Thai Turkey And Zucchini Meatballs

Servings: 4

Cooking Time: 12 Minutes

Ingredients:

- 1½ cups grated zucchini,
- squeezed dry in a clean kitchen towel (about 1 large zucchini)
- 3 scallions, finely chopped
- 2 cloves garlic, minced
- 1 tablespoon grated fresh ginger
- 1 tablespoon finely chopped fresh cilantro
- zest of 1 lime
- 1 teaspoon salt
- freshly ground black pepper
- 1½ pounds ground turkey (a mix of light and dark meat)
- 2 eggs, lightly beaten
- 1 cup Thai sweet chili sauce (spring roll sauce)
- lime wedges, for serving

Directions:

1. Combine the zucchini, scallions, garlic, ginger, cilantro, lime zest, salt, pepper, ground turkey and eggs in a bowl and mix the ingredients together. Gently shape the mixture into 24 balls, about the size of golf balls.

2. Preheat the air fryer to 380°F.
3. Working in batches, air-fry the meatballs for 12 minutes, turning the meatballs over halfway through the cooking time. As soon as the meatballs have finished cooking, toss them in a bowl with the Thai sweet chili sauce to coat.
4. Serve the meatballs over rice noodles or white rice with the remaining Thai sweet chili sauce and lime wedges to squeeze over the top.

Teriyaki Chicken Drumsticks

Servings: 2
Cooking Time: 17 Minutes

Ingredients:

- 2 tablespoons soy sauce*
- ¼ cup dry sherry
- 1 tablespoon brown sugar
- 2 tablespoons water
- 1 tablespoon rice wine vinegar
- 1 clove garlic, crushed
- 1-inch fresh ginger, peeled and sliced
- pinch crushed red pepper flakes
- 4 to 6 bone-in, skin-on chicken drumsticks
- 1 tablespoon cornstarch
- fresh cilantro leaves

Directions:

1. Make the marinade by combining the soy sauce, dry sherry, brown sugar, water, rice vinegar, garlic, ginger and crushed red pepper flakes. Pour the marinade over the chicken legs, cover and let the chicken marinate for 1 to 4 hours in the refrigerator.
2. Preheat the air fryer to 380°F.
3. Transfer the chicken from the marinade to the air fryer basket, transferring any extra marinade to a small saucepan. Air-fry at 380°F for 8 minutes. Flip the chicken over and continue to air-fry for another 6 minutes, watching to make sure it doesn't brown too much.
4. While the chicken is cooking, bring the reserved marinade to a simmer on the stovetop. Dissolve the cornstarch in 2 tablespoons of water and stir this into the saucepan. Bring to a boil to thicken the sauce. Remove the garlic clove and slices of ginger from the sauce and set aside.
5. When the time is up on the air fryer, brush the thickened sauce on the chicken and air-fry for 3 more minutes. Remove the chicken from the air fryer and brush with the remaining sauce.
6. Serve over rice and sprinkle the cilantro leaves on top.

Pickle Brined Fried Chicken

Servings: 4
Cooking Time: 47 Minutes

Ingredients:

- 4 bone-in, skin-on chicken legs, cut into drumsticks and thighs (about 3½ pounds)
- pickle juice from a 24-ounce jar of kosher dill pickles
- ½ cup flour
- salt and freshly ground black pepper
- 2 eggs
- 1 cup fine breadcrumbs
- 1 teaspoon salt
- 1 teaspoon freshly ground black pepper
- ½ teaspoon ground paprika
- ⅛ teaspoon ground cayenne pepper
- vegetable or canola oil in a spray bottle

Directions:

1. Place the chicken in a shallow dish and pour the pickle juice over the top. Cover and transfer the chicken to the refrigerator to brine in the pickle juice for 3 to 8 hours.
2. When you are ready to cook, remove the chicken from the refrigerator to let it come to room temperature while you set up a dredging station. Place the flour in a shallow dish and season well with salt and freshly ground black pepper. Whisk the eggs in a second shallow dish. In a third shallow dish, combine the breadcrumbs, salt, pepper, paprika and cayenne pepper.
3. Preheat the air fryer to 370°F.
4. Remove the chicken from the pickle brine and gently dry it with a clean kitchen towel. Dredge each piece of chicken in the flour, then dip it into the egg mixture, and finally press it into the breadcrumb mixture to coat all sides of the chicken. Place the breaded chicken

on a plate or baking sheet and spray each piece all over with vegetable oil.

5. Air-fry the chicken in two batches. Place two chicken thighs and two drumsticks into the air fryer basket. Air-fry for 10 minutes. Then, gently turn the chicken pieces over and air-fry for another 10 minutes. Remove the chicken pieces and let them rest on plate – do not cover. Repeat with the second batch of chicken, air-frying for 20 minutes, turning the chicken over halfway through.

6. Lower the temperature of the air fryer to 340°F. Place the first batch of chicken on top of the second batch already in the basket and air-fry for an additional 7 minutes. Serve warm and enjoy.

Nacho Chicken Fries

Servings: 4

Cooking Time: 7 Minutes

Ingredients:

- 1 pound chicken tenders
- salt
- ¼ cup flour
- 2 eggs
- ¾ cup panko breadcrumbs
- ¾ cup crushed organic nacho cheese tortilla chips
- oil for misting or cooking spray
- Seasoning Mix
- 1 tablespoon chili powder
- 1 teaspoon ground cumin
- ½ teaspoon garlic powder
- ½ teaspoon onion powder

Directions:

1. Stir together all seasonings in a small cup and set aside.
2. Cut chicken tenders in half crosswise, then cut into strips no wider than about ½ inch.
3. Preheat air fryer to 390°F.
4. Salt chicken to taste. Place strips in large bowl and sprinkle with 1 tablespoon of the seasoning mix. Stir well to distribute seasonings.
5. Add flour to chicken and stir well to coat all sides.
6. Beat eggs together in a shallow dish.
7. In a second shallow dish, combine the panko, crushed chips, and the remaining 2 teaspoons of seasoning mix.
8. Dip chicken strips in eggs, then roll in crumbs. Mist with oil or cooking spray.
9. Chicken strips will cook best if done in two batches. They can be crowded and overlapping a little but not stacked in double or triple layers.
10. Cook for 4minutes. Shake basket, mist with oil, and cook 3 moreminutes, until chicken juices run clear and outside is crispy.
11. Repeat step 10 to cook remaining chicken fries.

Turkey-hummus Wraps

Servings: 4

Cooking Time: 7 Minutes Per Batch

Ingredients:

- 4 large whole wheat wraps
- ½ cup hummus
- 16 thin slices deli turkey
- 8 slices provolone cheese
- 1 cup fresh baby spinach (or more to taste)

Directions:

1. To assemble, place 2 tablespoons of hummus on each wrap and spread to within about a half inch from edges. Top with 4 slices of turkey and 2 slices of provolone. Finish with ¼ cup of baby spinach—or pile on as much as you like.
2. Roll up each wrap. You don't need to fold or seal the ends.
3. Place 2 wraps in air fryer basket, seam side down.
4. Cook at 360°F for 4minutes to warm filling and melt cheese. If you like, you can continue cooking for 3 more minutes, until the wrap is slightly crispy.
5. Repeat step 4 to cook remaining wraps.

Coconut Curry Chicken With Coconut Rice

Servings: 4

Cooking Time: 56 Minutes

Ingredients:

- 1 (14-ounce) can coconut milk

- 2 tablespoons green or red curry paste
- zest and juice of one lime
- 1 clove garlic, minced
- 1 tablespoon grated fresh ginger
- 1 teaspoon ground cumin
- 1 (3- to 4-pound) chicken, cut into 8 pieces
- vegetable or olive oil
- salt and freshly ground black pepper
- fresh cilantro leaves
- For the rice:
- 1 cup basmati or jasmine rice
- 1 cup water
- 1 cup coconut milk
- ½ teaspoon salt
- freshly ground black pepper

Directions:

1. Make the marinade by combining the coconut milk, curry paste, lime zest and juice, garlic, ginger and cumin. Coat the chicken on all sides with the marinade and marinate the chicken for 1 hour to overnight in the refrigerator.
2. Preheat the air fryer to 380°F.
3. Brush the bottom of the air fryer basket with oil. Transfer the chicken thighs and drumsticks from the marinade to the air fryer basket, letting most of the marinade drip off. Season to taste with salt and freshly ground black pepper.
4. Air-fry the chicken drumsticks and thighs at 380°F for 12 minutes. Flip the chicken over and continue to air-fry for another 12 minutes. Set aside and air-fry the chicken breast pieces at 380°F for 15 minutes. Turn the chicken breast pieces over and air-fry for another 12 minutes. Return the chicken thighs and drumsticks to the air fryer and air-fry for an additional 5 minutes.
5. While the chicken is cooking, make the coconut rice. Rinse the rice kernels with water and drain well. Place the rice in a medium saucepan with a tight fitting lid, along with the water, coconut milk, salt and freshly ground black pepper. Bring the mixture to a boil and then cover, reduce the heat and let it cook gently for 20 minutes without lifting the lid. When the time is up, lift the lid, fluff with a fork and set aside.
6. Remove the chicken from the air fryer and serve warm with the coconut rice and fresh cilantro scattered around.

Parmesan Chicken Fingers

Servings: 2

Cooking Time: 19 Minutes

Ingredients:

- ½ cup flour
- 1 teaspoon salt
- freshly ground black pepper
- 2 eggs, beaten
- ¾ cup seasoned panko breadcrumbs
- ¾ cup grated Parmesan cheese
- 8 chicken tenders (about 1 pound)
- OR
- 2 to 3 boneless, skinless chicken breasts, cut into strips
- vegetable oil
- marinara sauce

Directions:

1. Set up a dredging station. Combine the flour, salt and pepper in a shallow dish. Place the beaten eggs in second shallow dish, and combine the panko breadcrumbs and Parmesan cheese in a third shallow dish.
2. Dredge the chicken tenders in the flour mixture. Then dip them into the egg, and finally place the chicken in the breadcrumb mixture. Press the coating onto both sides of the chicken tenders. Place the coated chicken tenders on a baking sheet until they are all coated. Spray both sides of the chicken fingers with vegetable oil.
3. Preheat the air fryer to 360°F.
4. Air-fry the chicken fingers in two batches. Transfer half the chicken fingers to the air fryer basket and air-fry for 9 minutes, turning the chicken over halfway through the cooking time. When the second batch of chicken fingers has finished cooking, return the first batch to the air fryer with the second batch and air-fry for one minute to heat everything through.
5. Serve immediately with marinara sauce, honey-mustard, ketchup or your favorite dipping sauce.

Quick Chicken For Filling

Servings: 2
Cooking Time: 8 Minutes

Ingredients:

- 1 pound chicken tenders, skinless and boneless
- ½ teaspoon ground cumin
- ½ teaspoon garlic powder
- cooking spray

Directions:

1. Sprinkle raw chicken tenders with seasonings.
2. Spray air fryer basket lightly with cooking spray to prevent sticking.
3. Place chicken in air fryer basket in single layer.
4. Cook at 390°F for 4minutes, turn chicken strips over, and cook for an additional 4minutes.
5. Test for doneness. Thick tenders may require an additional minute or two.

Chicken Nuggets

Servings: 20
Cooking Time: 14 Minutes Per Batch

Ingredients:

- 1 pound boneless, skinless chicken thighs, cut into 1-inch chunks
- ¾ teaspoon salt
- ½ teaspoon black pepper
- ½ teaspoon garlic powder
- ½ teaspoon onion powder
- ½ cup flour
- 2 eggs, beaten
- ½ cup panko breadcrumbs
- 3 tablespoons plain breadcrumbs
- oil for misting or cooking spray

Directions:

1. In the bowl of a food processor, combine chicken, ½ teaspoon salt, pepper, garlic powder, and onion powder. Process in short pulses until chicken is very finely chopped and well blended.
2. Place flour in one shallow dish and beaten eggs in another. In a third dish or plastic bag, mix together the panko crumbs, plain breadcrumbs, and ¼ teaspoon salt.
3. Shape chicken mixture into small nuggets. Dip nuggets in flour, then eggs, then panko crumb mixture.
4. Spray nuggets on both sides with oil or cooking spray and place in air fryer basket in a single layer, close but not overlapping.
5. Cook at 360°F for 10minutes. Spray with oil and cook 4 minutes, until chicken is done and coating is golden brown.
6. Repeat step 5 to cook remaining nuggets.

Chicken Fried Steak With Gravy

Servings: 4
Cooking Time: 10 Minutes Per Batch

Ingredients:

- ½ cup flour
- 2 teaspoons salt, divided
- freshly ground black pepper
- ¼ teaspoon garlic powder
- 1 cup buttermilk
- 1 cup fine breadcrumbs
- 4 tenderized top round steaks (about 6 to 8 ounces each; ½-inch thick)
- vegetable or canola oil
- For the Gravy:
- 2 tablespoons butter or bacon drippings
- ¼ onion, minced (about ¼ cup)
- 1 clove garlic, smashed
- ¼ teaspoon dried thyme
- 3 tablespoons flour
- 1 cup milk
- salt and lots of freshly ground black pepper
- a few dashes of Worcestershire sauce

Directions:

1. Set up a dredging station. Combine the flour, 1 teaspoon of salt, black pepper and garlic powder in a shallow bowl. Pour the buttermilk into a second shallow bowl. Finally, put the breadcrumbs and 1 teaspoon of salt in a third shallow bowl.
2. Dip the tenderized steaks into the flour, then the buttermilk, and then the breadcrumb mixture, pressing the crumbs onto the steak. Place them on a baking sheet and spray both sides generously with vegetable or canola oil.

3. Preheat the air fryer to 400°F.
4. Transfer the steaks to the air fryer basket, two at a time, and air-fry for 10 minutes, flipping the steaks over halfway through the cooking time. This will cook your steaks to medium. If you want the steaks cooked a little more or less, add or subtract a minute or two. Hold the first batch of steaks warm in a 170°F oven while you cook the second batch.
5. While the steaks are cooking, make the gravy. Melt the butter in a small saucepan over medium heat on the stovetop. Add the onion, garlic and thyme and cook for five minutes, until the onion is soft and just starting to brown. Stir in the flour and cook for another five minutes, stirring regularly, until the mixture starts to brown. Whisk in the milk and bring the mixture to a boil to thicken. Season to taste with salt, lots of freshly ground black pepper and a few dashes of Worcestershire sauce.
6. Plate the chicken fried steaks with mashed potatoes and vegetables and serve the gravy at the table to pour over the top.

Spicy Black Bean Turkey Burgers With Cumin-avocado Spread

Servings: 2

Cooking Time: 20 Minutes

Ingredients:

- 1 cup canned black beans, drained and rinsed
- ¾ pound lean ground turkey
- 2 tablespoons minced red onion
- 1 Jalapeño pepper, seeded and minced
- 2 tablespoons plain breadcrumbs
- ½ teaspoon chili powder
- ¼ teaspoon cayenne pepper
- salt, to taste
- olive or vegetable oil
- 2 slices pepper jack cheese
- toasted burger rolls, sliced tomatoes, lettuce leaves
- Cumin-Avocado Spread:
- 1 ripe avocado
- juice of 1 lime
- 1 teaspoon ground cumin
- ½ teaspoon salt
- 1 tablespoon chopped fresh cilantro
- freshly ground black pepper

Directions:

1. Place the black beans in a large bowl and smash them slightly with the back of a fork. Add the ground turkey, red onion, Jalapeño pepper, breadcrumbs, chili powder and cayenne pepper. Season with salt. Mix with your hands to combine all the ingredients and then shape them into 2 patties. Brush both sides of the burger patties with a little olive or vegetable oil.
2. Preheat the air fryer to 380°F.
3. Transfer the burgers to the air fryer basket and air-fry for 20 minutes, flipping them over halfway through the cooking process. Top the burgers with the pepper jack cheese (securing the slices to the burgers with a toothpick) for the last 2 minutes of the cooking process.
4. While the burgers are cooking, make the cumin avocado spread. Place the avocado, lime juice, cumin and salt in food processor and process until smooth. (For a chunkier spread, you can mash this by hand in a bowl.) Stir in the cilantro and season with freshly ground black pepper. Chill the spread until you are ready to serve.
5. When the burgers have finished cooking, remove them from the air fryer and let them rest on a plate, covered gently with aluminum foil. Brush a little olive oil on the insides of the burger rolls. Place the rolls, cut side up, into the air fryer basket and air-fry at 400°F for 1 minute to toast and warm them.
6. Spread the cumin-avocado spread on the rolls and build your burgers with lettuce and sliced tomatoes and any other ingredient you like. Serve warm with a side of sweet potato fries.

Mediterranean Stuffed Chicken Breasts

Servings: 4

Cooking Time: 24 Minutes

Ingredients:

- 4 boneless, skinless chicken breasts
- ½ teaspoon salt
- ½ teaspoon black pepper
- ½ teaspoon garlic powder
- ½ teaspoon paprika
- ½ cup canned artichoke hearts, chopped
- 4 ounces cream cheese
- ¼ cup grated Parmesan cheese

Directions:

1. Pat the chicken breasts with a paper towel. Using a sharp knife, cut a pouch in the side of each chicken breast for filling.
2. In a small bowl, mix the salt, pepper, garlic powder, and paprika. Season the chicken breasts with this mixture.
3. In a medium bowl, mix together the artichokes, cream cheese, and grated Parmesan cheese. Divide the filling between the 4 breasts, stuffing it inside the pouches. Use toothpicks to close the pouches and secure the filling.
4. Preheat the air fryer to 360°F.
5. Spray the air fryer basket liberally with cooking spray, add the stuffed chicken breasts to the basket, and spray liberally with cooking spray again. Cook for 14 minutes, carefully turn over the chicken breasts, and cook another 10 minutes. Check the temperature at 20 minutes cooking. Chicken breasts are fully cooked when the center measures 165°F. Cook in batches, if needed.

Chicken Cutlets With Broccoli Rabe And Roasted Peppers

Servings: 2

Cooking Time: 10 Minutes

Ingredients:

- ½ bunch broccoli rabe
- olive oil, in a spray bottle
- salt and freshly ground black pepper
- ⅔ cup roasted red pepper strips
- 2 (4-ounce) boneless, skinless chicken breasts
- 2 tablespoons all-purpose flour*
- 1 egg, beaten
- ⅓ cup seasoned breadcrumbs*
- 2 slices aged provolone cheese

Directions:

1. Bring a medium saucepot of salted water to a boil on the stovetop. Blanch the broccoli rabe for 3 minutes in the boiling water and then drain. When it has cooled a little, squeeze out as much water as possible, drizzle a little olive oil on top, season with salt and black pepper and set aside. Dry the roasted red peppers with a clean kitchen towel and set them aside as well.
2. Place each chicken breast between 2 pieces of plastic wrap. Use a meat pounder to flatten the chicken breasts to about ½-inch thick. Season the chicken on both sides with salt and pepper.
3. Preheat the air fryer to 400°F.
4. Set up a dredging station with three shallow dishes. Place the flour in one dish, the egg in a second dish and the breadcrumbs in a third dish. Coat the chicken on all sides with the flour. Shake off any excess flour and dip the chicken into the egg. Let the excess egg drip off and coat both sides of the chicken in the breadcrumbs. Spray the chicken with olive oil on both sides and transfer to the air fryer basket.
5. Air-fry the chicken at 400°F for 5 minutes. Turn the chicken over and air-fry for another minute. Then, top the chicken breast with the broccoli rabe and roasted peppers. Place a slice of the provolone cheese on top and secure it with a toothpick or two.
6. Air-fry at 360° for 3 to 4 minutes to melt the cheese and warm everything together.

Sweet Chili Spiced Chicken

Servings: 4

Cooking Time: 43 Minutes

Ingredients:

- Spice Rub:
- 2 tablespoons brown sugar
- 2 tablespoons paprika
- 1 teaspoon dry mustard powder
- 1 teaspoon chili powder

- 2 tablespoons coarse sea salt or kosher salt
- 2 teaspoons coarsely ground black pepper
- 1 tablespoon vegetable oil
- 1 (3½-pound) chicken, cut into 8 pieces

Directions:

1. Prepare the spice rub by combining the brown sugar, paprika, mustard powder, chili powder, salt and pepper. Rub the oil all over the chicken pieces and then rub the spice mix onto the chicken, covering completely. This is done very easily in a zipper sealable bag. You can do this ahead of time and let the chicken marinate in the refrigerator, or just proceed with cooking right away.
2. Preheat the air fryer to 370°F.
3. Air-fry the chicken in two batches. Place the two chicken thighs and two drumsticks into the air fryer basket. Air-fry at 370°F for 10 minutes. Then, gently turn the chicken pieces over and air-fry for another 10 minutes. Remove the chicken pieces and let them rest on a plate while you cook the chicken breasts. Air-fry the chicken breasts, skin side down for 8 minutes. Turn the chicken breasts over and air-fry for another 12 minutes.
4. Lower the temperature of the air fryer to 340°F. Place the first batch of chicken on top of the second batch already in the basket and air-fry for a final 3 minutes.
5. Let the chicken rest for 5 minutes and serve warm with some mashed potatoes and a green salad or vegetables.

Chicken Rochambeau

Servings: 4

Cooking Time: 20 Minutes

Ingredients:

- 1 tablespoon butter
- 4 chicken tenders, cut in half crosswise
- salt and pepper
- ¼ cup flour
- oil for misting
- 4 slices ham, ¼- to ⅜-inches thick and large enough to cover an English muffin
- 2 English muffins, split
- Sauce
- 2 tablespoons butter
- ½ cup chopped green onions
- ½ cup chopped mushrooms
- 2 tablespoons flour
- 1 cup chicken broth
- ¼ teaspoon garlic powder
- 1½ teaspoons Worcestershire sauce

Directions:

1. Place 1 tablespoon of butter in air fryer baking pan and cook at 390°F for 2minutes to melt.
2. Sprinkle chicken tenders with salt and pepper to taste, then roll in the ¼ cup of flour.
3. Place chicken in baking pan, turning pieces to coat with melted butter.
4. Cook at 390°F for 5minutes. Turn chicken pieces over, and spray tops lightly with olive oil. Cook 5minutes longer or until juices run clear. The chicken will not brown.
5. While chicken is cooking, make the sauce: In a medium saucepan, melt the 2 tablespoons of butter.
6. Add onions and mushrooms and sauté until tender, about 3minutes.
7. Stir in the flour. Gradually add broth, stirring constantly until you have a smooth gravy.
8. Add garlic powder and Worcestershire sauce and simmer on low heat until sauce thickens, about 5minutes.
9. When chicken is cooked, remove baking pan from air fryer and set aside.
10. Place ham slices directly into air fryer basket and cook at 390°F for 5minutes or until hot and beginning to sizzle a little. Remove and set aside on top of the chicken for now.
11. Place the English muffin halves in air fryer basket and cook at 390°F for 1 minute.
12. Open air fryer and place a ham slice on top of each English muffin half. Stack 2 pieces of chicken on top of each ham slice. Cook at 390°F for 1 to 2minutes to heat through.
13. Place each English muffin stack on a serving plate and top with plenty of sauce.

Air-fried Turkey Breast With Cherry Glaze

Servings: 6

Cooking Time: 54 Minutes

Ingredients:

- 1 (5-pound) turkey breast
- 2 teaspoons olive oil
- 1 teaspoon dried thyme
- ½ teaspoon dried sage
- 1 teaspoon salt
- ½ teaspoon freshly ground black pepper
- ½ cup cherry preserves
- 1 tablespoon chopped fresh thyme leaves
- 1 teaspoon soy sauce*
- freshly ground black pepper

Directions:

1. All turkeys are built differently, so depending on the turkey breast and how your butcher has prepared it, you may need to trim the bottom of the ribs in order to get the turkey to sit upright in the air fryer basket without touching the heating element. The key to this recipe is getting the right size turkey breast. Once you've managed that, the rest is easy, so make sure your turkey breast fits into the air fryer basket before you Preheat the air fryer.
2. Preheat the air fryer to 350°F.
3. Brush the turkey breast all over with the olive oil. Combine the thyme, sage, salt and pepper and rub the outside of the turkey breast with the spice mixture.
4. Transfer the seasoned turkey breast to the air fryer basket, breast side up, and air-fry at 350°F for 25 minutes. Turn the turkey breast on its side and air-fry for another 12 minutes. Turn the turkey breast on the opposite side and air-fry for 12 more minutes. The internal temperature of the turkey breast should reach 165°F when fully cooked.
5. While the turkey is air-frying, make the glaze by combining the cherry preserves, fresh thyme, soy sauce and pepper in a small bowl. When the cooking time is up, return the turkey breast to an upright position and brush the glaze all over the turkey. Air-fry for a final 5 minutes, until the skin is nicely browned and crispy. Let the turkey rest, loosely tented with foil, for at least 5 minutes before slicing and serving.

Jerk Chicken Drumsticks

Servings: 2

Cooking Time: 20 Minutes

Ingredients:

- 1 or 2 cloves garlic
- 1 inch of fresh ginger
- 2 serrano peppers, (with seeds if you like it spicy, seeds removed for less heat)
- 1 teaspoon ground allspice
- 1 teaspoon ground nutmeg
- 1 teaspoon chili powder
- ½ teaspoon dried thyme
- ½ teaspoon ground cinnamon
- ½ teaspoon paprika
- 1 tablespoon brown sugar
- 1 teaspoon soy sauce
- 2 tablespoons vegetable oil
- 6 skinless chicken drumsticks

Directions:

1. Combine all the ingredients except the chicken in a small chopper or blender and blend to a paste. Make slashes into the meat of the chicken drumsticks and rub the spice blend all over the chicken (a pair of plastic gloves makes this really easy). Transfer the rubbed chicken to a non-reactive covered container and let the chicken marinate for at least 30 minutes or overnight in the refrigerator.
2. Preheat the air fryer to 400°F.
3. Transfer the drumsticks to the air fryer basket. Air-fry for 10 minutes. Turn the drumsticks over and air-fry for another 10 minutes. Serve warm with some rice and vegetables or a green salad.

Lemon Sage Roast Chicken

Servings: 4

Cooking Time: 60 Minutes

Ingredients:

- 1 (4-pound) chicken
- 1 bunch sage, divided
- 1 lemon, zest and juice
- salt and freshly ground black pepper

Directions:

1. Preheat the air fryer to 350°F and pour a little water into the bottom of the air fryer drawer. (This will help prevent the grease that drips into the bottom drawer from burning and smoking.)
2. Run your fingers between the skin and flesh of the chicken breasts and thighs. Push a couple of sage leaves up underneath the skin of the chicken on each breast and each thigh.
3. Push some of the lemon zest up under the skin of the chicken next to the sage. Sprinkle some of the zest inside the chicken cavity, and reserve any leftover zest. Squeeze the lemon juice all over the chicken and in the cavity as well.
4. Season the chicken, inside and out, with the salt and freshly ground black pepper. Set a few sage leaves aside for the final garnish. Crumple up the remaining sage leaves and push them into the cavity of the chicken, along with one of the squeezed lemon halves.
5. Place the chicken breast side up into the air fryer basket and air-fry for 20 minutes at 350°F. Flip the chicken over so that it is breast side down and continue to air-fry for another 20 minutes. Return the chicken to breast side up and finish air-frying for 20 more minutes. The internal temperature of the chicken should register 165°F in the thickest part of the thigh when fully cooked. Remove the chicken from the air fryer and let it rest on a cutting board for at least 5 minutes.
6. Cut the rested chicken into pieces, sprinkle with the reserved lemon zest and garnish with the reserved sage leaves.

Philly Chicken Cheesesteak Stromboli

Servings: 2

Cooking Time: 28 Minutes

Ingredients:

- ½ onion, sliced
- 1 teaspoon vegetable oil
- 2 boneless, skinless chicken breasts, partially frozen and sliced very thin on the bias (about 1 pound)
- 1 tablespoon Worcestershire sauce
- salt and freshly ground black pepper
- ½ recipe of Blue Jean Chef pizza dough (see page 229), or 14 ounces of store-bought pizza dough
- 1½ cups grated Cheddar cheese
- ½ cup Cheese Whiz® (or other jarred cheese sauce), warmed gently in the microwave
- tomato ketchup for serving

Directions:

1. Preheat the air fryer to 400°F.
2. Toss the sliced onion with oil and air-fry for 8 minutes, stirring halfway through the cooking time. Add the sliced chicken and Worcestershire sauce to the air fryer basket, and toss to evenly distribute the ingredients. Season the mixture with salt and freshly ground black pepper and air-fry for 8 minutes, stirring a couple of times during the cooking process. Remove the chicken and onion from the air fryer and let the mixture cool a little.
3. On a lightly floured surface, roll or press the pizza dough out into a 13-inch by 11-inch rectangle, with the long side closest to you. Sprinkle half of the Cheddar cheese over the dough leaving an empty 1-inch border from the edge farthest away from you. Top the cheese with the chicken and onion mixture, spreading it out evenly. Drizzle the cheese sauce over the meat and sprinkle the remaining Cheddar cheese on top.
4. Start rolling the stromboli away from you and toward the empty border. Make sure the filling stays tightly tucked inside the roll. Finally, tuck the ends of the dough in and pinch the seam shut. Place the seam side down and shape the Stromboli into a U-shape to fit in the air-fry basket. Cut 4 small slits with the tip of a sharp knife evenly in the top of the dough and lightly brush the stromboli with a little oil.
5. Preheat the air fryer to 370°F.

6. Spray or brush the air fryer basket with oil and transfer the U-shaped stromboli to the air fryer basket. Air-fry for 12 minutes, turning the stromboli over halfway through the cooking time. (Use a plate to invert the stromboli out of the air fryer basket and then slide it back into the basket off the plate.)
7. To remove, carefully flip stromboli over onto a cutting board. Let it rest for a couple of minutes before serving. Slice the stromboli into 3-inch pieces and serve with ketchup for dipping, if desired.

Parmesan Crusted Chicken Cordon Bleu

Servings: 2
Cooking Time: 14 Minutes

Ingredients:

- 2 (6-ounce) boneless, skinless chicken breasts
- salt and freshly ground black pepper
- 1 tablespoon Dijon mustard
- 4 slices Swiss cheese
- 4 slices deli-sliced ham
- ¼ cup all-purpose flour*
- 1 egg, beaten
- ¾ cup panko breadcrumbs*
- ⅓ cup grated Parmesan cheese
- olive oil, in a spray bottle

Directions:

1. Butterfly the chicken breasts. Place the chicken breast on a cutting board and press down on the breast with the palm of your hand. Slice into the long side of the chicken breast, parallel to the cutting board, but not all the way through to the other side. Open the chicken breast like a "book". Place a piece of plastic wrap over the chicken breast and gently pound it with a meat mallet to make it evenly thick.
2. Season the chicken with salt and pepper. Spread the Dijon mustard on the inside of each chicken breast. Layer one slice of cheese on top of the mustard, then top with the 2 slices of ham and the other slice of cheese.
3. Starting with the long edge of the chicken breast, roll the chicken up to the other side. Secure it shut with 1 or 2 toothpicks.
4. Preheat the air fryer to 350°F.
5. Set up a dredging station with three shallow dishes. Place the flour in the first dish. Place the beaten egg in the second shallow dish. Combine the panko breadcrumbs and Parmesan cheese together in the third shallow dish. Dip the stuffed and rolled chicken breasts in the flour, then the beaten egg and then roll in the breadcrumb-cheese mixture to cover on all sides. Press the crumbs onto the chicken breasts with your hands to make sure they are well adhered. Spray the chicken breasts with olive oil and transfer to the air fryer basket.
6. Air-fry at 350°F for 14 minutes, flipping the breasts over halfway through the cooking time. Let the chicken rest for a few minutes before removing the toothpicks, slicing and serving.

Honey Lemon Thyme Glazed Cornish Hen

Servings: 2
Cooking Time: 20 Minutes

Ingredients:

- 1 (2-pound) Cornish game hen, split in half
- olive oil
- salt and freshly ground black pepper
- ¼ teaspoon dried thyme
- ¼ cup honey
- 1 tablespoon lemon zest
- juice of 1 lemon
- 1½ teaspoons chopped fresh thyme leaves
- ½ teaspoon soy sauce
- freshly ground black pepper

Directions:

1. Split the game hen in half by cutting down each side of the backbone and then cutting through the breast. Brush or spray both halves of the game hen with the olive oil and then season with the salt, pepper and dried thyme.
2. Preheat the air fryer to 390°F.
3. Place the game hen, skin side down, into the air fryer and air-fry for 5 minutes. Turn the hen halves over and air-fry for 10 minutes.

4. While the hen is cooking, combine the honey, lemon zest and juice, fresh thyme, soy sauce and pepper in a small bowl.
5. When the air fryer timer rings, brush the honey glaze onto the game hen and continue to air-fry for another 3 to 5 minutes, just until the hen is nicely glazed, browned and has an internal temperature of 165°F.
6. Let the hen rest for 5 minutes and serve warm.

Nashville Hot Chicken

Servings: 4
Cooking Time: 27 Minutes

Ingredients:

- 1 (4-pound) chicken, cut into 6 pieces (2 breasts, 2 thighs and 2 drumsticks)
- 2 eggs
- 1 cup buttermilk
- 2 cups all-purpose flour
- 2 tablespoons paprika
- 1 teaspoon garlic powder
- 1 teaspoon onion powder
- 2 teaspoons salt
- 1 teaspoon freshly ground black pepper
- vegetable oil, in a spray bottle
- Nashville Hot Sauce:
- 1 tablespoon cayenne pepper
- 1 teaspoon salt
- ¼ cup vegetable oil
- 4 slices white bread
- dill pickle slices

Directions:

1. Cut the chicken breasts into 2 pieces so that you have a total of 8 pieces of chicken.
2. Set up a two-stage dredging station. Whisk the eggs and buttermilk together in a bowl. Combine the flour, paprika, garlic powder, onion powder, salt and black pepper in a zipper-sealable plastic bag. Dip the chicken pieces into the egg-buttermilk mixture, then toss them in the seasoned flour, coating all sides. Repeat this procedure (egg mixture and then flour mixture) one more time. This can be a little messy, but make sure all sides of the chicken are completely covered. Spray the chicken with vegetable oil and set aside.
3. Preheat the air fryer to 370°F. Spray or brush the bottom of the air-fryer basket with a little vegetable oil.
4. Air-fry the chicken in two batches at 370°F for 20 minutes, flipping the pieces over halfway through the cooking process. Transfer the chicken to a plate, but do not cover. Repeat with the second batch of chicken.
5. Lower the temperature on the air fryer to 340°F. Flip the chicken back over and place the first batch of chicken on top of the second batch already in the basket. Air-fry for another 7 minutes.
6. While the chicken is air-frying, combine the cayenne pepper and salt in a bowl. Heat the vegetable oil in a small saucepan and when it is very hot, add it to the spice mix, whisking until smooth. It will sizzle briefly when you add it to the spices. Place the fried chicken on top of the white bread slices and brush the hot sauce all over chicken. Top with the pickle slices and serve warm. Enjoy the heat and the flavor!

Southern-style Chicken Legs

Servings: 6
Cooking Time: 20 Minutes

Ingredients:

- 2 cups buttermilk
- 1 tablespoon hot sauce
- 12 chicken legs
- ½ teaspoon salt
- ½ teaspoon pepper
- 1 teaspoon paprika
- ½ teaspoon onion powder
- 1 teaspoon garlic powder
- 1 cup all-purpose flour

Directions:

1. In an airtight container, place the buttermilk, hot sauce, and chicken legs and refrigerate for 4 to 8 hours.
2. In a medium bowl, whisk together the salt, pepper, paprika, onion powder, garlic powder, and flour. Drain the chicken legs from the buttermilk and dip the chicken legs into the flour mixture, stirring to coat well.
3. Preheat the air fryer to 390°F.
4. Place the chicken legs in the air fryer basket and spray with cooking spray. Cook for 10 minutes, turn the

chicken legs over, and cook for another 8 to 10 minutes. Check for an internal temperature of 165°F.

Crispy Fried Onion Chicken Breasts

Servings: 2

Cooking Time: 13 Minutes

Ingredients:

- ¼ cup all-purpose flour*
- salt and freshly ground black pepper
- 1 egg
- 2 tablespoons Dijon mustard
- 1½ cups crispy fried onions (like French's®)
- ½ teaspoon paprika
- 2 (5-ounce) boneless, skinless chicken breasts
- vegetable or olive oil, in a spray bottle

Directions:

1. Preheat the air fryer to 380°F.
2. Set up a dredging station with three shallow dishes. Place the flour in the first shallow dish and season well with salt and freshly ground black pepper. Combine the egg and Dijon mustard in a second shallow dish and whisk until smooth. Place the fried onions in a sealed bag and using a rolling pin, crush them into coarse crumbs. Combine these crumbs with the paprika in the third shallow dish.
3. Dredge the chicken breasts in the flour. Shake off any excess flour and dip them into the egg mixture. Let any excess egg drip off. Then coat both sides of the chicken breasts with the crispy onions. Press the crumbs onto the chicken breasts with your hands to make sure they are well adhered.
4. Spray or brush the bottom of the air fryer basket with oil. Transfer the chicken breasts to the air fryer basket and air-fry at 380°F for 13 minutes, turning the chicken over halfway through the cooking time.
5. Serve immediately.

Chicken Chunks

Servings: 4

Cooking Time: 10 Minutes

Ingredients:

- 1 pound chicken tenders cut in large chunks, about 1½ inches
- salt and pepper
- ½ cup cornstarch
- 2 eggs, beaten
- 1 cup panko breadcrumbs
- oil for misting or cooking spray

Directions:

1. Season chicken chunks to your liking with salt and pepper.
2. Dip chicken chunks in cornstarch. Then dip in egg and shake off excess. Then roll in panko crumbs to coat well.
3. Spray all sides of chicken chunks with oil or cooking spray.
4. Place chicken in air fryer basket in single layer and cook at 390°F for 5minutes. Spray with oil, turn chunks over, and spray other side.
5. Cook for an additional 5minutes or until chicken juices run clear and outside is golden brown.
6. Repeat steps 4 and 5 to cook remaining chicken.

Maple Bacon Wrapped Chicken Breasts

Servings: 2

Cooking Time: 18 Minutes

Ingredients:

- 2 (6-ounce) boneless, skinless chicken breasts
- 2 tablespoons maple syrup, divided
- freshly ground black pepper
- 6 slices thick-sliced bacon
- fresh celery or parsley leaves
- Ranch Dressing:
- ¼ cup mayonnaise
- ¼ cup buttermilk
- ¼ cup Greek yogurt
- 1 tablespoon chopped fresh chives
- 1 tablespoon chopped fresh parsley
- 1 tablespoon chopped fresh dill
- 1 tablespoon lemon juice
- salt and freshly ground black pepper

Directions:

1. Brush the chicken breasts with half the maple syrup and season with freshly ground black pepper. Wrap three

slices of bacon around each chicken breast, securing the ends with toothpicks.

2. Preheat the air fryer to 380°F.

3. Air-fry the chicken for 6 minutes. Then turn the chicken breasts over, pour more maple syrup on top and air-fry for another 6 minutes. Turn the chicken breasts one more time, brush the remaining maple syrup all over and continue to air-fry for a final 6 minutes.

4. While the chicken is cooking, prepare the dressing by combining all the dressing ingredients together in a bowl.

5. When the chicken has finished cooking, remove the toothpicks and serve each breast with a little dressing drizzled over each one. Scatter lots of fresh celery or parsley leaves on top.

Pecan Turkey Cutlets

Servings: 4

Cooking Time: 12 Minutes

Ingredients:

- ¾ cup panko breadcrumbs
- ¼ teaspoon salt
- ¼ teaspoon pepper
- ¼ teaspoon dry mustard
- ¼ teaspoon poultry seasoning
- ½ cup pecans
- ¼ cup cornstarch
- 1 egg, beaten
- 1 pound turkey cutlets, ½-inch thick
- salt and pepper
- oil for misting or cooking spray

Directions:

1. Place the panko crumbs, ¼ teaspoon salt, ¼ teaspoon pepper, mustard, and poultry seasoning in food processor. Process until crumbs are finely crushed. Add pecans and process in short pulses just until nuts are finely chopped. Go easy so you don't overdo it!
2. Preheat air fryer to 360°F.
3. Place cornstarch in one shallow dish and beaten egg in another. Transfer coating mixture from food processor into a third shallow dish.
4. Sprinkle turkey cutlets with salt and pepper to taste.
5. Dip cutlets in cornstarch and shake off excess. Then dip in beaten egg and roll in crumbs, pressing to coat well. Spray both sides with oil or cooking spray.
6. Place 2 cutlets in air fryer basket in a single layer and cook for 12 minutes or until juices run clear.
7. Repeat step 6 to cook remaining cutlets.

Crispy Duck With Cherry Sauce

Servings: 2

Cooking Time: 33 Minutes

Ingredients:

- 1 whole duck (up to 5 pounds), split in half, back and rib bones removed
- 1 teaspoon olive oil
- salt and freshly ground black pepper
- Cherry Sauce:
- 1 tablespoon butter
- 1 shallot, minced
- ½ cup sherry
- ¾ cup cherry preserves 1 cup chicken stock
- 1 teaspoon white wine vinegar
- 1 teaspoon fresh thyme leaves
- salt and freshly ground black pepper

Directions:

1. Preheat the air fryer to 400°F.
2. Trim some of the fat from the duck. Rub olive oil on the duck and season with salt and pepper. Place the duck halves in the air fryer basket, breast side up and facing the center of the basket.
3. Air-fry the duck for 20 minutes. Turn the duck over and air-fry for another 6 minutes.
4. While duck is air-frying, make the cherry sauce. Melt the butter in a large sauté pan. Add the shallot and sauté until it is just starting to brown – about 2 to 3 minutes. Add the sherry and deglaze the pan by scraping up any brown bits from the bottom of the pan. Simmer the liquid for a few minutes, until it has reduced by half. Add the cherry preserves, chicken stock and white wine vinegar. Whisk well to combine all the ingredients. Simmer the sauce until it thickens and coats the back of a spoon – about 5 to 7 minutes. Season with salt and pepper and stir in the fresh thyme leaves.

5. When the air fryer timer goes off, spoon some cherry sauce over the duck and continue to air-fry at 400°F for 4 more minutes. Then, turn the duck halves back over so that the breast side is facing up. Spoon more cherry sauce over the top of the duck, covering the skin completely. Air-fry for 3 more minutes and then remove the duck to a plate to rest for a few minutes.
6. Serve the duck in halves, or cut each piece in half again for a smaller serving. Spoon any additional sauce over the duck or serve it on the side.

Chicken Strips

Servings: 4
Cooking Time: 8 Minutes

Ingredients:

- 1 pound chicken tenders
- Marinade
- ¼ cup olive oil
- 2 tablespoons water
- 2 tablespoons honey
- 2 tablespoons white vinegar
- ½ teaspoon salt
- ½ teaspoon crushed red pepper
- 1 teaspoon garlic powder
- 1 teaspoon onion powder
- ½ teaspoon paprika

Directions:

1. Combine all marinade ingredients and mix well.
2. Add chicken and stir to coat. Cover tightly and let marinate in refrigerator for 30minutes.
3. Remove tenders from marinade and place them in a single layer in the air fryer basket.
4. Cook at 390°F for 3minutes. Turn tenders over and cook for 5 minutes longer or until chicken is done and juices run clear.
5. Repeat step 4 to cook remaining tenders.

Fiesta Chicken Plate

Servings: 4
Cooking Time: 15 Minutes

Ingredients:

- 1 pound boneless, skinless chicken breasts (2 large breasts)
- 2 tablespoons lime juice
- 1 teaspoon cumin
- ½ teaspoon salt
- ½ cup grated Pepper Jack cheese
- 1 16-ounce can refried beans
- ½ cup salsa
- 2 cups shredded lettuce
- 1 medium tomato, chopped
- 2 avocados, peeled and sliced
- 1 small onion, sliced into thin rings
- sour cream
- tortilla chips (optional)

Directions:

1. Split each chicken breast in half lengthwise.
2. Mix lime juice, cumin, and salt together and brush on all surfaces of chicken breasts.
3. Place in air fryer basket and cook at 390°F for 15 minutes, until well done.
4. Divide the cheese evenly over chicken breasts and cook for an additional minute to melt cheese.
5. While chicken is cooking, heat refried beans on stovetop or in microwave.
6. When ready to serve, divide beans among 4 plates. Place chicken breasts on top of beans and spoon salsa over. Arrange the lettuce, tomatoes, and avocados artfully on each plate and scatter with the onion rings.
7. Pass sour cream at the table and serve with tortilla chips if desired.

Simple Buttermilk Fried Chicken

Servings: 4
Cooking Time: 27 Minutes

Ingredients:

- 1 (4-pound) chicken, cut into 8 pieces
- 2 cups buttermilk
- hot sauce (optional)
- 1½ cups flour*
- 2 teaspoons paprika
- 1 teaspoon salt
- freshly ground black pepper
- 2 eggs, lightly beaten

- vegetable oil, in a spray bottle

Directions:

1. Cut the chicken into 8 pieces and submerge them in the buttermilk and hot sauce, if using. A zipper-sealable plastic bag works well for this. Let the chicken soak in the buttermilk for at least one hour or even overnight in the refrigerator.
2. Set up a dredging station. Mix the flour, paprika, salt and black pepper in a clean zipper-sealable plastic bag. Whisk the eggs and place them in a shallow dish. Remove four pieces of chicken from the buttermilk and transfer them to the bag with the flour. Shake them around to coat on all sides. Remove the chicken from the flour, shaking off any excess flour, and dip them into the beaten egg. Return the chicken to the bag of seasoned flour and shake again. Set the coated chicken aside and repeat with the remaining four pieces of chicken.
3. Preheat the air fryer to 370°F.
4. Spray the chicken on all sides with the vegetable oil and then transfer one batch to the air fryer basket. Air-fry the chicken at 370°F for 20 minutes, flipping the pieces over halfway through the cooking process, taking care not to knock off the breading. Transfer the chicken to a plate, but do not cover. Repeat with the second batch of chicken.
5. Lower the temperature on the air fryer to 340°F. Flip the chicken back over and place the first batch of chicken on top of the second batch already in the basket. Air-fry for another 7 minutes and serve warm.

Chicken Flautas

Servings: 6

Cooking Time: 8 Minutes

Ingredients:

- 6 tablespoons whipped cream cheese
- 1 cup shredded cooked chicken
- 6 tablespoons mild pico de gallo salsa
- ⅓ cup shredded Mexican cheese
- ½ teaspoon taco seasoning
- Six 8-inch flour tortillas
- 2 cups shredded lettuce
- ½ cup guacamole

Directions:

1. Preheat the air fryer to 370°F.
2. In a large bowl, mix the cream cheese, chicken, salsa, shredded cheese, and taco seasoning until well combined.
3. Lay the tortillas on a flat surface. Divide the cheese-and-chicken mixture into 6 equal portions; then place the mixture in the center of the tortillas, spreading evenly, leaving about 1 inch from the edge of the tortilla.
4. Spray the air fryer basket with olive oil spray. Roll up the flautas and place them edge side down into the basket. Lightly mist the top of the flautas with olive oil spray.
5. Repeat until the air fryer basket is full. You may need to cook these in batches, depending on the size of your air fryer.
6. Cook for 7 minutes, or until the outer edges are browned.
7. Remove from the air fryer basket and serve warm over a bed of shredded lettuce with guacamole on top.

Asian Meatball Tacos

Servings: 4

Cooking Time: 10 Minutes

Ingredients:

- 1 pound lean ground turkey
- 3 tablespoons soy sauce
- 1 tablespoon brown sugar
- ½ teaspoon onion powder
- ½ teaspoon garlic powder
- 1 tablespoon sesame seeds
- 1 English cucumber
- 4 radishes
- 2 tablespoons white wine vinegar
- 1 lime, juiced and divided
- 1 tablespoon avocado oil
- Salt, to taste
- ½ cup Greek yogurt
- 1 to 3 teaspoons Sriracha, based on desired spiciness
- 1 cup shredded cabbage
- ¼ cup chopped cilantro
- Eight 6-inch flour tortillas

Directions:

1. Preheat the air fryer to 360°F.

2. In a large bowl, mix the ground turkey, soy sauce, brown sugar, onion powder, garlic powder, and sesame seeds. Form the meat into 1-inch meatballs and place in the air fryer basket. Cook for 5 minutes, shake the basket, and cook another 5 minutes. Using a food thermometer, make sure the internal temperature of the meatballs is 165°F.

3. Meanwhile, dice the cucumber and radishes and place in a medium bowl. Add the white wine vinegar, 1 teaspoon of the lime juice, and the avocado oil, and stir to coat. Season with salt to desired taste.

4. In a large bowl, mix the Greek yogurt, Sriracha, and the remaining lime juice, and stir. Add in the cabbage and cilantro; toss well to create a slaw.

5. In a heavy skillet, heat the tortillas over medium heat for 1 to 2 minutes on each side, or until warmed.

6. To serve, place a tortilla on a plate, top with 5 meatballs, then with cucumber and radish salad, and finish with 2 tablespoons of cabbage slaw.

Sesame Orange Chicken

Servings: 2

Cooking Time: 9 Minutes

Ingredients:

- 1 pound boneless, skinless chicken breasts, cut into cubes
- salt and freshly ground black pepper
- ¼ cup cornstarch
- 2 eggs, beaten
- 1½ cups panko breadcrumbs
- vegetable or peanut oil, in a spray bottle
- 12 ounces orange marmalade
- 1 tablespoon soy sauce
- 1 teaspoon minced ginger
- 2 tablespoons hoisin sauce
- 1 tablespoon sesame oil
- sesame seeds, toasted

Directions:

1. Season the chicken pieces with salt and pepper. Set up a dredging station. Put the cornstarch in a zipper-sealable plastic bag. Place the beaten eggs in a bowl and put the panko breadcrumbs in a shallow dish. Transfer the seasoned chicken to the bag with the cornstarch and shake well to completely coat the chicken on all sides. Remove the chicken from the bag, shaking off any excess cornstarch and dip the pieces into the egg. Let any excess egg drip from the chicken and transfer into the breadcrumbs, pressing the crumbs onto the chicken pieces with your hands. Spray the chicken pieces with vegetable or peanut oil.

2. Preheat the air fryer to 400°F.

3. Combine the orange marmalade, soy sauce, ginger, hoisin sauce and sesame oil in a saucepan. Bring the mixture to a boil on the stovetop, lower the heat and simmer for 10 minutes, until the sauce has thickened. Set aside and keep warm.

4. Transfer the coated chicken to the air fryer basket and air-fry at 400°F for 9 minutes, shaking the basket a few times during the cooking process to help the chicken cook evenly.

5. Right before serving, toss the browned chicken pieces with the sesame orange sauce. Serve over white rice with steamed broccoli. Sprinkle the sesame seeds on top.

Taquitos

Servings: 12

Cooking Time: 6 Minutes Per Batch

Ingredients:

- 1 teaspoon butter
- 2 tablespoons chopped green onions
- 1 cup cooked chicken, shredded
- 2 tablespoons chopped green chiles
- 2 ounces Pepper Jack cheese, shredded
- 4 tablespoons salsa
- ½ teaspoon lime juice
- ¼ teaspoon cumin
- ½ teaspoon chile powder
- ⅛ teaspoon garlic powder
- 12 corn tortillas
- oil for misting or cooking spray

Directions:

1. Melt butter in a saucepan over medium heat. Add green onions and sauté a minute or two, until tender.

2. Remove from heat and stir in the chicken, green chiles, cheese, salsa, lime juice, and seasonings.

3. Preheat air fryer to 390°F.
4. To soften refrigerated tortillas, wrap in damp paper towels and microwave for 30 to 60 seconds, until slightly warmed.
5. Remove one tortilla at a time, keeping others covered with the damp paper towels. Place a heaping tablespoon of filling into tortilla, roll up and secure with toothpick. Spray all sides with oil or cooking spray.
6. Place taquitos in air fryer basket, either in a single layer or stacked. To stack, leave plenty of space between taquitos and alternate the direction of the layers, 4 on the bottom lengthwise, then 4 more on top crosswise.
7. Cook for 6minutes or until brown and crispy.
8. Repeat steps 6 and 7 to cook remaining taquitos.
9. Serve hot with guacamole, sour cream, salsa or all three!

Crispy "fried" Chicken

Servings: 4
Cooking Time: 14 Minutes

Ingredients:

- ¾ cup all-purpose flour
- ½ teaspoon paprika
- ¼ teaspoon black pepper
- ¼ teaspoon salt
- 2 large eggs
- 1½ cups panko breadcrumbs
- 1 pound boneless, skinless chicken tenders

Directions:

1. Preheat the air fryer to 400°F.
2. In a shallow bowl, mix the flour with the paprika, pepper, and salt.
3. In a separate bowl, whisk the eggs; set aside.
4. In a third bowl, place the breadcrumbs.
5. Liberally spray the air fryer basket with olive oil spray.
6. Pat the chicken tenders dry with a paper towel. Dredge the tenders one at a time in the flour, then dip them in the egg, and toss them in the breadcrumb coating. Repeat until all tenders are coated.
7. Set each tender in the air fryer, leaving room on each side of the tender to allow for flipping.
8. When the basket is full, cook 4 to 7 minutes, flip, and cook another 4 to 7 minutes.
9. Remove the tenders and let cool 5 minutes before serving. Repeat until all tenders are cooked.

Peachy Chicken Chunks With Cherries

Servings: 4
Cooking Time: 16 Minutes

Ingredients:

- ⅓ cup peach preserves
- 1 teaspoon ground rosemary
- ½ teaspoon black pepper
- ½ teaspoon salt
- ½ teaspoon marjoram
- 1 teaspoon light olive oil
- 1 pound boneless chicken breasts, cut in 1½-inch chunks
- oil for misting or cooking spray
- 10-ounce package frozen unsweetened dark cherries, thawed and drained

Directions:

1. In a medium bowl, mix together peach preserves, rosemary, pepper, salt, marjoram, and olive oil.
2. Stir in chicken chunks and toss to coat well with the preserve mixture.
3. Spray air fryer basket with oil or cooking spray and lay chicken chunks in basket.
4. Cook at 390°F for 7minutes. Stir. Cook for 8 more minutes or until chicken juices run clear.
5. When chicken has cooked through, scatter the cherries over and cook for additional minute to heat cherries.

Spinach And Feta Stuffed Chicken Breasts

Servings: 4
Cooking Time: 27 Minutes

Ingredients:

- 1 (10-ounce) package frozen spinach, thawed and drained well
- 1 cup feta cheese, crumbled
- ½ teaspoon freshly ground black pepper

- 4 boneless chicken breasts
- salt and freshly ground black pepper
- 1 tablespoon olive oil

Directions:

1. Prepare the filling. Squeeze out as much liquid as possible from the thawed spinach. Rough chop the spinach and transfer it to a mixing bowl with the feta cheese and the freshly ground black pepper.
2. Prepare the chicken breast. Place the chicken breast on a cutting board and press down on the chicken breast with one hand to keep it stabilized. Make an incision about 1-inch long in the fattest side of the breast. Move the knife up and down inside the chicken breast, without poking through either the top or the bottom, or the other side of the breast. The inside pocket should be about 3-inches long, but the opening should only be about 1-inch wide. If this is too difficult, you can make the incision longer, but you will have to be more careful when cooking the chicken breast since this will expose more of the stuffing.
3. Once you have prepared the chicken breasts, use your fingers to stuff the filling into each pocket, spreading the mixture down as far as you can.
4. Preheat the air fryer to 380°F.
5. Lightly brush or spray the air fryer basket and the chicken breasts with olive oil. Transfer two of the stuffed chicken breasts to the air fryer. Air-fry for 12 minutes, turning the chicken breasts over halfway through the cooking time. Remove the chicken to a resting plate and air-fry the second two breasts for 12 minutes. Return the first batch of chicken to the air fryer with the second batch and air-fry for 3 more minutes. When the chicken is cooked, an instant read thermometer should register 165°F in the thickest part of the chicken, as well as in the stuffing.
6. Remove the chicken breasts and let them rest on a cutting board for 2 to 3 minutes. Slice the chicken on the bias and serve with the slices fanned out.

Southern-fried Chicken Livers

Servings: 4

Cooking Time: 12 Minutes

Ingredients:

- 2 eggs
- 2 tablespoons water
- ¾ cup flour
- 1½ cups panko breadcrumbs
- ½ cup plain breadcrumbs
- 1 teaspoon salt
- ½ teaspoon black pepper
- 20 ounces chicken livers, salted to taste
- oil for misting or cooking spray

Directions:

1. Beat together eggs and water in a shallow dish. Place the flour in a separate shallow dish.
2. In the bowl of a food processor, combine the panko, plain breadcrumbs, salt, and pepper. Process until well mixed and panko crumbs are finely crushed. Place crumbs in a third shallow dish.
3. Dip livers in flour, then egg wash, and then roll in panko mixture to coat well with crumbs.
4. Spray both sides of livers with oil or cooking spray. Cooking in two batches, place livers in air fryer basket in single layer.
5. Cook at 390°F for 7minutes. Spray livers, turn over, and spray again. Cook for 5 more minutes, until done inside and coating is golden brown.
6. Repeat to cook remaining livers.

Chicken Schnitzel Dogs

Servings: 4

Cooking Time: 10 Minutes

Ingredients:

- ½ cup flour
- ½ teaspoon salt
- 1 teaspoon marjoram
- 1 teaspoon dried parsley flakes
- ½ teaspoon thyme
- 1 egg
- 1 teaspoon lemon juice
- 1 teaspoon water
- 1 cup breadcrumbs
- 4 chicken tenders, pounded thin
- oil for misting or cooking spray
- 4 whole-grain hotdog buns
- 4 slices Gouda cheese

- 1 small Granny Smith apple, thinly sliced
- ½ cup shredded Napa cabbage
- coleslaw dressing

Directions:

1. In a shallow dish, mix together the flour, salt, marjoram, parsley, and thyme.
2. In another shallow dish, beat together egg, lemon juice, and water.
3. Place breadcrumbs in a third shallow dish.
4. Cut each of the flattened chicken tenders in half lengthwise.
5. Dip flattened chicken strips in flour mixture, then egg wash. Let excess egg drip off and roll in breadcrumbs. Spray both sides with oil or cooking spray.
6. Cook at 390°F for 5minutes. Spray with oil, turn over, and spray other side.
7. Cook for 3 to 5minutes more, until well done and crispy brown.
8. To serve, place 2 schnitzel strips on bottom of each hot dog bun. Top with cheese, sliced apple, and cabbage. Drizzle with coleslaw dressing and top with other half of bun.

Teriyaki Chicken Legs

Servings: 2

Cooking Time: 20 Minutes

Ingredients:

- 4 tablespoons teriyaki sauce
- 1 tablespoon orange juice
- 1 teaspoon smoked paprika
- 4 chicken legs
- cooking spray

Directions:

1. Mix together the teriyaki sauce, orange juice, and smoked paprika. Brush on all sides of chicken legs.
2. Spray air fryer basket with nonstick cooking spray and place chicken in basket.
3. Cook at 360°F for 6minutes. Turn and baste with sauce. Cook for 6 moreminutes, turn and baste. Cook for 8 minutes more, until juices run clear when chicken is pierced with a fork.

Chicken Adobo

Servings: 6

Cooking Time: 12 Minutes

Ingredients:

- 6 boneless chicken thighs
- ¼ cup soy sauce or tamari
- ½ cup rice wine vinegar
- 4 cloves garlic, minced
- ⅛ teaspoon crushed red pepper flakes
- ½ teaspoon black pepper

Directions:

1. Place the chicken thighs into a resealable plastic bag with the soy sauce or tamari, the rice wine vinegar, the garlic, and the crushed red pepper flakes. Seal the bag and let the chicken marinate at least 1 hour in the refrigerator.
2. Preheat the air fryer to 400°F.
3. Drain the chicken and pat dry with a paper towel. Season the chicken with black pepper and liberally spray with cooking spray.
4. Place the chicken in the air fryer basket and cook for 9 minutes, turn over at 9 minutes and check for an internal temperature of 165°F, and cook another 3 minutes.

Cornish Hens With Honey-lime Glaze

Servings: 2

Cooking Time: 30 Minutes

Ingredients:

- 1 Cornish game hen (1½–2 pounds)
- 1 tablespoon honey
- 1 tablespoon lime juice
- 1 teaspoon poultry seasoning
- salt and pepper
- cooking spray

Directions:

1. To split the hen into halves, cut through breast bone and down one side of the backbone.
2. Mix the honey, lime juice, and poultry seasoning together and brush or rub onto all sides of the hen. Season to taste with salt and pepper.

3. Spray air fryer basket with cooking spray and place hen halves in the basket, skin-side down.
4. Cook at 330°F for 30 minutes. Hen will be done when juices run clear when pierced at leg joint with a fork. Let hen rest for 5 to 10minutes before cutting.

Jerk Turkey Meatballs

Servings: 7
Cooking Time: 8 Minutes

Ingredients:

- 1 pound lean ground turkey
- ¼ cup chopped onion
- 1 teaspoon minced garlic
- ½ teaspoon dried thyme
- ¼ teaspoon ground cinnamon
- 1 teaspoon cayenne pepper
- ½ teaspoon paprika
- ½ teaspoon salt
- ⅛ teaspoon black pepper
- ¼ teaspoon red pepper flakes
- 2 teaspoons brown sugar
- 1 large egg, whisked
- ⅓ cup panko breadcrumbs
- 2⅓ cups cooked brown Jasmine rice
- 2 green onions, chopped
- ¾ cup sweet onion dressing

Directions:

1. Preheat the air fryer to 350°F.
2. In a medium bowl, mix the ground turkey with the onion, garlic, thyme, cinnamon, cayenne pepper, paprika, salt, pepper, red pepper flakes, and brown sugar. Add the whisked egg and stir in the breadcrumbs until the turkey starts to hold together.
3. Using a 1-ounce scoop, portion the turkey into meatballs. You should get about 28 meatballs.
4. Spray the air fryer basket with olive oil spray.
5. Place the meatballs into the air fryer basket and cook for 5 minutes, shake the basket, and cook another 2 to 4 minutes (or until the internal temperature of the meatballs reaches 165°F).
6. Remove the meatballs from the basket and repeat for the remaining meatballs.
7. Serve warm over a bed of rice with chopped green onions and spicy Caribbean jerk dressing.

Gluten-free Nutty Chicken Fingers

Servings: 4
Cooking Time: 10 Minutes

Ingredients:

- ½ cup gluten-free flour
- ½ teaspoon garlic powder
- ¼ teaspoon onion powder
- ¼ teaspoon black pepper
- ¼ teaspoon salt
- 1 cup walnuts, pulsed into coarse flour
- ½ cup gluten-free breadcrumbs
- 2 large eggs
- 1 pound boneless, skinless chicken tenders

Directions:

1. Preheat the air fryer to 400°F.
2. In a medium bowl, mix the flour, garlic, onion, pepper, and salt. Set aside.
3. In a separate bowl, mix the walnut flour and breadcrumbs.
4. In a third bowl, whisk the eggs.
5. Liberally spray the air fryer basket with olive oil spray.
6. Pat the chicken tenders dry with a paper towel. Dredge the tenders one at a time in the flour, then dip them in the egg, and toss them in the breadcrumb coating. Repeat until all tenders are coated.
7. Set each tender in the air fryer, leaving room on each side of the tender to allow for flipping.
8. When the basket is full, cook 5 minutes, flip, and cook another 5 minutes. Check the internal temperature after cooking completes; it should read 165°F. If it does not, cook another 2 to 4 minutes.
9. Remove the tenders and let cool 5 minutes before serving. Repeat until all the tenders are cooked.

Tandoori Chicken Legs

Servings: 2

Cooking Time: 30 Minutes

Ingredients:

- 1 cup plain yogurt
- 2 cloves garlic, minced
- 1 tablespoon grated fresh ginger
- 2 teaspoons paprika
- 2 teaspoons ground coriander
- 1 teaspoon ground turmeric
- 1 teaspoon salt
- ¼ teaspoon ground cayenne pepper
- juice of 1 lime
- 2 bone-in, skin-on chicken legs
- fresh cilantro leaves

Directions:

1. Make the marinade by combining the yogurt, garlic, ginger, spices and lime juice. Make slashes into the chicken legs to help the marinade penetrate the meat. Pour the marinade over the chicken legs, cover and let the chicken marinate for at least an hour or overnight in the refrigerator.
2. Preheat the air fryer to 380°F.
3. Transfer the chicken legs from the marinade to the air fryer basket, reserving any extra marinade. Air-fry for 15 minutes. Flip the chicken over and pour the remaining marinade over the top. Air-fry for another 15 minutes, watching to make sure it doesn't brown too much. If it does start to get too brown, you can loosely tent the chicken with aluminum foil, tucking the ends of the foil under the chicken to stop it from blowing around.
4. Serve over rice with some fresh cilantro on top.

Buttermilk-fried Drumsticks

Servings: 2

Cooking Time: 25 Minutes

Ingredients:

- 1 egg
- ½ cup buttermilk
- ¾ cup self-rising flour
- ¾ cup seasoned panko breadcrumbs
- 1 teaspoon salt
- ¼ teaspoon ground black pepper (to mix into coating)
- 4 chicken drumsticks, skin on
- oil for misting or cooking spray

Directions:

1. Beat together egg and buttermilk in shallow dish.
2. In a second shallow dish, combine the flour, panko crumbs, salt, and pepper.
3. Sprinkle chicken legs with additional salt and pepper to taste.
4. Dip legs in buttermilk mixture, then roll in panko mixture, pressing in crumbs to make coating stick. Mist with oil or cooking spray.
5. Spray air fryer basket with cooking spray.
6. Cook drumsticks at 360°F for 10minutes. Turn pieces over and cook an additional 10minutes.
7. Turn pieces to check for browning. If you have any white spots that haven't begun to brown, spritz them with oil or cooking spray. Continue cooking for 5 more minutes or until crust is golden brown and juices run clear. Larger, meatier drumsticks will take longer to cook than small ones.

Thai Chicken Drumsticks

Servings: 4

Cooking Time: 20 Minutes

Ingredients:

- 2 tablespoons soy sauce
- ¼ cup rice wine vinegar
- 2 tablespoons chili garlic sauce
- 2 tablespoons sesame oil
- 1 teaspoon minced fresh ginger
- 2 teaspoons sugar
- ½ teaspoon ground coriander
- juice of 1 lime
- 8 chicken drumsticks (about 2½ pounds)
- ¼ cup chopped peanuts
- chopped fresh cilantro
- lime wedges

Directions:

1. Combine the soy sauce, rice wine vinegar, chili sauce, sesame oil, ginger, sugar, coriander and lime juice in a large bowl and mix together. Add the chicken drumsticks and marinate for 30 minutes.

2. Preheat the air fryer to 370°F.
3. Place the chicken in the air fryer basket. It's ok if the ends of the drumsticks overlap a little. Spoon half of the marinade over the chicken, and reserve the other half.
4. Air-fry for 10 minutes. Turn the chicken over and pour the rest of the marinade over the chicken. Air-fry for an additional 10 minutes.
5. Transfer the chicken to a plate to rest and cool to an edible temperature. Pour the marinade from the bottom of the air fryer into a small saucepan and bring it to a simmer over medium-high heat. Simmer the liquid for 2 minutes so that it thickens enough to coat the back of a spoon.
6. Transfer the chicken to a serving platter, pour the sauce over the chicken and sprinkle the chopped peanuts on top. Garnish with chopped cilantro and lime wedges.

Southwest Gluten-free Turkey Meatloaf

Servings: 8
Cooking Time: 35 Minutes

Ingredients:

- 1 pound lean ground turkey
- ¼ cup corn grits
- ¼ cup diced onion
- 1 teaspoon minced garlic
- ½ teaspoon black pepper
- ½ teaspoon salt
- 1 large egg
- ½ cup ketchup
- 4 teaspoons chipotle hot sauce
- ⅓ cup shredded cheddar cheese

Directions:

1. Preheat the air fryer to 350°F.
2. In a large bowl, mix together the ground turkey, corn grits, onion, garlic, black pepper, and salt.
3. In a small bowl, whisk the egg. Add the egg to the turkey mixture and combine.
4. In a small bowl, mix the ketchup and hot sauce. Set aside.
5. Liberally spray a 9-x-4-inch loaf pan with olive oil spray. Depending on the size of your air fryer, you may need to use 2 or 3 mini loaf pans.
6. Spoon the ground turkey mixture into the loaf pan and evenly top with half of the ketchup mixture. Cover with foil and place the meatloaf into the air fryer. Cook for 30 minutes; remove the foil and discard. Check the internal temperature (it should be nearing 165°F).
7. Coat the top of the meatloaf with the remaining ketchup mixture, and sprinkle the cheese over the top. Place the meatloaf back in the air fryer for the remaining 5 minutes (or until the internal temperature reaches 165°F).
8. Remove from the oven and let cool 5 minutes before serving. Serve warm with desired sides.

Vegetarians Recipes

Rigatoni With Roasted Onions, Fennel, Spinach And Lemon Pepper Ricotta

Servings: 2

Cooking Time: 13 Minutes

Ingredients:

- 1 red onion, rough chopped into large chunks
- 2 teaspoons olive oil, divided
- 1 bulb fennel, sliced ¼-inch thick
- ¾ cup ricotta cheese
- 1½ teaspoons finely chopped lemon zest, plus more for garnish
- 1 teaspoon lemon juice
- salt and freshly ground black pepper
- 8 ounces (½ pound) dried rigatoni pasta
- 3 cups baby spinach leaves

Directions:

1. Bring a large stockpot of salted water to a boil on the stovetop and Preheat the air fryer to 400°F.
2. While the water is coming to a boil, toss the chopped onion in 1 teaspoon of olive oil and transfer to the air fryer basket. Air-fry at 400°F for 5 minutes. Toss the sliced fennel with 1 teaspoon of olive oil and add this to the air fryer basket with the onions. Continue to air-fry at 400°F for 8 minutes, shaking the basket a few times during the cooking process.
3. Combine the ricotta cheese, lemon zest and juice, ¼ teaspoon of salt and freshly ground black pepper in a bowl and stir until smooth.
4. Add the dried rigatoni to the boiling water and cook according to the package directions. When the pasta is cooked al dente, reserve one cup of the pasta water and drain the pasta into a colander.
5. Place the spinach in a serving bowl and immediately transfer the hot pasta to the bowl, wilting the spinach. Add the roasted onions and fennel and toss together. Add a little pasta water to the dish if it needs moistening. Then, dollop the lemon pepper ricotta cheese on top and nestle it into the hot pasta. Garnish with more lemon zest if desired.

Parmesan Portobello Mushroom Caps

Servings: 2

Cooking Time: 14 Minutes

Ingredients:

- ¼ cup flour*
- 1 egg, lightly beaten
- 1 cup seasoned breadcrumbs*
- 2 large portobello mushroom caps, stems and gills removed
- olive oil, in a spray bottle
- ½ cup tomato sauce
- ¾ cup grated mozzarella cheese
- 1 tablespoon grated Parmesan cheese
- 1 tablespoon chopped fresh basil or parsley

Directions:

1. Set up a dredging station with three shallow dishes. Place the flour in the first shallow dish, egg in the second dish and breadcrumbs in the last dish. Dredge the mushrooms in flour, then dip them into the egg and finally press them into the breadcrumbs to coat on all sides. Spray both sides of the coated mushrooms with olive oil.
2. Preheat the air fryer to 400°F.
3. Air-fry the mushrooms at 400°F for 10 minutes, turning them over halfway through the cooking process.
4. Fill the underside of the mushrooms with the tomato sauce and then top the sauce with the mozzarella and Parmesan cheeses. Reset the air fryer temperature to 350°F and air-fry for an additional 4 minutes, until the cheese has melted and is slightly browned.
5. Serve the mushrooms with pasta tossed with tomato sauce and garnish with some chopped fresh basil or parsley.

Spicy Vegetable And Tofu Shake Fry

Servings: 4
Cooking Time: 17 Minutes

Ingredients:

- 4 teaspoons canola oil, divided
- 2 tablespoons rice wine vinegar
- 1 tablespoon sriracha chili sauce
- ¼ cup soy sauce*
- ½ teaspoon toasted sesame oil
- 1 teaspoon minced garlic
- 1 tablespoon minced fresh ginger
- 8 ounces extra firm tofu
- ½ cup vegetable stock or water
- 1 tablespoon honey
- 1 tablespoon cornstarch
- ½ red onion, chopped
- 1 red or yellow bell pepper, chopped
- 1 cup green beans, cut into 2-inch lengths
- 4 ounces mushrooms, sliced
- 2 scallions, sliced
- 2 tablespoons fresh cilantro leaves
- 2 teaspoons toasted sesame seeds

Directions:

1. Combine 1 tablespoon of the oil, vinegar, sriracha sauce, soy sauce, sesame oil, garlic and ginger in a small bowl. Cut the tofu into bite-sized cubes and toss the tofu in with the marinade while you prepare the other vegetables. When you are ready to start cooking, remove the tofu from the marinade and set it aside. Add the water, honey and cornstarch to the marinade and bring to a simmer on the stovetop, just until the sauce thickens. Set the sauce aside.
2. Preheat the air fryer to 400°F.
3. Toss the onion, pepper, green beans and mushrooms in a bowl with a little canola oil and season with salt. Air-fry at 400°F for 11 minutes, shaking the basket and tossing the vegetables every few minutes. When the vegetables are cooked to your preferred doneness, remove them from the air fryer and set aside.
4. Add the tofu to the air fryer basket and air-fry at 400°F for 6 minutes, shaking the basket a few times during the cooking process. Add the vegetables back to the basket and air-fry for another minute. Transfer the vegetables and tofu to a large bowl, add the scallions and cilantro leaves and toss with the sauce. Serve over rice with sesame seeds sprinkled on top.

Black Bean Empanadas

Servings: 12
Cooking Time: 35 Minutes

Ingredients:

- 1½ cups all-purpose flour
- 1 cup whole-wheat flour
- 1 teaspoon salt
- ½ cup cold unsalted butter
- 1 egg
- ½ cup milk
- One 14.5-ounce can black beans, drained and rinsed
- ¼ cup chopped cilantro
- 1 cup shredded purple cabbage
- 1 cup shredded Monterey jack cheese
- ¼ cup salsa

Directions:

1. In a food processor, place the all-purpose flour, whole-wheat flour, salt, and butter into processor and process for 2 minutes, scraping down the sides of the food processor every 30 seconds. Add in the egg and blend for 30 seconds. Using the pulse button, add in the milk 1 tablespoon at a time, or until dough is moist enough to handle and be rolled into a ball. Let the dough rest at room temperature for 30 minutes.
2. Meanwhile, in a large bowl, mix together the black beans, cilantro, cabbage, Monterey Jack cheese, and salsa.
3. On a floured surface, cut the dough in half; then form a ball and cut each ball into 6 equal pieces, totaling 12 equal pieces. Work with one piece at a time, and cover the remaining dough with a towel.
4. Roll out a piece of dough into a 6-inch round, much like a tortilla, ¼ inch thick. Place 4 tablespoons of filling in the center of the round, and fold over to form a half-circle. Using a fork, crimp the edges together and pierce the top for air holes. Repeat with the remaining dough and filling.
5. Preheat the air fryer to 350°F.

6. Working in batches, place 3 to 4 empanadas in the air fryer basket and spray with cooking spray. Cook for 4 minutes, flip over the empanadas and spray with cooking spray, and cook another 4 minutes.

Spicy Sesame Tempeh Slaw With Peanut Dressing

Servings: 2
Cooking Time: 8 Minutes

Ingredients:

- 2 cups hot water
- 1 teaspoon salt
- 8 ounces tempeh, sliced into 1-inch-long pieces
- 2 tablespoons low-sodium soy sauce
- 2 tablespoons rice vinegar
- 1 tablespoon filtered water
- 2 teaspoons sesame oil
- ½ teaspoon fresh ginger
- 1 clove garlic, minced
- ¼ teaspoon black pepper
- ½ jalapeño, sliced
- 4 cups cabbage slaw
- 4 tablespoons Peanut Dressing (see the following recipe)
- 2 tablespoons fresh chopped cilantro
- 2 tablespoons chopped peanuts

Directions:

1. Mix the hot water with the salt and pour over the tempeh in a glass bowl. Stir and cover with a towel for 10 minutes.
2. Discard the water and leave the tempeh in the bowl.
3. In a medium bowl, mix the soy sauce, rice vinegar, filtered water, sesame oil, ginger, garlic, pepper, and jalapeño. Pour over the tempeh and cover with a towel. Place in the refrigerator to marinate for at least 2 hours.
4. Preheat the air fryer to 370°F. Remove the tempeh from the bowl and discard the remaining marinade.
5. Liberally spray the metal trivet that goes into the air fryer basket and place the tempeh on top of the trivet.
6. Cook for 4 minutes, flip, and cook another 4 minutes.
7. In a large bowl, mix the cabbage slaw with the Peanut Dressing and toss in the cilantro and chopped peanuts.
8. Portion onto 4 plates and place the cooked tempeh on top when cooking completes. Serve immediately.

Cauliflower Steaks Gratin

Servings: 2
Cooking Time: 13 Minutes

Ingredients:

- 1 head cauliflower
- 1 tablespoon olive oil
- salt and freshly ground black pepper
- ½ teaspoon chopped fresh thyme leaves
- 3 tablespoons grated Parmigiano-Reggiano cheese
- 2 tablespoons panko breadcrumbs

Directions:

1. Preheat the air-fryer to 370°F.
2. Cut two steaks out of the center of the cauliflower. To do this, cut the cauliflower in half and then cut one slice about 1-inch thick off each half. The rest of the cauliflower will fall apart into florets, which you can roast on their own or save for another meal.
3. Brush both sides of the cauliflower steaks with olive oil and season with salt, freshly ground black pepper and fresh thyme. Place the cauliflower steaks into the air fryer basket and air-fry for 6 minutes. Turn the steaks over and air-fry for another 4 minutes. Combine the Parmesan cheese and panko breadcrumbs and sprinkle the mixture over the tops of both steaks and air-fry for another 3 minutes until the cheese has melted and the breadcrumbs have browned. Serve this with some sautéed bitter greens and air-fried blistered tomatoes.

Veggie Burgers

Servings: 4
Cooking Time: 15 Minutes

Ingredients:

- 2 cans black beans, rinsed and drained
- ½ cup cooked quinoa
- ½ cup shredded raw sweet potato
- ¼ cup diced red onion
- 2 teaspoons ground cumin
- 1 teaspoon coriander powder
- ½ teaspoon salt
- oil for misting or cooking spray
- 8 slices bread
- suggested toppings: lettuce, tomato, red onion, Pepper Jack cheese, guacamole

Directions:

1. In a medium bowl, mash the beans with a fork.
2. Add the quinoa, sweet potato, onion, cumin, coriander, and salt and mix well with the fork.
3. Shape into 4 patties, each ¾-inch thick.
4. Mist both sides with oil or cooking spray and also mist the basket.
5. Cook at 390°F for 15minutes.
6. Follow the recipe for Toast, Plain & Simple.
7. Pop the veggie burgers back in the air fryer for a minute or two to reheat if necessary.
8. Serve on the toast with your favorite burger toppings.

Quinoa Burgers With Feta Cheese And Dill

Servings: 6
Cooking Time: 10 Minutes

Ingredients:

- 1 cup quinoa (red, white or multi-colored)
- 1½ cups water
- 1 teaspoon salt
- freshly ground black pepper
- 1½ cups rolled oats
- 3 eggs, lightly beaten
- ¼ cup minced white onion
- ½ cup crumbled feta cheese
- ¼ cup chopped fresh dill
- salt and freshly ground black pepper
- vegetable or canola oil, in a spray bottle
- whole-wheat hamburger buns (or gluten-free hamburger buns*)
- arugula
- tomato, sliced
- red onion, sliced
- mayonnaise

Directions:

1. Make the quinoa: Rinse the quinoa in cold water in a saucepan, swirling it with your hand until any dry husks rise to the surface. Drain the quinoa as well as you can and then put the saucepan on the stovetop to dry and toast the quinoa. Turn the heat to medium-high and shake the pan regularly until you see the quinoa moving easily and can hear the seeds moving in the pan, indicating that they are dry. Add the water, salt and pepper. Bring the liquid to a boil and then reduce the heat to low or medium-low. You should see just a few bubbles, not a boil. Cover with a lid, leaving it askew and simmer for 20 minutes. Turn the heat off and fluff the quinoa with a fork. If there's any liquid left in the bottom of the pot, place it back on the burner for another 3 minutes or so. Spread the cooked quinoa out on a sheet pan to cool.
2. Combine the room temperature quinoa in a large bowl with the oats, eggs, onion, cheese and dill. Season with salt and pepper and mix well (remember that feta cheese is salty). Shape the mixture into 6 patties with flat sides (so they fit more easily into the air fryer). Add a little water or a few more rolled oats if necessary to get the mixture to be the right consistency to make patties.
3. Preheat the air-fryer to 400°F.
4. Spray both sides of the patties generously with oil and transfer them to the air fryer basket in one layer (you will probably have to cook these burgers in batches, depending on the size of your air fryer). Air-fry each batch at 400°F for 10 minutes, flipping the burgers over halfway through the cooking time.
5. Build your burger on the whole-wheat hamburger buns with arugula, tomato, red onion and mayonnaise.

Roasted Vegetable Thai Green Curry

Servings: 4

Cooking Time: 16 Minutes

Ingredients:

- 1 (13-ounce) can coconut milk
- 3 tablespoons green curry paste
- 1 tablespoon soy sauce*
- 1 tablespoon rice wine vinegar
- 1 teaspoon sugar
- 1 teaspoon minced fresh ginger
- ½ onion, chopped
- 3 carrots, sliced
- 1 red bell pepper, chopped
- olive oil
- 10 stalks of asparagus, cut into 2-inch pieces
- 3 cups broccoli florets
- basmati rice for serving
- fresh cilantro
- crushed red pepper flakes (optional)

Directions:

1. Combine the coconut milk, green curry paste, soy sauce, rice wine vinegar, sugar and ginger in a medium saucepan and bring to a boil on the stovetop. Reduce the heat and simmer for 20 minutes while you cook the vegetables. Set aside.
2. Preheat the air fryer to 400°F.
3. Toss the onion, carrots, and red pepper together with a little olive oil and transfer the vegetables to the air fryer basket. Air-fry at 400°F for 10 minutes, shaking the basket a few times during the cooking process. Add the asparagus and broccoli florets and air-fry for an additional 6 minutes, again shaking the basket for even cooking.
4. When the vegetables are cooked to your liking, toss them with the green curry sauce and serve in bowls over basmati rice. Garnish with fresh chopped cilantro and crushed red pepper flakes.

Roasted Vegetable Stromboli

Servings: 2

Cooking Time: 29 Minutes

Ingredients:

- ½ onion, thinly sliced
- ½ red pepper, julienned
- ½ yellow pepper, julienned
- olive oil
- 1 small zucchini, thinly sliced
- 1 cup thinly sliced mushrooms
- 1½ cups chopped broccoli
- 1 teaspoon Italian seasoning
- salt and freshly ground black pepper
- ½ recipe of Blue Jean Chef Pizza dough (page 231)

OR 1 (14-ounce) tube refrigerated pizza dough

- 2 cups grated mozzarella cheese
- ¼ cup grated Parmesan cheese
- ½ cup sliced black olives, optional
- dried oregano
- pizza or marinara sauce

Directions:

1. Preheat the air fryer to 400°F.
2. Toss the onions and peppers with a little olive oil and air-fry the vegetables for 7 minutes, shaking the basket once or twice while the vegetables cook. Add the zucchini, mushrooms, broccoli and Italian seasoning to the basket. Add a little more olive oil and season with salt and freshly ground black pepper. Air-fry for an additional 7 minutes, shaking the basket halfway through. Let the vegetables cool slightly while you roll out the pizza dough.
3. On a lightly floured surface, roll or press the pizza dough out into a 13-inch by 11-inch rectangle, with the long side closest to you. Sprinkle half of the mozzarella and Parmesan cheeses over the dough leaving an empty 1-inch border from the edge farthest away from you. Spoon the roasted vegetables over the cheese, sprinkle the olives over everything and top with the remaining cheese.
4. Start rolling the stromboli away from you and toward the empty border. Make sure the filling stays tightly tucked inside the roll. Finally, tuck the ends of the dough in and pinch the seam shut. Place the seam side down and shape the stromboli into a U-shape to fit into the air fryer basket. Cut 4 small slits with the tip of a sharp knife evenly in the top of the dough, lightly

brush the stromboli with a little oil and sprinkle with some dried oregano.

5. Preheat the air fryer to 360°F.

6. Spray or brush the air fryer basket with oil and transfer the U-shaped stromboli to the air fryer basket. Air-fry for 15 minutes, flipping the stromboli over after the first 10 minutes. (Use a plate to invert the Stromboli out of the air fryer basket and then slide it back into the basket off the plate.)

7. To remove, carefully flip the stromboli over onto a cutting board. Let it rest for a couple of minutes before serving. Cut it into 2-inch slices and serve with pizza or marinara sauce.

Roasted Vegetable, Brown Rice And Black Bean Burrito

Servings: 2

Cooking Time: 20 Minutes

Ingredients:

- ½ zucchini, sliced ¼-inch thick
- ½ red onion, sliced
- 1 yellow bell pepper, sliced
- 2 teaspoons olive oil
- salt and freshly ground black pepper
- 2 burrito size flour tortillas
- 1 cup grated pepper jack cheese
- ½ cup cooked brown rice
- ½ cup canned black beans, drained and rinsed
- ¼ teaspoon ground cumin
- 1 tablespoon chopped fresh cilantro
- fresh salsa, guacamole and sour cream, for serving

Directions:

1. Preheat the air fryer to 400°F.

2. Toss the vegetables in a bowl with the olive oil, salt and freshly ground black pepper. Air-fry at 400°F for 12 to 15 minutes, shaking the basket a few times during the cooking process. The vegetables are done when they are cooked to your liking.

3. In the meantime, start building the burritos. Lay the tortillas out on the counter. Sprinkle half of the cheese in the center of the tortillas. Combine the rice, beans, cumin and cilantro in a bowl, season to taste with salt and freshly ground black pepper and then divide the mixture between the two tortillas. When the vegetables have finished cooking, transfer them to the two tortillas, placing the vegetables on top of the rice and beans. Sprinkle the remaining cheese on top and then roll the burritos up, tucking in the sides of the tortillas as you roll. Brush or spray the outside of the burritos with olive oil and transfer them to the air fryer.

4. Air-fry at 360°F for 8 minutes, turning them over when there are about 2 minutes left. The burritos will have slightly brown spots, but will still be pliable.

5. Serve with some fresh salsa, guacamole and sour cream.

Asparagus, Mushroom And Cheese Soufflés

Servings: 3

Cooking Time: 21 Minutes

Ingredients:

- butter
- grated Parmesan cheese
- 3 button mushrooms, thinly sliced
- 8 spears asparagus, sliced ½-inch long
- 1 teaspoon olive oil
- 1 tablespoon butter
- 4½ teaspoons flour
- pinch paprika
- pinch ground nutmeg
- salt and freshly ground black pepper
- ½ cup milk
- ½ cup grated Gruyère cheese or other Swiss cheese (about 2 ounces)
- 2 eggs, separated

Directions:

1. Butter three 6-ounce ramekins and dust with grated Parmesan cheese. (Butter the ramekins and then coat the butter with Parmesan by shaking it around in the ramekin and dumping out any excess.)

2. Preheat the air fryer to 400°F.

3. Toss the mushrooms and asparagus in a bowl with the olive oil. Transfer the vegetables to the air fryer and

air-fry for 7 minutes, shaking the basket once or twice to redistribute the Ingredients while they cook.

4. While the vegetables are cooking, make the soufflé base. Melt the butter in a saucepan on the stovetop over medium heat. Add the flour, stir and cook for a minute or two. Add the paprika, nutmeg, salt and pepper. Whisk in the milk and bring the mixture to a simmer to thicken. Remove the pan from the heat and add the cheese, stirring to melt. Let the mixture cool for just a few minutes and then whisk the egg yolks in, one at a time. Stir in the cooked mushrooms and asparagus. Let this soufflé base cool.
5. In a separate bowl, whisk the egg whites to soft peak stage (the point at which the whites can almost stand up on the end of your whisk). Fold the whipped egg whites into the soufflé base, adding a little at a time.
6. Preheat the air fryer to 330°F.
7. Transfer the batter carefully to the buttered ramekins, leaving about ½-inch at the top. Place the ramekins into the air fryer basket and air-fry for 14 minutes. The soufflés should have risen nicely and be brown on top. Serve immediately.

Broccoli Cheddar Stuffed Potatoes

Servings: 2

Cooking Time: 42 Minutes

Ingredients:

- 2 large russet potatoes, scrubbed
- 1 tablespoon olive oil
- salt and freshly ground black pepper
- 2 tablespoons butter
- ¼ cup sour cream
- 3 tablespoons half-and-half (or milk)
- 1¼ cups grated Cheddar cheese, divided
- ¾ teaspoon salt
- freshly ground black pepper
- 1 cup frozen baby broccoli florets, thawed and drained

Directions:

1. Preheat the air fryer to 400°F.
2. Rub the potatoes all over with olive oil and season generously with salt and freshly ground black pepper. Transfer the potatoes into the air fryer basket and air-fry for 30 minutes, turning the potatoes over halfway through the cooking process.
3. Remove the potatoes from the air fryer and let them rest for 5 minutes. Cut a large oval out of the top of both potatoes. Leaving half an inch of potato flesh around the edge of the potato, scoop the inside of the potato out and into a large bowl to prepare the potato filling. Mash the scooped potato filling with a fork and add the butter, sour cream, half-and-half, 1 cup of the grated Cheddar cheese, salt and pepper to taste. Mix well and then fold in the broccoli florets.
4. Stuff the hollowed out potato shells with the potato and broccoli mixture. Mound the filling high in the potatoes – you will have more filling than room in the potato shells.
5. Transfer the stuffed potatoes back to the air fryer basket and air-fry at 360°F for 10 minutes. Sprinkle the remaining Cheddar cheese on top of each stuffed potato, lower the heat to 330°F and air-fry for an additional minute or two to melt cheese.

Thai Peanut Veggie Burgers

Servings: 6

Cooking Time: 14 Minutes

Ingredients:

- One 15.5-ounce can cannellini beans
- 1 teaspoon minced garlic
- ¼ cup chopped onion
- 1 Thai chili pepper, sliced
- 2 tablespoons natural peanut butter
- ½ teaspoon black pepper
- ½ teaspoon salt
- ⅓ cup all-purpose flour (optional)
- ½ cup cooked quinoa
- 1 large carrot, grated
- 1 cup shredded red cabbage
- ¼ cup peanut dressing
- ¼ cup chopped cilantro
- 6 Hawaiian rolls
- 6 butterleaf lettuce leaves

Directions:

1. Preheat the air fryer to 350°F.

2. To a blender or food processor fitted with a metal blade, add the beans, garlic, onion, chili pepper, peanut butter, pepper, and salt. Pulse for 5 to 10 seconds. Do not over process. The mixture should be coarse, not smooth.
3. Remove from the blender or food processor and spoon into a large bowl. Mix in the cooked quinoa and carrots. At this point, the mixture should begin to hold together to form small patties. If the dough appears to be too sticky (meaning you likely processed a little too long), add the flour to hold the patties together.
4. Using a large spoon, form 8 equal patties out of the batter.
5. Liberally spray a metal trivet with olive oil spray and set in the air fryer basket. Place the patties into the basket, leaving enough space to be able to turn them with a spatula.
6. Cook for 7 minutes, flip, and cook another 7 minutes.
7. Remove from the heat and repeat with additional patties.
8. To serve, place the red cabbage in a bowl and toss with peanut dressing and cilantro. Place the veggie burger on a bun, and top with a slice of lettuce and cabbage slaw.

Mexican Twice Air-fried Sweet Potatoes

Servings: 2
Cooking Time: 42 Minutes

Ingredients:

- 2 large sweet potatoes
- olive oil
- salt and freshly ground black pepper
- ⅓ cup diced red onion
- ⅓ cup diced red bell pepper
- ½ cup canned black beans, drained and rinsed
- ½ cup corn kernels, fresh or frozen
- ½ teaspoon chili powder
- 1½ cups grated pepper jack cheese, divided
- Jalapeño peppers, sliced

Directions:

1. Preheat the air fryer to 400°F.
2. Rub the outside of the sweet potatoes with olive oil and season with salt and freshly ground black pepper. Transfer the potatoes into the air fryer basket and air-fry at 400°F for 30 minutes, rotating the potatoes a few times during the cooking process.
3. While the potatoes are air-frying, start the potato filling. Preheat a large sauté pan over medium heat on the stovetop. Add the onion and pepper and sauté for a few minutes, until the vegetables start to soften. Add the black beans, corn, and chili powder and sauté for another 3 minutes. Set the mixture aside.
4. Remove the sweet potatoes from the air fryer and let them rest for 5 minutes. Slice off one inch of the flattest side of both potatoes. Scrape the potato flesh out of the potatoes, leaving half an inch of potato flesh around the edge of the potato. Place all the potato flesh into a large bowl and mash it with a fork. Add the black bean mixture and 1 cup of the pepper jack cheese to the mashed sweet potatoes. Season with salt and freshly ground black pepper and mix well. Stuff the hollowed out potato shells with the black bean and sweet potato mixture, mounding the filling high in the potatoes.
5. Transfer the stuffed potatoes back into the air fryer basket and air-fry at 370°F for 10 minutes. Sprinkle the remaining cheese on top of each stuffed potato, lower the heat to 340°F and air-fry for an additional 2 minutes to melt the cheese. Top with a couple slices of Jalapeño pepper and serve warm with a green salad.

Falafels

Servings: 12
Cooking Time: 10 Minutes

Ingredients:

- 1 pouch falafel mix
- 2–3 tablespoons plain breadcrumbs
- oil for misting or cooking spray

Directions:

1. Prepare falafel mix according to package directions.
2. Preheat air fryer to 390°F.
3. Place breadcrumbs in shallow dish or on wax paper.
4. Shape falafel mixture into 12 balls and flatten slightly. Roll in breadcrumbs to coat all sides and mist with oil or cooking spray.
5. Place falafels in air fryer basket in single layer and cook for 5minutes. Shake basket, and continue cooking for 5minutes, until they brown and are crispy.

Basic Fried Tofu

Servings: 4

Cooking Time: 17 Minutes

Ingredients:

- 14 ounces extra-firm tofu, drained and pressed
- 1 tablespoon sesame oil
- 2 tablespoons low-sodium soy sauce
- ¼ cup rice vinegar
- 1 tablespoon fresh grated ginger
- 1 clove garlic, minced
- 3 tablespoons cornstarch
- ¼ teaspoon black pepper
- ⅛ teaspoon salt

Directions:

1. Cut the tofu into 16 cubes. Set aside in a glass container with a lid.
2. In a medium bowl, mix the sesame oil, soy sauce, rice vinegar, ginger, and garlic. Pour over the tofu and secure the lid. Place in the refrigerator to marinate for an hour.
3. Preheat the air fryer to 350°F.
4. In a small bowl, mix the cornstarch, black pepper, and salt.
5. Transfer the tofu to a large bowl and discard the leftover marinade. Pour the cornstarch mixture over the tofu and toss until all the pieces are coated.
6. Liberally spray the air fryer basket with olive oil mist and set the tofu pieces inside. Allow space between the tofu so it can cook evenly. Cook in batches if necessary.
7. Cook 15 to 17 minutes, shaking the basket every 5 minutes to allow the tofu to cook evenly on all sides. When it's done cooking, the tofu will be crisped and browned on all sides.
8. Remove the tofu from the air fryer basket and serve warm.

Tacos

Servings: 24

Cooking Time: 8 Minutes Per Batch

Ingredients:

- 1 24-count package 4-inch corn tortillas
- 1½ cups refried beans (about ¾ of a 15-ounce can)
- 4 ounces sharp Cheddar cheese, grated
- ½ cup salsa
- oil for misting or cooking spray

Directions:

1. Preheat air fryer to 390°F.
2. Wrap refrigerated tortillas in damp paper towels and microwave for 30 to 60 seconds to warm. If necessary, rewarm tortillas as you go to keep them soft enough to fold without breaking.
3. Working with one tortilla at a time, top with 1 tablespoon of beans, 1 tablespoon of grated cheese, and 1 teaspoon of salsa. Fold over and press down very gently on the center. Press edges firmly all around to seal. Spray both sides with oil or cooking spray.
4. Cooking in two batches, place half the tacos in the air fryer basket. To cook 12 at a time, you may need to stand them upright and lean some against the sides of basket. It's okay if they're crowded as long as you leave a little room for air to circulate around them.
5. Cook for 8 minutes or until golden brown and crispy.
6. Repeat steps 4 and 5 to cook remaining tacos.

Curried Potato, Cauliflower And Pea Turnovers

Servings: 4

Cooking Time: 40 Minutes

Ingredients:

- Dough:
- 2 cups all-purpose flour
- ½ teaspoon baking powder
- 1 teaspoon salt
- freshly ground black pepper
- ¼ teaspoon dried thyme
- ¼ cup canola oil
- ½ to ⅔ cup water
- Turnover Filling:
- 1 tablespoon canola or vegetable oil
- 1 onion, finely chopped
- 1 clove garlic, minced
- 1 tablespoon grated fresh ginger
- ½ teaspoon cumin seeds
- ½ teaspoon fennel seeds

- 1 teaspoon curry powder
- 2 russet potatoes, diced
- 2 cups cauliflower florets
- ½ cup frozen peas
- 2 tablespoons chopped fresh cilantro
- salt and freshly ground black pepper
- 2 tablespoons butter, melted
- mango chutney, for serving

Directions:

1. Start by making the dough. Combine the flour, baking powder, salt, pepper and dried thyme in a mixing bowl or the bowl of a stand mixer. Drizzle in the canola oil and pinch it together with your fingers to turn the flour into a crumby mixture. Stir in the water (enough to bring the dough together). Knead the dough for 5 minutes or so until it is smooth. Add a little more water or flour as needed. Let the dough rest while you make the turnover filling.
2. Preheat a large skillet on the stovetop over medium-high heat. Add the oil and sauté the onion until it starts to become tender – about 4 minutes. Add the garlic and ginger and continue to cook for another minute. Add the dried spices and toss everything to coat. Add the potatoes and cauliflower to the skillet and pour in 1½ cups of water. Simmer everything together for 20 to 25 minutes, or until the potatoes are soft and most of the water has evaporated. If the water has evaporated and the vegetables still need more time, just add a little water and continue to simmer until everything is tender. Stir well, crushing the potatoes and cauliflower a little as you do so. Stir in the peas and cilantro, season to taste with salt and freshly ground black pepper and set aside to cool.
3. Divide the dough into 4 balls. Roll the dough balls out into ¼-inch thick circles. Divide the cooled potato filling between the dough circles, placing a mound of the filling on one side of each piece of dough, leaving an empty border around the edge of the dough. Brush the edges of the dough with a little water and fold one edge of circle over the filling to meet the other edge of the circle, creating a half moon. Pinch the edges together with your fingers and then press the edge with the tines of a fork to decorate and seal.
4. Preheat the air fryer to 380°F.
5. Spray or brush the air fryer basket with oil. Brush the turnovers with the melted butter and place 2 turnovers into the air fryer basket. Air-fry for 15 minutes. Flip the turnovers over and air-fry for another 5 minutes. Repeat with the remaining 2 turnovers.
6. These will be very hot when they come out of the air fryer. Let them cool for at least 20 minutes before serving warm with mango chutney.

Vegetable Couscous

Servings: 4

Cooking Time: 10 Minutes

Ingredients:

- 4 ounces white mushrooms, sliced
- ½ medium green bell pepper, julienned
- 1 cup cubed zucchini
- ¼ small onion, slivered
- 1 stalk celery, thinly sliced
- ¼ teaspoon ground coriander
- ¼ teaspoon ground cumin
- salt and pepper
- 1 tablespoon olive oil
- Couscous
- ¾ cup uncooked couscous
- 1 cup vegetable broth or water
- ½ teaspoon salt (omit if using salted broth)

Directions:

1. Combine all vegetables in large bowl. Sprinkle with coriander, cumin, and salt and pepper to taste. Stir well, add olive oil, and stir again to coat vegetables evenly.
2. Place vegetables in air fryer basket and cook at 390°F for 5minutes. Stir and cook for 5 more minutes, until tender.
3. While vegetables are cooking, prepare the couscous: Place broth or water and salt in large saucepan. Heat to boiling, stir in couscous, cover, and remove from heat.
4. Let couscous sit for 5minutes, stir in cooked vegetables, and serve hot.

Spinach And Cheese Calzone

Servings: 2
Cooking Time: 10 Minutes

Ingredients:

- ⅔ cup frozen chopped spinach, thawed
- 1 cup grated mozzarella cheese
- 1 cup ricotta cheese
- ½ teaspoon Italian seasoning
- ½ teaspoon salt
- freshly ground black pepper
- 1 store-bought or homemade pizza dough* (about 12 to 16 ounces)
- 2 tablespoons olive oil
- pizza or marinara sauce (optional)

Directions:

1. Drain and squeeze all the water out of the thawed spinach and set it aside. Mix the mozzarella cheese, ricotta cheese, Italian seasoning, salt and freshly ground black pepper together in a bowl. Stir in the chopped spinach.
2. Divide the dough in half. With floured hands or on a floured surface, stretch or roll one half of the dough into a 10-inch circle. Spread half of the cheese and spinach mixture on half of the dough, leaving about one inch of dough empty around the edge.
3. Fold the other half of the dough over the cheese mixture, almost to the edge of the bottom dough to form a half moon. Fold the bottom edge of dough up over the top edge and crimp the dough around the edges in order to make the crust and seal the calzone. Brush the dough with olive oil. Repeat with the second half of dough to make the second calzone.
4. Preheat the air fryer to 360°F.
5. Brush or spray the air fryer basket with olive oil. Air-fry the calzones one at a time for 10 minutes, flipping the calzone over half way through. Serve with warm pizza or marinara sauce if desired.

Cheese Ravioli

Servings: 4
Cooking Time: 9 Minutes

Ingredients:

- 1 egg
- ¼ cup milk
- 1 cup breadcrumbs
- 2 teaspoons Italian seasoning
- ⅛ teaspoon ground rosemary
- ¼ teaspoon basil
- ¼ teaspoon parsley
- 9-ounce package uncooked cheese ravioli
- ¼ cup flour
- oil for misting or cooking spray

Directions:

1. Preheat air fryer to 390°F.
2. In a medium bowl, beat together egg and milk.
3. In a large plastic bag, mix together the breadcrumbs, Italian seasoning, rosemary, basil, and parsley.
4. Place all the ravioli and the flour in a bag or a bowl with a lid and shake to coat.
5. Working with a handful at a time, drop floured ravioli into egg wash. Remove ravioli, letting excess drip off, and place in bag with breadcrumbs.
6. When all ravioli are in the breadcrumbs' bag, shake well to coat all pieces.
7. Dump enough ravioli into air fryer basket to form one layer. Mist with oil or cooking spray. Dump the remaining ravioli on top of the first layer and mist with oil.
8. Cook for 5minutes. Shake well and spray with oil. Break apart any ravioli stuck together and spray any spots you missed the first time.
9. Cook 4 minutes longer, until ravioli puff up and are crispy golden brown.

Lentil Fritters

Servings: 9
Cooking Time: 12 Minutes

Ingredients:

- 1 cup cooked red lentils
- 1 cup riced cauliflower
- ½ medium zucchini, shredded (about 1 cup)
- ¼ cup finely chopped onion
- ¼ teaspoon salt
- ¼ teaspoon black pepper
- ½ teaspoon garlic powder

- ¼ teaspoon paprika
- 1 large egg
- ⅓ cup quinoa flour

Directions:

1. Preheat the air fryer to 370°F.
2. In a large bowl, mix the lentils, cauliflower, zucchini, onion, salt, pepper, garlic powder, and paprika. Mix in the egg and flour until a thick dough forms.
3. Using a large spoon, form the dough into 9 large fritters.
4. Liberally spray the air fryer basket with olive oil. Place the fritters into the basket, leaving space around each fritter so you can flip them.
5. Cook for 6 minutes, flip, and cook another 6 minutes.
6. Remove from the air fryer and repeat with the remaining fritters. Serve warm with desired sauce and sides.

Roasted Vegetable Pita Pizza

Servings: 4

Cooking Time: 20 Minutes

Ingredients:

- 1 medium red bell pepper, seeded and cut into quarters
- 1 teaspoon extra-virgin olive oil
- ⅛ teaspoon black pepper
- ⅛ teaspoon salt
- Two 6-inch whole-grain pita breads
- 6 tablespoons pesto sauce
- ¼ small red onion, thinly sliced
- ½ cup shredded part-skim mozzarella cheese

Directions:

1. Preheat the air fryer to 400°F.
2. In a small bowl, toss the bell peppers with the olive oil, pepper, and salt.
3. Place the bell peppers in the air fryer and cook for 15 minutes, shaking every 5 minutes to prevent burning.
4. Remove the peppers and set aside. Turn the air fryer temperature down to 350°F.
5. Lay the pita bread on a flat surface. Cover each with half the pesto sauce; then top with even portions of the red bell peppers and onions. Sprinkle cheese over the top. Spray the air fryer basket with olive oil mist.
6. Carefully lift the pita bread into the air fryer basket with a spatula.
7. Cook for 5 to 8 minutes, or until the outer edges begin to brown and the cheese is melted.
8. Serve warm with desired sides.

Spaghetti Squash And Kale Fritters With Pomodoro Sauce

Servings: 3

Cooking Time: 45 Minutes

Ingredients:

- 1½-pound spaghetti squash (about half a large or a whole small squash)
- olive oil
- ½ onion, diced
- ½ red bell pepper, diced
- 2 cloves garlic, minced
- 4 cups coarsely chopped kale
- salt and freshly ground black pepper
- 1 egg
- ⅓ cup breadcrumbs, divided*
- ⅓ cup grated Parmesan cheese
- ½ teaspoon dried rubbed sage
- pinch nutmeg
- Pomodoro Sauce:
- 2 tablespoons olive oil
- ½ onion, chopped
- 1 to 2 cloves garlic, minced
- 1 (28-ounce) can peeled tomatoes
- ¼ cup red wine
- 1 teaspoon Italian seasoning
- 2 tablespoons chopped fresh basil, plus more for garnish
- salt and freshly ground black pepper
- ½ teaspoon sugar (optional)

Directions:

1. Preheat the air fryer to 370°F.
2. Cut the spaghetti squash in half lengthwise and remove the seeds. Rub the inside of the squash with olive oil and season with salt and pepper. Place the squash, cut

side up, into the air fryer basket and air-fry for 30 minutes, flipping the squash over halfway through the cooking process.

3. While the squash is cooking, Preheat a large sauté pan over medium heat on the stovetop. Add a little olive oil and sauté the onions for 3 minutes, until they start to soften. Add the red pepper and garlic and continue to sauté for an additional 4 minutes. Add the kale and season with salt and pepper. Cook for 2 more minutes, or until the kale is soft. Transfer the mixture to a large bowl and let it cool.
4. While the squash continues to cook, make the Pomodoro sauce. Preheat the large sauté pan again over medium heat on the stovetop. Add the olive oil and sauté the onion and garlic for 2 to 3 minutes, until the onion begins to soften. Crush the canned tomatoes with your hands and add them to the pan along with the red wine and Italian seasoning and simmer for 20 minutes. Add the basil and season to taste with salt, pepper and sugar (if using).
5. When the spaghetti squash has finished cooking, use a fork to scrape the inside flesh of the squash onto a sheet pan. Spread the squash out and let it cool.
6. Once cool, add the spaghetti squash to the kale mixture, along with the egg, breadcrumbs, Parmesan cheese, sage, nutmeg, salt and freshly ground black pepper. Stir to combine well and then divide the mixture into 6 thick portions. You can shape the portions into patties, but I prefer to keep them a little random and unique in shape. Spray or brush the fritters with olive oil.
7. Preheat the air fryer to 370°F.
8. Brush the air fryer basket with a little olive oil and transfer the fritters to the basket. Air-fry the squash and kale fritters at 370°F for 15 minutes, flipping them over halfway through the cooking process.
9. Serve the fritters warm with the Pomodoro sauce spooned over the top or pooled on your plate. Garnish with the fresh basil leaves.

Charred Cauliflower Tacos

Servings: 4

Cooking Time: 10 Minutes

Ingredients:

- 1 head cauliflower, washed and cut into florets
- 2 tablespoons avocado oil
- 2 teaspoons taco seasoning
- 1 medium avocado
- ½ teaspoon garlic powder
- ¼ teaspoon black pepper
- ¼ teaspoon salt
- 2 tablespoons chopped red onion
- 2 teaspoons fresh squeezed lime juice
- ¼ cup chopped cilantro
- Eight 6-inch corn tortillas
- ½ cup cooked corn
- ½ cup shredded purple cabbage

Directions:

1. Preheat the air fryer to 390°F.
2. In a large bowl, toss the cauliflower with the avocado oil and taco seasoning. Set the metal trivet inside the air fryer basket and liberally spray with olive oil.
3. Place the cauliflower onto the trivet and cook for 10 minutes, shaking every 3 minutes to allow for an even char.
4. While the cauliflower is cooking, prepare the avocado sauce. In a medium bowl, mash the avocado; then mix in the garlic powder, pepper, salt, and onion. Stir in the lime juice and cilantro; set aside.
5. Remove the cauliflower from the air fryer basket.
6. Place 1 tablespoon of avocado sauce in the middle of a tortilla, and top with corn, cabbage, and charred cauliflower. Repeat with the remaining tortillas. Serve immediately.

Pizza Portobello Mushrooms

Servings: 2

Cooking Time: 18 Minutes

Ingredients:

- 2 portobello mushroom caps, gills removed (see Figure 13-1)
- 1 teaspoon extra-virgin olive oil
- ¼ cup diced onion
- 1 teaspoon minced garlic
- 1 medium zucchini, shredded
- 1 teaspoon dried oregano
- ½ teaspoon black pepper

- ¼ teaspoon salt
- ⅓ cup marinara sauce
- ¼ cup shredded part-skim mozzarella cheese
- ¼ teaspoon red pepper flakes
- 2 tablespoons Parmesan cheese
- 2 tablespoons chopped basil

Directions:

1. Preheat the air fryer to 370°F.
2. Lightly spray the mushrooms with an olive oil mist and place into the air fryer to cook for 10 minutes, cap side up.
3. Add the olive oil to a pan and sauté the onion and garlic together for about 2 to 4 minutes. Stir in the zucchini, oregano, pepper, and salt, and continue to cook. When the zucchini has cooked down (usually about 4 to 6 minutes), add in the marinara sauce. Remove from the heat and stir in the mozzarella cheese.
4. Remove the mushrooms from the air fryer basket when cooking completes. Reset the temperature to 350°F.
5. Using a spoon, carefully stuff the mushrooms with the zucchini marinara mixture.
6. Return the stuffed mushrooms to the air fryer basket and cook for 5 to 8 minutes, or until the cheese is lightly browned. You should be able to easily insert a fork into the mushrooms when they're cooked.
7. Remove the mushrooms and sprinkle the red pepper flakes, Parmesan cheese, and fresh basil over the top.
8. Serve warm.

Stuffed Zucchini Boats

Servings: 2

Cooking Time: 20 Minutes

Ingredients:

- olive oil
- ½ cup onion, finely chopped
- 1 clove garlic, finely minced
- ½ teaspoon dried oregano
- ¼ teaspoon dried thyme
- ¾ cup couscous
- 1½ cups chicken stock, divided
- 1 tomato, seeds removed and finely chopped
- ½ cup coarsely chopped Kalamata olives
- ½ cup grated Romano cheese
- ¼ cup pine nuts, toasted
- 1 tablespoon chopped fresh parsley
- 1 teaspoon salt
- freshly ground black pepper
- 1 egg, beaten
- 1 cup grated mozzarella cheese, divided
- 2 thick zucchini

Directions:

1. Preheat a sauté pan on the stovetop over medium-high heat. Add the olive oil and sauté the onion until it just starts to soften–about 4 minutes. Stir in the garlic, dried oregano and thyme. Add the couscous and sauté for just a minute. Add 1¼ cups of the chicken stock and simmer over low heat for 3 to 5 minutes, until liquid has been absorbed and the couscous is soft. Remove the pan from heat and set it aside to cool slightly.
2. Fluff the couscous and add the tomato, Kalamata olives, Romano cheese, pine nuts, parsley, salt and pepper. Mix well. Add the remaining chicken stock, the egg and ½ cup of the mozzarella cheese. Stir to ensure everything is combined.
3. Cut each zucchini in half lengthwise. Then, trim each half of the zucchini into four 5-inch lengths. (Save the trimmed ends of the zucchini for another use.) Use a spoon to scoop out the center of the zucchini, leaving some flesh around the sides. Brush both sides of the zucchini with olive oil and season the cut side with salt and pepper.
4. Preheat the air fryer to 380°F.
5. Divide the couscous filling between the four zucchini boats. Use your hands to press the filling together and fill the inside of the zucchini. The filling should be mounded into the boats and rounded on top.
6. Transfer the zucchini boats to the air fryer basket and drizzle the stuffed zucchini boats with olive oil. Air-fry for 19 minutes. Then, sprinkle the remaining mozzarella cheese on top of the zucchini, pressing it down onto the filling lightly to prevent it from blowing around in the air fryer. Air-fry for one more minute to melt the cheese. Transfer the finished zucchini boats to a serving platter and garnish with the chopped parsley.

Roasted Vegetable Lasagna

Servings: 6
Cooking Time: 55 Minutes

Ingredients:

- 1 zucchini, sliced
- 1 yellow squash, sliced
- 8 ounces mushrooms, sliced
- 1 red bell pepper, cut into 2-inch strips
- 1 tablespoon olive oil
- 2 cups ricotta cheese
- 2 cups grated mozzarella cheese, divided
- 1 egg
- 1 teaspoon salt
- freshly ground black pepper
- ¼ cup shredded carrots
- ½ cup chopped fresh spinach
- 8 lasagna noodles, cooked
- Béchamel Sauce:
- 3 tablespoons butter
- 3 tablespoons flour
- 2½ cups milk
- ½ cup grated Parmesan cheese
- ½ teaspoon salt
- freshly ground black pepper
- pinch of ground nutmeg

Directions:

1. Preheat the air fryer to 400°F.
2. Toss the zucchini, yellow squash, mushrooms and red pepper in a large bowl with the olive oil and season with salt and pepper. Air-fry for 10 minutes, shaking the basket once or twice while the vegetables cook.
3. While the vegetables are cooking, make the béchamel sauce and cheese filling. Melt the butter in a medium saucepan over medium-high heat on the stovetop. Add the flour and whisk, cooking for a couple of minutes. Add the milk and whisk vigorously until smooth. Bring the mixture to a boil and simmer until the sauce thickens. Stir in the Parmesan cheese and season with the salt, pepper and nutmeg. Set the sauce aside.
4. Combine the ricotta cheese, 1¼ cups of the mozzarella cheese, egg, salt and pepper in a large bowl and stir until combined. Fold in the carrots and spinach.
5. When the vegetables have finished cooking, build the lasagna. Use a baking dish that is 6 inches in diameter and 4 inches high. Cover the bottom of the baking dish with a little béchamel sauce. Top with two lasagna noodles, cut to fit the dish and overlapping each other a little. Spoon a third of the ricotta cheese mixture and then a third of the roasted veggies on top of the noodles. Pour ½ cup of béchamel sauce on top and then repeat these layers two more times: noodles – cheese mixture – vegetables – béchamel sauce. Sprinkle the remaining mozzarella cheese over the top. Cover the dish with aluminum foil, tenting it loosely so the aluminum doesn't touch the cheese.
6. Lower the dish into the air fryer basket using an aluminum foil sling (fold a piece of aluminum foil into a strip about 2-inches wide by 24-inches long). Fold the ends of the aluminum foil over the top of the dish before returning the basket to the air fryer. Air-fry for 45 minutes, removing the foil for the last 2 minutes, to slightly brown the cheese on top.
7. Let the lasagna rest for at least 20 minutes to set up a little before slicing into it and serving.

Arancini With Marinara

Servings: 6
Cooking Time: 15 Minutes

Ingredients:

- 2 cups cooked rice
- 1 cup grated Parmesan cheese
- 1 egg, whisked
- ¼ teaspoon dried thyme
- ½ teaspoon dried oregano
- ½ teaspoon dried basil
- ½ teaspoon dried parsley
- 1 teaspoon salt
- ¼ teaspoon paprika
- 1 cup breadcrumbs
- 4 ounces mozzarella, cut into 24 cubes
- 2 cups marinara sauce

Directions:

1. In a large bowl, mix together the rice, Parmesan cheese, and egg.

2. In another bowl, mix together the thyme, oregano, basil, parsley, salt, paprika, and breadcrumbs.
3. Form 24 rice balls with the rice mixture. Use your thumb to make an indentation in the center and stuff 1 cube of mozzarella in the center of the rice; close the ball around the cheese.
4. Roll the rice balls in the seasoned breadcrumbs until all are coated.
5. Preheat the air fryer to 400°F.
6. Place the rice balls in the air fryer basket and coat with cooking spray. Cook for 8 minutes, shake the basket, and cook another 7 minutes.
7. Heat the marinara sauce in a saucepan until warm. Serve sauce as a dip for arancini.

Tandoori Paneer Naan Pizza

Servings: 4
Cooking Time: 10 Minutes

Ingredients:

- 6 tablespoons plain Greek yogurt, divided
- 1¼ teaspoons garam marsala, divided
- ½ teaspoon turmeric, divided
- ¼ teaspoon garlic powder
- ½ teaspoon paprika, divided
- ½ teaspoon black pepper, divided
- 3 ounces paneer, cut into small cubes
- 1 tablespoon extra-virgin olive oil
- 2 teaspoons minced garlic
- 4 cups baby spinach
- 2 tablespoons marinara sauce
- ¼ teaspoon salt
- 2 plain naan breads (approximately 6 inches in diameter)
- ½ cup shredded part-skim mozzarella cheese

Directions:

1. Preheat the air fryer to 350°F.
2. In a small bowl, mix 2 tablespoons of the yogurt, ½ teaspoon of the garam marsala, ¼ teaspoon of the turmeric, the garlic powder, ¼ teaspoon of the paprika, and ¼ teaspoon of the black pepper. Toss the paneer cubes in the mixture and let marinate for at least an hour.
3. Meanwhile, in a pan, heat the olive oil over medium heat. Add in the minced garlic and sauté for 1 minute. Stir in the spinach and begin to cook until it wilts. Add in the remaining 4 tablespoons of yogurt and the marinara sauce. Stir in the remaining ¾ teaspoon of garam masala, the remaining ¼ teaspoon of turmeric, the remaining ¼ teaspoon of paprika, the remaining ¼ teaspoon of black pepper, and the salt. Let simmer a minute or two, and then remove from the heat.
4. Equally divide the spinach mixture amongst the two naan breads. Place 1½ ounces of the marinated paneer on each naan.
5. Liberally spray the air fryer basket with olive oil mist.
6. Use a spatula to pick up one naan and place it in the air fryer basket.
7. Cook for 4 minutes, open the basket and sprinkle ¼ cup of mozzarella cheese on top, and cook another 4 minutes.
8. Remove from the air fryer and repeat with the remaining naan.
9. Serve warm.

Egg Rolls

Servings: 4
Cooking Time: 8 Minutes

Ingredients:

- 1 clove garlic, minced
- 1 teaspoon sesame oil
- 1 teaspoon olive oil
- ½ cup chopped celery
- ½ cup grated carrots
- 2 green onions, chopped
- 2 ounces mushrooms, chopped
- 2 cups shredded Napa cabbage
- 1 teaspoon low-sodium soy sauce
- 1 teaspoon cornstarch
- salt
- 1 egg
- 1 tablespoon water
- 4 egg roll wraps
- olive oil for misting or cooking spray

Directions:

1. In a large skillet, sauté garlic in sesame and olive oils over medium heat for 1 minute.

2. Add celery, carrots, onions, and mushrooms to skillet. Cook 1 minute, stirring.
3. Stir in cabbage, cover, and cook for 1 minute or just until cabbage slightly wilts.
4. In a small bowl, mix soy sauce and cornstarch. Stir into vegetables to thicken. Remove from heat. Salt to taste if needed.
5. Beat together egg and water in a small bowl.
6. Divide filling into 4 portions and roll up in egg roll wraps. Brush all over with egg wash to seal.
7. Mist egg rolls very lightly with olive oil or cooking spray and place in air fryer basket.
8. Cook at 390°F for 4minutes. Turn over and cook 4 more minutes, until golden brown and crispy.

Mushroom, Zucchini And Black Bean Burgers

Servings: 4
Cooking Time: 18 Minutes

Ingredients:

- 1 cup diced zucchini, (about ½ medium zucchini)
- 1 tablespoon olive oil
- salt and freshly ground black pepper
- 1 cup chopped brown mushrooms (about 3 ounces)
- 1 small clove garlic
- 1 (15-ounce) can black beans, drained and rinsed
- 1 teaspoon lemon zest
- 1 tablespoon chopped fresh cilantro
- ½ cup plain breadcrumbs
- 1 egg, beaten
- ½ teaspoon salt
- freshly ground black pepper
- whole-wheat pita bread, burger buns or brioche buns
- mayonnaise, tomato, avocado and lettuce, for serving

Directions:

1. Preheat the air fryer to 400°F.
2. Toss the zucchini with the olive oil, season with salt and freshly ground black pepper and air-fry for 6 minutes, shaking the basket once or twice while it cooks.
3. Transfer the zucchini to a food processor with the mushrooms, garlic and black beans and process until still a little chunky but broken down and pasty. Transfer the mixture to a bowl. Add the lemon zest, cilantro, breadcrumbs and egg and mix well. Season again with salt and freshly ground black pepper. Shape the mixture into four burger patties and refrigerate for at least 15 minutes.
4. Preheat the air fryer to 370°F. Transfer two of the veggie burgers to the air fryer basket and air-fry for 12 minutes, flipping the burgers gently halfway through the cooking time. Keep the burgers warm by loosely tenting them with foil while you cook the remaining two burgers. Return the first batch of burgers back into the air fryer with the second batch for the last two minutes of cooking to re-heat.
5. Serve on toasted whole-wheat pita bread, burger buns or brioche buns with some mayonnaise, tomato, avocado and lettuce.

Mushroom And Fried Onion Quesadilla

Servings: 2
Cooking Time: 33 Minutes

Ingredients:

- 1 onion, sliced
- 2 tablespoons butter, melted
- 10 ounces button mushrooms, sliced
- 2 tablespoons Worcestershire sauce
- salt and freshly ground black pepper
- 4 (8-inch) flour tortillas
- 2 cups grated Fontina cheese
- vegetable or olive oil

Directions:

1. Preheat the air fryer to 400°F.
2. Toss the onion slices with the melted butter and transfer them to the air fryer basket. Air-fry at 400°F for 15 minutes, shaking the basket several times during the cooking process. Add the mushrooms and Worcestershire sauce to the onions and stir to combine. Air-fry at 400°F for an additional 10 minutes. Season with salt and freshly ground black pepper.
3. Lay two of the tortillas on a cutting board. Top each tortilla with ½ cup of the grated cheese, half of the onion and mushroom mixture and then finally another ½ cup of the cheese. Place the remaining tortillas on top of the cheese and press down firmly.

4. Brush the air fryer basket with a little oil. Place a quesadilla in the basket and brush the top with a little oil. Secure the top tortilla to the bottom with three toothpicks and air-fry at 400°F for 5 minutes. Flip the quesadilla over by inverting it onto a plate and sliding it back into the basket. Remove the toothpicks and brush the other side with oil. Air-fry for an additional 3 minutes.

5. Invert the quesadilla onto a cutting board and cut it into 4 or 6 triangles. Serve immediately.

Cheesy Enchilada Stuffed Baked Potatoes

Servings: 4

Cooking Time: 37 Minutes

Ingredients:

- 2 medium russet potatoes, washed
- One 15-ounce can mild red enchilada sauce
- One 15-ounce can low-sodium black beans, rinsed and drained
- 1 teaspoon taco seasoning
- ½ cup shredded cheddar cheese
- 1 medium avocado, halved
- ½ teaspoon garlic powder
- ¼ teaspoon black pepper
- ¼ teaspoon salt
- 2 teaspoons fresh lime juice
- 2 tablespoon chopped red onion
- ¼ cup chopped cilantro

Directions:

1. Preheat the air fryer to 390°F.
2. Puncture the outer surface of the potatoes with a fork.
3. Set the potatoes inside the air fryer basket and cook for 20 minutes, rotate, and cook another 10 minutes.
4. In a large bowl, mix the enchilada sauce, black beans, and taco seasoning.
5. When the potatoes have finished cooking, carefully remove them from the air fryer basket and let cool for 5 minutes.
6. Using a pair of tongs to hold the potato if it's still too hot to touch, slice the potato in half lengthwise. Use a spoon to scoop out the potato flesh and add it into the bowl with the enchilada sauce. Mash the potatoes with the enchilada sauce mixture, creating a uniform stuffing.
7. Place the potato skins into an air-fryer-safe pan and stuff the halves with the enchilada stuffing. Sprinkle the cheese over the top of each potato.
8. Set the air fryer temperature to 350°F, return the pan to the air fryer basket, and cook for another 5 to 7 minutes to heat the potatoes and melt the cheese.
9. While the potatoes are cooking, take the avocado and scoop out the flesh into a small bowl. Mash it with the back of a fork; then mix in the garlic powder, pepper, salt, lime juice, and onion. Set aside.
10. When the potatoes have finished cooking, remove the pan from the air fryer and place the potato halves on a plate. Top with avocado mash and fresh cilantro. Serve immediately.

Pinto Taquitos

Servings: 4

Cooking Time: 8 Minutes

Ingredients:

- 12 corn tortillas (6- to 7-inch size)
- Filling
- ½ cup refried pinto beans
- ½ cup grated sharp Cheddar or Pepper Jack cheese
- ¼ cup corn kernels (if frozen, measure after thawing and draining)
- 2 tablespoons chopped green onion
- 2 tablespoons chopped jalapeño pepper (seeds and ribs removed before chopping)
- ½ teaspoon lime juice
- ½ teaspoon chile powder, plus extra for dusting
- ½ teaspoon cumin
- ½ teaspoon garlic powder
- oil for misting or cooking spray
- salsa, sour cream, or guacamole for dipping

Directions:

1. Mix together all filling Ingredients.
2. Warm refrigerated tortillas for easier rolling. (Wrap in damp paper towels and microwave for 30 to 60 seconds.)

3. Working with one at a time, place 1 tablespoon of filling on tortilla and roll up. Spray with oil or cooking spray and dust outside with chile powder to taste.
4. Place 6 taquitos in air fryer basket (4 on bottom layer, 2 stacked crosswise on top). Cook at 390°F for 8 minutes, until crispy and brown.
5. Repeat step 4 to cook remaining taquitos.
6. Serve plain or with salsa, sour cream, or guacamole for dipping.

Falafel

Servings: 4
Cooking Time: 10 Minutes

Ingredients:

- 1 cup dried chickpeas
- ½ onion, chopped
- 1 clove garlic
- ¼ cup fresh parsley leaves
- 1 teaspoon salt
- ¼ teaspoon crushed red pepper flakes
- 1 teaspoon ground cumin
- ½ teaspoon ground coriander
- 1 to 2 tablespoons flour
- olive oil
- Tomato Salad
- 2 tomatoes, seeds removed and diced
- ½ cucumber, finely diced
- ¼ red onion, finely diced and rinsed with water
- 1 teaspoon red wine vinegar
- 1 tablespoon olive oil
- salt and freshly ground black pepper
- 2 tablespoons chopped fresh parsley

Directions:

1. Cover the chickpeas with water and let them soak overnight on the counter. Then drain the chickpeas and put them in a food processor, along with the onion, garlic, parsley, spices and 1 tablespoon of flour. Pulse in the food processor until the mixture has broken down into a coarse paste consistency. The mixture should hold together when you pinch it. Add more flour as needed, until you get this consistency.
2. Scoop portions of the mixture (about 2 tablespoons in size) and shape into balls. Place the balls on a plate and refrigerate for at least 30 minutes. You should have between 12 and 14 balls.
3. Preheat the air fryer to 380°F.
4. Spray the falafel balls with oil and place them in the air fryer. Air-fry for 10 minutes, rolling them over and spraying them with oil again halfway through the cooking time so that they cook and brown evenly.
5. Serve with pita bread, hummus, cucumbers, hot peppers, tomatoes or any other fillings you might like.

Eggplant Parmesan

Servings: 4
Cooking Time: 8 Minutes Per Batch

Ingredients:

- 1 medium eggplant, 6–8 inches long
- salt
- 1 large egg
- 1 tablespoon water
- ⅔ cup panko breadcrumbs
- ⅓ cup grated Parmesan cheese, plus more for serving
- 1 tablespoon Italian seasoning
- ¾ teaspoon oregano
- oil for misting or cooking spray
- 1 24-ounce jar marinara sauce
- 8 ounces spaghetti, cooked
- pepper

Directions:

1. Preheat air fryer to 390°F.
2. Leaving peel intact, cut eggplant into 8 round slices about ¾-inch thick. Salt to taste.
3. Beat egg and water in a shallow dish.
4. In another shallow dish, combine panko, Parmesan, Italian seasoning, and oregano.
5. Dip eggplant slices in egg wash and then crumbs, pressing lightly to coat.
6. Mist slices with oil or cooking spray.
7. Place 4 eggplant slices in air fryer basket and cook for 8 minutes, until brown and crispy.
8. While eggplant is cooking, heat marinara sauce.
9. Repeat step 7 to cook remaining eggplant slices.
10. To serve, place cooked spaghetti on plates and top with marinara and eggplant slices. At the table, pass extra Parmesan cheese and freshly ground black pepper.

Corn And Pepper Jack Chile Rellenos With Roasted Tomato Sauce

Servings: 3

Cooking Time: 30 Minutes

Ingredients:

- 3 Poblano peppers
- 1 cup all-purpose flour*
- salt and freshly ground black pepper
- 2 eggs, lightly beaten
- 1 cup plain breadcrumbs*
- olive oil, in a spray bottle
- Sauce
- 2 cups cherry tomatoes
- 1 Jalapeño pepper, halved and seeded
- 1 clove garlic
- ¼ red onion, broken into large pieces
- 1 tablespoon olive oil
- salt, to taste
- 2 tablespoons chopped fresh cilantro
- Filling
- olive oil
- ¼ red onion, finely chopped
- 1 teaspoon minced garlic
- 1 cup corn kernels, fresh or frozen
- 2 cups grated pepper jack cheese

Directions:

1. Start by roasting the peppers. Preheat the air fryer to 400°F. Place the peppers into the air fryer basket and air-fry at 400°F for 10 minutes, turning them over halfway through the cooking time. Remove the peppers from the basket and cover loosely with foil.
2. While the peppers are cooling, make the roasted tomato sauce. Place all sauce Ingredients except for the cilantro into the air fryer basket and air-fry at 400°F for 10 minutes, shaking the basket once or twice. When the sauce Ingredients have finished air-frying, transfer everything to a blender or food processor and blend or process to a smooth sauce, adding a little warm water to get the desired consistency. Season to taste with salt, add the cilantro and set aside.
3. While the sauce Ingredients are cooking in the air fryer, make the filling. Heat a skillet on the stovetop over medium heat. Add the olive oil and sauté the red onion and garlic for 4 to 5 minutes. Transfer the onion and garlic to a bowl, stir in the corn and cheese, and set aside.
4. Set up a dredging station with three shallow dishes. Place the flour, seasoned with salt and pepper, in the first shallow dish. Place the eggs in the second dish, and fill the third shallow dish with the breadcrumbs. When the peppers have cooled, carefully slice into one side of the pepper to create an opening. Pull the seeds out of the peppers and peel away the skins, trying not to tear the pepper. Fill each pepper with some of the corn and cheese filling and close the pepper up again by folding one side of the opening over the other. Carefully roll each pepper in the seasoned flour, then into the egg and finally into the breadcrumbs to coat on all sides, trying not to let the pepper fall open. Spray the peppers on all sides with a little olive oil.
5. Air-fry two peppers at a time at 350°F for 6 minutes. Turn the peppers over and air-fry for another 4 minutes. Serve the peppers warm on a bed of the roasted tomato sauce.

Vegetable Hand Pies

Servings: 8

Cooking Time: 10 Minutes Per Batch

Ingredients:

- ¾ cup vegetable broth
- 8 ounces potatoes
- ¾ cup frozen chopped broccoli, thawed
- ¼ cup chopped mushrooms
- 1 tablespoon cornstarch
- 1 tablespoon milk
- 1 can organic flaky biscuits (8 large biscuits)
- oil for misting or cooking spray

Directions:

1. Place broth in medium saucepan over low heat.
2. While broth is heating, grate raw potato into a bowl of water to prevent browning. You will need ¾ cup grated potato.
3. Roughly chop the broccoli.
4. Drain potatoes and put them in the broth along with the broccoli and mushrooms. Cook on low for 5 minutes.

5. Dissolve cornstarch in milk, then stir the mixture into the broth. Cook about a minute, until mixture thickens a little. Remove from heat and cool slightly.
6. Separate each biscuit into 2 rounds. Divide vegetable mixture evenly over half the biscuit rounds, mounding filling in the center of each.
7. Top the four rounds with filling, then the other four rounds and crimp the edges together with a fork.
8. Spray both sides with oil or cooking spray and place 4 pies in a single layer in the air fryer basket.
9. Cook at 330°F for approximately 10 minutes.
10. Repeat with the remaining biscuits. The second batch may cook more quickly because the fryer will be hot.

Veggie Fried Rice

Servings: 4
Cooking Time: 25 Minutes

Ingredients:

- 1 cup cooked brown rice
- ⅓ cup chopped onion
- ½ cup chopped carrots
- ½ cup chopped bell peppers
- ½ cup chopped broccoli florets
- 3 tablespoons low-sodium soy sauce
- 1 tablespoon sesame oil
- 1 teaspoon ground ginger
- 1 teaspoon ground garlic powder
- ½ teaspoon black pepper
- ⅛ teaspoon salt
- 2 large eggs

Directions:

1. Preheat the air fryer to 370°F.
2. In a large bowl, mix together the brown rice, onions, carrots, bell pepper, and broccoli.
3. In a small bowl, whisk together the soy sauce, sesame oil, ginger, garlic powder, pepper, salt, and eggs.
4. Pour the egg mixture into the rice and vegetable mixture and mix together.
5. Liberally spray a 7-inch springform pan (or compatible air fryer dish) with olive oil. Add the rice mixture to the pan and cover with aluminum foil.
6. Place a metal trivet into the air fryer basket and set the pan on top. Cook for 15 minutes. Carefully remove the pan from basket, discard the foil, and mix the rice. Return the rice to the air fryer basket, turning down the temperature to 350°F and cooking another 10 minutes.
7. Remove and let cool 5 minutes. Serve warm.

Appetizers And Snacks

Avocado Fries

Servings: 8

Cooking Time: 8 Minutes

Ingredients:

- 2 medium avocados, firm but ripe
- 1 large egg
- ½ teaspoon garlic powder
- ¼ teaspoon cayenne pepper
- ¼ teaspoon salt
- ¾ cup almond flour
- ½ cup finely grated Parmesan cheese
- ½ cup gluten-free breadcrumbs

Directions:

1. Preheat the air fryer to 370°F.
2. Rinse the outside of the avocado with water. Slice the avocado in half, slice it in half again, and then slice it in half once more to get 8 slices. Remove the outer skin. Repeat for the other avocado. Set the avocado slices aside.
3. In a small bowl, whisk the egg, garlic powder, cayenne pepper, and salt in a small bowl. Set aside.
4. In a separate bowl, pour the almond flour.
5. In a third bowl, mix the Parmesan cheese and breadcrumbs.
6. Carefully roll the avocado slices in the almond flour, then dip them in the egg wash, and coat them in the cheese and breadcrumb topping. Repeat until all 16 fries are coated.
7. Liberally spray the air fryer basket with olive oil spray and place the avocado fries into the basket, leaving a little space around the sides between fries. Depending on the size of your air fryer, you may need to cook these in batches.
8. Cook fries for 8 minutes, or until the outer coating turns light brown.
9. Carefully remove, repeat with remaining slices, and then serve warm.

Cheese Straws

Servings: 8

Cooking Time: 7 Minutes

Ingredients:

- For dusting All-purpose flour
- Two quarters of one thawed sheet (that is, a half of the sheet cut into two even pieces; wrap and refreeze the remainder) A 17.25-ounce box frozen puff pastry
- 1 Large egg(s)
- 2 tablespoons Water
- ¼ cup (about ¾ ounce) Finely grated Parmesan cheese
- up to 1 teaspoon Ground black pepper

Directions:

1. Preheat the air fryer to 400°F.
2. Dust a clean, dry work surface with flour. Set one of the pieces of puff pastry on top, dust the pastry lightly with flour, and roll with a rolling pin to a 6-inch square.
3. Whisk the egg(s) and water in a small or medium bowl until uniform. Brush the pastry square(s) generously with this mixture. Sprinkle each square with 2 tablespoons grated cheese and up to ½ teaspoon ground black pepper.
4. Cut each square into 4 even strips. Grasp each end of 1 strip with clean, dry hands; twist it into a cheese straw. Place the twisted straws on a baking sheet.
5. Lay as many straws as will fit in the air-fryer basket—as a general rule, 4 of them in a small machine, 5 in a medium model, or 6 in a large. There should be space for air to circulate around the straws. Set the baking sheet with any remaining straws in the fridge.
6. Air-fry undisturbed for 7 minutes, or until puffed and crisp. Use tongs to transfer the cheese straws to a wire rack, then make subsequent batches in the same way (keeping the baking sheet with the remaining straws in the fridge as each batch cooks). Serve warm.

Garlic Breadsticks

Servings: 12

Cooking Time: 7 Minutes

Ingredients:

- 1½ tablespoons Olive oil
- 1½ teaspoons Minced garlic
- ¼ teaspoon Table salt
- ¼ teaspoon Ground black pepper
- 6 ounces Purchased pizza dough (vegan dough, if that's a concern)

Directions:

1. Preheat the air fryer to 400°F. Mix the oil, garlic, salt, and pepper in a small bowl.
2. Divide the pizza dough into 4 balls for a small air fryer, 6 for a medium machine, or 8 for a large, each ball about the size of a walnut in its shell. (Each should weigh 1 ounce, if you want to drag out a scale and get obsessive.) Roll each ball into a 5-inch-long stick under your clean palms on a clean, dry work surface. Brush the sticks with the oil mixture.
3. When the machine is at temperature, place the prepared dough sticks in the basket, leaving a 1-inch space between them. Air-fry undisturbed for 7 minutes, or until puffed, golden, and set to the touch.
4. Use kitchen tongs to gently transfer the breadsticks to a wire rack and repeat step 3 with the remaining dough sticks.

Shrimp Egg Rolls

Servings: 8

Cooking Time: 10 Minutes

Ingredients:

- 1 tablespoon vegetable oil
- ½ head green or savoy cabbage, finely shredded
- 1 cup shredded carrots
- 1 cup canned bean sprouts, drained
- 1 tablespoon soy sauce
- ½ teaspoon sugar
- 1 teaspoon sesame oil
- ¼ cup hoisin sauce
- freshly ground black pepper
- 1 pound cooked shrimp, diced
- ¼ cup scallions
- 8 egg roll wrappers
- vegetable oil
- duck sauce

Directions:

1. Preheat a large sauté pan over medium-high heat. Add the oil and cook the cabbage, carrots and bean sprouts until they start to wilt – about 3 minutes. Add the soy sauce, sugar, sesame oil, hoisin sauce and black pepper. Sauté for a few more minutes. Stir in the shrimp and scallions and cook until the vegetables are just tender. Transfer the mixture to a colander in a bowl to cool. Press or squeeze out any excess water from the filling so that you don't end up with soggy egg rolls.
2. To make the egg rolls, place the egg roll wrappers on a flat surface with one of the points facing towards you so they look like diamonds. Dividing the filling evenly between the eight wrappers, spoon the mixture onto the center of the egg roll wrappers. Spread the filling across the center of the wrappers from the left corner to the right corner, but leave 2 inches from each corner empty. Brush the empty sides of the wrapper with a little water. Fold the bottom corner of the wrapper tightly up over the filling, trying to avoid making any air pockets. Fold the left corner in toward the center and then the right corner toward the center. It should now look like an envelope. Tightly roll the egg roll from the bottom to the top open corner. Press to seal the egg roll together, brushing with a little extra water if need be. Repeat this technique with all 8 egg rolls.
3. Preheat the air fryer to 370°F.
4. Spray or brush all sides of the egg rolls with vegetable oil. Air-fry four egg rolls at a time for 10 minutes, turning them over halfway through the cooking time.
5. Serve hot with duck sauce or your favorite dipping sauce.

Granola Three Ways

Servings: 4
Cooking Time: 10 Minutes

Ingredients:

- Nantucket Granola
- ¼ cup maple syrup
- ¼ cup dark brown sugar
- 1 tablespoon butter
- 1 teaspoon vanilla extract
- 1 cup rolled oats
- ½ cup dried cranberries
- ½ cup walnuts, chopped
- ¼ cup pumpkin seeds
- ¼ cup shredded coconut
- Blueberry Delight
- ¼ cup honey
- ¼ cup light brown sugar
- 1 tablespoon butter
- 1 teaspoon lemon extract
- 1 cup rolled oats
- ½ cup sliced almonds
- ½ cup dried blueberries
- ¼ cup pumpkin seeds
- ¼ cup sunflower seeds
- Cherry Black Forest Mix
- ¼ cup honey
- ¼ cup light brown sugar
- 1 tablespoon butter
- 1 teaspoon almond extract
- 1 cup rolled oats
- ½ cup sliced almonds
- ½ cup dried cherries
- ¼ cup shredded coconut
- ¼ cup dark chocolate chips
- oil for misting or cooking spray

Directions:

1. Combine the syrup or honey, brown sugar, and butter in a small saucepan or microwave-safe bowl. Heat and stir just until butter melts and sugar dissolves. Stir in the extract.
2. Place all other dry ingredients in a large bowl. (For the Cherry Black Forest Mix, don't add the chocolate chips yet.)
3. Pour melted butter mixture over dry ingredients and stir until oat mixture is well coated.
4. Lightly spray a baking pan with oil or cooking spray.
5. Pour granola into pan and cook at 390°F for 5minutes. Stir. Continue cooking for 5minutes, stirring every minute or two, until golden brown. Watch closely. Once the mixture begins to brown, it will cook quickly.
6. Remove granola from pan and spread on wax paper. It will become crispier as it cools.
7. For the Cherry Black Forest Mix, stir in chocolate chips after granola has cooled completely.
8. Store in an airtight container.

Dill Fried Pickles With Light Ranch Dip

Servings: 4
Cooking Time: 8 Minutes

Ingredients:

- 4 to 6 large dill pickles, sliced in half or quartered lengthwise
- ½ cup all-purpose flour*
- 2 eggs, lightly beaten
- 1 cup plain breadcrumbs*
- 1 teaspoon salt
- ⅛ teaspoon cayenne pepper
- 2 tablespoons fresh dill leaves, dried well
- vegetable oil, in a spray bottle
- Light Ranch Dip
- ¼ cup reduced-fat mayonnaise
- ¼ cup buttermilk
- ¼ cup non-fat Greek yogurt
- 1 tablespoon chopped fresh chives
- 1 tablespoon chopped fresh parsley
- 1 tablespoon lemon juice
- salt and freshly ground black pepper

Directions:

1. Dry the dill pickle spears very well with a clean kitchen towel.
2. Set up a dredging station using three shallow dishes. Place the flour in the first shallow dish. Place the eggs into the second dish. Combine the breadcrumbs, salt,

cayenne and fresh dill in a food processor and process until everything is combined and the crumbs are very fine. Place the crumb mixture in the third dish.

3. Preheat the air fryer to 400°F.
4. Coat the pickles by dredging them first in the flour, then the egg, and then the breadcrumbs, pressing the crumbs on gently with your hands. Set the coated pickles on a tray and spray them on all sides with vegetable oil.
5. Air-fry one layer of pickles at a time at 400°F for 8 minutes, turning them over halfway through the cooking process and spraying lightly again if necessary. The crumbs should be nicely browned on all sides.
6. While the pickles are air-frying, make the light ranch dip by mixing everything together in a bowl. Serve the pickles warm with the dip on the side.

Turkey Bacon Dates

Servings: 16
Cooking Time: 7 Minutes

Ingredients:

- 16 whole, pitted dates
- 16 whole almonds
- 6 to 8 strips turkey bacon

Directions:

1. Stuff each date with a whole almond.
2. Depending on the size of your stuffed dates, cut bacon strips into halves or thirds. Each strip should be long enough to wrap completely around a date.
3. Wrap each date in a strip of bacon with ends overlapping and secure with toothpicks.
4. Place in air fryer basket and cook at 390°F for 7 minutes, until bacon is as crispy as you like.
5. Drain on paper towels or wire rack. Serve hot or at room temperature.

Blistered Shishito Peppers

Servings: 3
Cooking Time: 5 Minutes

Ingredients:

- 6 ounces (about 18) Shishito peppers
- Vegetable oil spray
- For garnishing Coarse sea or kosher salt and lemon wedges

Directions:

1. Preheat the air fryer to 400°F.
2. Put the peppers in a bowl and lightly coat them with vegetable oil spray. Toss gently, spray again, and toss until the peppers are glistening but not drenched.
3. Pour the peppers into the basket, spread them into as close to one layer as you can, and air-fry for 5 minutes, tossing and rearranging the peppers at the 2- and 4-minute marks, until the peppers are blistered and even blackened in spots.
4. Pour the peppers into a bowl, add salt to taste, and toss gently. Serve the peppers with lemon wedges to squeeze over them.

Parmesan Crackers

Servings: 6
Cooking Time: 6 Minutes

Ingredients:

- 2 cups finely grated Parmesan cheese
- ¼ teaspoon paprika
- ¼ teaspoon garlic powder
- ½ teaspoon dried thyme
- 1 tablespoon all-purpose flour

Directions:

1. Preheat the air fryer to 380°F.
2. In a medium bowl, stir together the Parmesan, paprika, garlic powder, thyme, and flour.
3. Line the air fryer basket with parchment paper.
4. Using a tablespoon measuring tool, create 1-tablespoon mounds of seasoned cheese on the parchment paper, leaving 2 inches between the mounds to allow for spreading.
5. Cook the crackers for 6 minutes. Allow the cheese to harden and cool before handling. Repeat in batches with the remaining cheese.

Caponata Salsa

Servings: 6
Cooking Time: 16 Minutes

Ingredients:

- 4 cups (one 1-pound eggplant) Purple Italian eggplant(s), stemmed and diced (no need to peel)
- Olive oil spray
- 1½ cups Celery, thinly sliced
- 16 (about ½ pound) Cherry or grape tomatoes, halved
- 1 tablespoon Drained and rinsed capers, chopped
- Up to 1 tablespoon Minced fresh rosemary leaves
- 1½ tablespoons Red wine vinegar
- 1½ teaspoons Granulated white sugar
- ¾ teaspoon Table salt
- ¾ teaspoon Ground black pepper

Directions:

1. Preheat the air fryer to 350°F .
2. Put the eggplant pieces in a bowl and generously coat them with olive oil spray. Toss and stir, spray again, and toss some more, until the pieces are glistening.
3. When the machine is at temperature, pour the eggplant pieces into the basket and spread them out into an even layer. Air-fry for 8 minutes, tossing and rearranging the pieces twice.
4. Meanwhile, put the celery and tomatoes in the same bowl the eggplant pieces had been in. Generously coat them with olive oil spray; then toss well, spray again, and toss some more, until the vegetables are well coated.
5. When the eggplant has cooked for 8 minutes, pour the celery and tomatoes on top in the basket. Air-fry undisturbed for 8 minutes more, until the tomatoes have begun to soften.
6. Pour the contents of the basket back into the same bowl. Add the capers, rosemary, vinegar, sugar, salt, and pepper. Toss well to blend, breaking up the tomatoes a bit to create more moisture in the mixture.
7. Cover and refrigerate for 2 hours to blend the flavors. Serve chilled or at room temperature. The caponata salsa can stay in its covered bowl in the fridge for up to 2 days before the vegetables weep too much moisture and the dish becomes too wet.

Eggplant Fries

Servings: 4
Cooking Time: 8 Minutes

Ingredients:

- 1 medium eggplant
- 1 teaspoon ground coriander
- 1 teaspoon cumin
- 1 teaspoon garlic powder
- ½ teaspoon salt
- 1 cup crushed panko breadcrumbs
- 1 large egg
- 2 tablespoons water
- oil for misting or cooking spray

Directions:

1. Peel and cut the eggplant into fat fries, ⅜- to ½-inch thick.
2. Preheat air fryer to 390°F.
3. In a small cup, mix together the coriander, cumin, garlic, and salt.
4. Combine 1 teaspoon of the seasoning mix and panko crumbs in a shallow dish.
5. Place eggplant fries in a large bowl, sprinkle with remaining seasoning, and stir well to combine.
6. Beat eggs and water together and pour over eggplant fries. Stir to coat.
7. Remove eggplant from egg wash, shaking off excess, and roll in panko crumbs.
8. Spray with oil.
9. Place half of the fries in air fryer basket. You should have only a single layer, but it's fine if they overlap a little.
10. Cook for 5minutes. Shake basket, mist lightly with oil, and cook 3 minutes longer, until browned and crispy.
11. Repeat step 10 to cook remaining eggplant.

Sugar-glazed Walnuts

Servings: 6

Cooking Time: 5 Minutes

Ingredients:

- 1 Large egg white(s)
- 2 tablespoons Granulated white sugar
- ⅛ teaspoon Table salt
- 2 cups (7 ounces) Walnut halves

Directions:

1. Preheat the air fryer to 400°F.
2. Use a whisk to beat the egg white(s) in a large bowl until quite foamy, more so than just well combined but certainly not yet a meringue.
3. If you're working with the quantities for a small batch, remove half of the foamy egg white.
4. If you're working with the quantities for a large batch, remove a quarter of it. It's fine to eyeball the amounts.
5. You can store the removed egg white in a sealed container to save for another use.
6. Stir in the sugar and salt. Add the walnut halves and toss to coat evenly and well, including the nuts' crevasses.
7. When the machine is at temperature, use a slotted spoon to transfer the walnut halves to the basket, taking care not to dislodge any coating. Gently spread the nuts into as close to one layer as you can. Air-fry undisturbed for 2 minutes.
8. Break up any clumps, toss the walnuts gently but well, and air-fry for 3 minutes more, tossing after 1 minute, then every 30 seconds thereafter, until the nuts are browned in spots and very aromatic. Watch carefully so they don't burn.
9. Gently dump the nuts onto a lipped baking sheet and spread them into one layer. Cool for at least 10 minutes before serving, separating any that stick together. The walnuts can be stored in a sealed container at room temperature for up to 5 days.

Buffalo Cauliflower

Servings: 6

Cooking Time: 12 Minutes

Ingredients:

- 1 large head of cauliflower, washed and cut into medium-size florets
- ½ cup all-purpose flour
- ¼ cup melted butter
- 3 tablespoons hot sauce
- ½ teaspoon garlic powder
- ½ cup blue cheese dip or ranch dressing (optional)

Directions:

1. Preheat the air fryer to 350°F.
2. Make sure the cauliflower florets are dry, and then coat them in flour.
3. Liberally spray the air fryer basket with an olive oil mist. Place the cauliflower into the basket, making sure not to stack them on top of each other. Depending on the size of your air fryer, you may need to do this in two batches.
4. Cook for 6 minutes, then shake the basket, and cook another 6 minutes.
5. While cooking, mix the melted butter, hot sauce, and garlic powder in a large bowl.
6. Carefully remove the cauliflower from the air fryer. Toss the cauliflower into the butter mixture to coat. Repeat Steps 2–4 for any leftover cauliflower. Serve warm with the dip of your choice.

Fried Pickles

Servings: 2

Cooking Time: 15 Minutes

Ingredients:

- 1 egg
- 1 tablespoon milk
- ¼ teaspoon hot sauce
- 2 cups sliced dill pickles, well drained
- ¾ cup breadcrumbs
- oil for misting or cooking spray

Directions:

1. Preheat air fryer to 390°F.
2. Beat together egg, milk, and hot sauce in a bowl large enough to hold all the pickles.
3. Add pickles to the egg wash and stir well to coat.
4. Place breadcrumbs in a large plastic bag or container with lid.

5. Drain egg wash from pickles and place them in bag with breadcrumbs. Shake to coat.
6. Pile pickles into air fryer basket and spray with oil.
7. Cook for 5minutes. Shake basket and spray with oil.
8. Cook 5 more minutes. Shake and spray again. Separate any pickles that have stuck together and mist any spots you've missed.
9. Cook for 5minutes longer or until dark golden brown and crispy.

Fried Wontons

Servings: 24
Cooking Time: 6 Minutes

Ingredients:

- 6 ounces Lean ground beef, pork, or turkey
- 1 tablespoon Regular or reduced-sodium soy sauce or tamari sauce
- 1½ teaspoons Minced garlic
- ¾ teaspoon Ground dried ginger
- ½ teaspoon Ground white pepper
- 24 Wonton wrappers (thawed, if necessary)
- Vegetable oil spray

Directions:

1. Preheat the air fryer to 350°F .
2. Stir the ground meat, soy or tamari sauce, garlic, ginger, and white pepper in a bowl until the spices are uniformly distributed in the mixture.
3. Set a small bowl of water on a clean, dry surface or next to a clean, dry cutting board. Set one wonton wrapper on the surface. Dip your clean finger in the water, then run it along the edges of the wrapper. Set 1 teaspoon of the ground meat mixture in the center of the wrapper. Fold it over, corner to corner, to create a filled triangle. Press to seal the edges, then pull the corners on the longest side up and together over the filling to create the classic wonton shape. Press the corners together to seal. Set aside and continue filling and making more filled wontons.
4. Generously coat the filled wontons on all sides with vegetable oil spray. Arrange them in the basket in one layer and air-fry for 6 minutes, shaking the basket gently at the 2- and 4-minute marks to rearrange the wontons (but always making sure they're still in one layer), until golden brown and crisp.
5. Pour the wontons in the basket onto a wire rack or even into a serving bowl. Cool for 2 or 3 minutes (but not much longer) and serve hot.

Garlic Parmesan Kale Chips

Servings: 2
Cooking Time: 6 Minutes

Ingredients:

- 16 large kale leaves, washed and thick stems removed
- 1 tablespoon avocado oil
- ½ teaspoon garlic powder
- 1 teaspoon soy sauce or tamari
- ¼ cup grated Parmesan cheese

Directions:

1. Preheat the air fryer to 370°F.
2. Make a stack of kale leaves and cut them into 4 pieces.
3. Place the kale pieces into a large bowl. Drizzle the avocado oil onto the kale and rub to coat. Add the garlic powder, soy sauce or tamari, and cheese, tossing to coat.
4. Pour the chips into the air fryer basket and cook for 3 minutes, shake the basket, and cook another 3 minutes, checking for crispness every minute. When done cooking, pour the kale chips onto paper towels and cool at least 5 minutes before serving.

Shrimp Pirogues

Servings: 8
Cooking Time: 5 Minutes

Ingredients:

- 12 ounces small, peeled, and deveined raw shrimp
- 3 ounces cream cheese, room temperature
- 2 tablespoons plain yogurt
- 1 teaspoon lemon juice
- 1 teaspoon dried dill weed, crushed
- salt
- 4 small hothouse cucumbers, each approximately 6 inches long

Directions:

1. Pour 4 tablespoons water in bottom of air fryer drawer.
2. Place shrimp in air fryer basket in single layer and cook at 390°F for 5 minutes, just until done. Watch carefully because shrimp cooks quickly, and overcooking makes it tough.
3. Chop shrimp into small pieces, no larger than ½ inch. Refrigerate while mixing the remaining ingredients.
4. With a fork, mash and whip the cream cheese until smooth.
5. Stir in the yogurt and beat until smooth. Stir in lemon juice, dill weed, and chopped shrimp.
6. Taste for seasoning. If needed, add ¼ to ½ teaspoon salt to suit your taste.
7. Store in refrigerator until serving time.
8. When ready to serve, wash and dry cucumbers and split them lengthwise. Scoop out the seeds and turn cucumbers upside down on paper towels to drain for 10minutes.
9. Just before filling, wipe centers of cucumbers dry. Spoon the shrimp mixture into the pirogues and cut in half crosswise. Serve immediately.

Asian Rice Logs

Servings: 8

Cooking Time: 5 Minutes

Ingredients:

- 1½ cups cooked jasmine or sushi rice
- ¼ teaspoon salt
- 2 teaspoons five-spice powder
- 2 teaspoons diced shallots
- 1 tablespoon tamari sauce
- 1 egg, beaten
- 1 teaspoon sesame oil
- 2 teaspoons water
- ⅓ cup plain breadcrumbs
- ¾ cup panko breadcrumbs
- 2 tablespoons sesame seeds
- Orange Marmalade Dipping Sauce
- ½ cup all-natural orange marmalade
- 1 tablespoon soy sauce

Directions:

1. Make the rice according to package instructions. While the rice is cooking, make the dipping sauce by combining the marmalade and soy sauce and set aside.
2. Stir together the cooked rice, salt, five-spice powder, shallots, and tamari sauce.
3. Divide rice into 8 equal pieces. With slightly damp hands, mold each piece into a log shape. Chill in freezer for 10 to 15minutes.
4. Mix the egg, sesame oil, and water together in a shallow bowl.
5. Place the plain breadcrumbs on a sheet of wax paper.
6. Mix the panko breadcrumbs with the sesame seeds and place on another sheet of wax paper.
7. Roll the rice logs in plain breadcrumbs, then dip in egg wash, and then dip in the panko and sesame seeds.
8. Cook the logs at 390°F for approximately 5minutes, until golden brown.
9. Cool slightly before serving with Orange Marmalade Dipping Sauce.

Onion Puffs

Servings: 14

Cooking Time: 8 Minutes

Ingredients:

- Vegetable oil spray
- ¾ cup Chopped yellow or white onion
- ½ cup Seasoned Italian-style panko bread crumbs
- 4½ tablespoons All-purpose flour
- 4½ tablespoons Whole, low-fat, or fat-free milk
- 1½ tablespoons Yellow cornmeal
- 1¼ teaspoons Granulated white sugar
- ½ teaspoon Baking powder
- ¼ teaspoon Table salt

Directions:

1. Cut or tear a piece of aluminum foil so that it lines the air fryer's basket with a ½-inch space on each of its four sides. Lightly coat the foil with vegetable oil spray, then set the foil sprayed side up inside the basket.
2. Preheat the air fryer to 400°F.
3. Stir the onion, bread crumbs, flour, milk, cornmeal, sugar, baking powder, and salt in a bowl to form a thick batter.

4. Remove the basket from the machine. Drop the onion batter by 2-tablespoon measures onto the foil, spacing the mounds evenly across its surface. Return the basket to the machine and air-fry undisturbed for 4 minutes.

5. Remove the basket from the machine. Lightly coat the puffs with vegetable oil spray. Use kitchen tongs to pick up a corner of the foil, then gently pull it out of the basket, letting the puffs slip onto the basket directly. Return the basket to the machine and continue air-frying undisturbed for 8 minutes, or until brown and crunchy.

6. Use kitchen tongs to transfer the puffs to a wire rack or a serving platter. Cool for 5 minutes before serving.

Barbecue Chicken Nachos

Servings: 3

Cooking Time: 5 Minutes

Ingredients:

- 3 heaping cups (a little more than 3 ounces) Corn tortilla chips (gluten-free, if a concern)
- ¾ cup Shredded deboned and skinned rotisserie chicken meat (gluten-free, if a concern)
- 3 tablespoons Canned black beans, drained and rinsed
- 9 rings Pickled jalapeño slices
- 4 Small pickled cocktail onions, halved
- 3 tablespoons Barbecue sauce (any sort)
- ¾ cup (about 3 ounces) Shredded Cheddar cheese

Directions:

1. Preheat the air fryer to 400°F.
2. Cut a circle of parchment paper to line a 6-inch round cake pan for a small air fryer, a 7-inch round cake pan for a medium air fryer, or an 8-inch round cake pan for a large machine.
3. Fill the pan with an even layer of about two-thirds of the chips. Sprinkle the chicken evenly over the chips. Set the pan in the basket and air-fry undisturbed for 2 minutes.
4. Remove the basket from the machine. Scatter the beans, jalapeño rings, and pickled onion halves over the chicken. Drizzle the barbecue sauce over everything, then sprinkle the cheese on top.
5. Return the basket to the machine and air-fry undisturbed for 3 minutes, or until the cheese has melted and is bubbly. Remove the pan from the machine and cool for a couple of minutes before serving.

Smoked Whitefish Spread

Servings: 1

Cooking Time: 10 Minutes

Ingredients:

- ¾ pound Boneless skinless white-flesh fish fillets, such as hake or trout
- 3 tablespoons Liquid smoke
- 3 tablespoons Regular, low-fat, or fat-free mayonnaise (gluten-free, if a concern)
- 2 teaspoons Jarred prepared white horseradish (optional)
- ¼ teaspoon Onion powder
- ¼ teaspoon Celery seeds
- ¼ teaspoon Table salt
- ¼ teaspoon Ground black pepper

Directions:

1. Put the fish fillets in a zip-closed bag, add the liquid smoke, and seal closed. Rub the liquid smoke all over the fish , then refrigerate the sealed bag for 2 hours.
2. Preheat the air fryer to 400°F.
3. Set a 12-inch piece of aluminum foil on your work surface. Remove the fish fillets from the bag and set them in the center of this piece of foil (the fillets can overlap). Fold the long sides of the foil together and crimp them closed. Make a tight seam so no steam can escape. Fold up the ends and crimp to seal well.
4. Set the packet in the basket and air-fry undisturbed for 10 minutes.
5. Use kitchen tongs to transfer the foil packet to a wire rack. Cool for a minute or so. Open the packet, transfer the fish to a plate, and refrigerate for 30 minutes.
6. Put the cold fish in a food processor. Add the mayonnaise, horseradish (if using), onion powder, celery seeds, salt, and pepper. Cover and pulse to a slightly coarse spread, certainly not fully smooth.
7. For a more traditional texture, put the fish fillets in a bowl, add the other ingredients, and stir with a wooden

spoon, mashing the fish with everything else to make a coarse paste.

8. Scrape the spread into a bowl and serve at once, or cover with plastic wrap and store in the fridge for up to 4 days.

Classic Chicken Wings

Servings: 8

Cooking Time: 20 Minutes

Ingredients:

- 16 chicken wings
- ¼ cup all-purpose flour
- ¼ teaspoon garlic powder
- ¼ teaspoon paprika
- ½ teaspoon salt
- ½ teaspoon black pepper
- ¼ cup butter
- ½ cup hot sauce
- ½ teaspoon Worcestershire sauce
- 2 ounces crumbled blue cheese, for garnish

Directions:

1. Preheat the air fryer to 380°F.
2. Pat the chicken wings dry with paper towels.
3. In a medium bowl, mix together the flour, garlic powder, paprika, salt, and pepper. Toss the chicken wings with the flour mixture, dusting off any excess.
4. Place the chicken wings in the air fryer basket, making sure that the chicken wings aren't touching. Cook the chicken wings for 10 minutes, turn over, and cook another 5 minutes. Raise the temperature to 400°F and continue crisping the chicken wings for an additional 3 to 5 minutes.
5. Meanwhile, in a microwave-safe bowl, melt the butter and hot sauce for 1 to 2 minutes in the microwave. Remove from the microwave and stir in the Worcestershire sauce.
6. When the chicken wings have cooked, immediately transfer the chicken wings into the hot sauce mixture. Serve the coated chicken wings on a plate, and top with crumbled blue cheese.

Parmesan Pizza Nuggets

Servings: 8

Cooking Time: 6 Minutes

Ingredients:

- ¾ cup warm filtered water
- 1 package fast-rising yeast
- ½ teaspoon salt
- 2 cups all-purpose flour
- ¼ cup finely grated Parmesan cheese
- 1 teaspoon Italian seasoning
- 2 tablespoon extra-virgin olive oil
- 1 teaspoon kosher salt

Directions:

1. Preheat the air fryer to 370°F.
2. In a large microwave-safe bowl, add the water. Heat for 40 seconds in the microwave. Remove and mix in the yeast and salt. Let sit 5 minutes.
3. Meanwhile, in a medium bowl, mix the flour with the Parmesan cheese and Italian seasoning. Set aside.
4. Using a stand mixer with a dough hook attachment, add the yeast liquid and then mix in the flour mixture ⅓ cup at a time until all the flour mixture is added and a dough is formed.
5. Remove the bowl from the stand, and then let the dough rise for 1 hour in a warm space, covered with a kitchen towel.
6. After the dough has doubled in size, remove it from the bowl and punch it down a few times on a lightly floured flat surface.
7. Divide the dough into 4 balls, and then roll each ball out into a long, skinny, sticklike shape.
8. Using a sharp knife, cut each dough stick into 6 pieces. Repeat for the remaining dough balls until you have about 24 nuggets formed.
9. Lightly brush the top of each bite with the egg whites and cover with a pinch of sea salt.
10. Spray the air fryer basket with olive oil spray and place the pizza nuggets on top. Cook for 6 minutes, or until lightly browned. Remove and keep warm.
11. Repeat until all the nuggets are cooked.
12. Serve warm.

Crunchy Tortellini Bites

Servings: 5
Cooking Time: 10 Minutes

Ingredients:

- 10 ounces (about 2½ cups) Cheese tortellini
- ⅓ cup Yellow cornmeal
- ⅓ cup Seasoned Italian-style dried bread crumbs
- ⅓ cup (about 1 ounce) Finely grated Parmesan cheese
- 1 Large egg
- Olive oil spray

Directions:

1. Bring a large pot of water to a boil over high heat. Add the tortellini and cook for 3 minutes. Drain in a colander set in the sink, then spread out the tortellini on a large baking sheet and cool for 15 minutes.
2. Preheat the air fryer to 400°F.
3. Mix the cornmeal, bread crumbs, and cheese in a large zip-closed plastic bag.
4. Whisk the egg in a medium bowl until uniform. Add the tortellini and toss well to coat, even along the inside curve of the pasta. Use a slotted spoon or kitchen tongs to transfer 5 or 6 tortellini to the plastic bag, seal, and shake gently to coat thoroughly and evenly. Set the coated tortellini aside on a cutting board and continue coating the rest in the same way.
5. Generously coat the tortellini on all sides with the olive oil spray, then set them in one layer in the basket. Air-fry undisturbed for 10 minutes, gently tossing the basket and rearranging the tortellini at the 4- and 7-minute marks, until brown and crisp.
6. Pour the contents of the basket onto a wire rack. Cool for 5 minutes before serving.

Grilled Ham & Muenster Cheese On Raisin Bread

Servings: 1
Cooking Time: 10 Minutes

Ingredients:

- 2 slices raisin bread
- 2 tablespoons butter, softened
- 2 teaspoons honey mustard
- 3 slices thinly sliced honey ham (about 3 ounces)
- 4 slices Muenster cheese (about 3 ounces)
- 2 toothpicks

Directions:

1. Preheat the air fryer to 370°F.
2. Spread the softened butter on one side of both slices of raisin bread and place the bread, buttered side down on the counter. Spread the honey mustard on the other side of each slice of bread. Layer 2 slices of cheese, the ham and the remaining 2 slices of cheese on one slice of bread and top with the other slice of bread. Remember to leave the buttered side of the bread on the outside.
3. Transfer the sandwich to the air fryer basket and secure the sandwich with toothpicks.
4. Air-fry at 370°F for 5 minutes. Flip the sandwich over, remove the toothpicks and air-fry for another 5 minutes. Cut the sandwich in half and enjoy!!

Baba Ghanouj

Servings: 2
Cooking Time: 40 Minutes

Ingredients:

- 2 Small (12-ounce) purple Italian eggplant(s)
- ¼ cup Olive oil
- ¼ cup Tahini
- ½ teaspoon Ground black pepper
- ¼ teaspoon Onion powder
- ¼ teaspoon Mild smoked paprika (optional)
- Up to 1 teaspoon Table salt

Directions:

1. Preheat the air fryer to 400°F.
2. Prick the eggplant(s) on all sides with a fork. When the machine is at temperature, set the eggplant(s) in the basket in one layer. Air-fry undisturbed for 40 minutes, or until blackened and soft.
3. Remove the basket from the machine. Cool the eggplant(s) in the basket for 20 minutes.
4. Use a nonstick-safe spatula, and perhaps a flatware tablespoon for balance, to gently transfer the eggplant(s) to a bowl. The juices will run out. Make sure the bowl is close to the basket. Split the eggplant(s) open.
5. Scrape the soft insides of half an eggplant into a food processor. Repeat with the remaining piece(s). Add

any juices from the bowl to the eggplant in the food processor, but discard the skins and stems.

6. Add the olive oil, tahini, pepper, onion powder, and smoked paprika (if using). Add about half the salt, then cover and process until smooth, stopping the machine at least once to scrape down the inside of the canister. Check the spread for salt and add more as needed. Scrape the baba ghanouj into a bowl and serve warm, or set aside at room temperature for up to 2 hours, or cover and store in the refrigerator for up to 4 days.

Pizza Bagel Bites

Servings: 2

Cooking Time: 5 Minutes

Ingredients:

- 2 Mini bagel(s), split into two rings
- ¼ cup Purchased pizza sauce
- ½ cup Finely grated or shredded cheese, such as Parmesan cheese, semi-firm mozzarella, fontina, or (preferably) a cheese blend

Directions:

1. Preheat the air fryer to 375°F .
2. Spread the cut side of each bagel half with 1 tablespoon pizza sauce; top each half with 2 tablespoons shredded cheese.
3. When the machine is at temperature, put the bagels cheese side up in the basket in one layer. Air-fry undisturbed for 4 minutes, or until the cheese has melted and is gooey. You may need to air-fry the pizza bagel bites for 1 minute extra if the temperature is at 360°F.
4. Use a nonstick-safe spatula to transfer the topped bagel halves to a wire rack. Cool for at least 5 minutes before serving.

Grilled Cheese Sandwich Deluxe

Servings: 4

Cooking Time: 6 Minutes

Ingredients:

- 8 ounces Brie
- 8 slices oat nut bread
- 1 large ripe pear, cored and cut into ½-inch-thick slices
- 2 tablespoons butter, melted

Directions:

1. Spread a quarter of the Brie on each of four slices of bread.
2. Top Brie with thick slices of pear, then the remaining 4 slices of bread.
3. Lightly brush both sides of each sandwich with melted butter.
4. Cooking 2 at a time, place sandwiches in air fryer basket and cook at 360°F for 6minutes or until cheese melts and outside looks golden brown.

Warm And Salty Edamame

Servings: 4

Cooking Time: 10 Minutes

Ingredients:

- 1 pound Unshelled edamame
- Vegetable oil spray
- ¾ teaspoon Coarse sea salt or kosher salt

Directions:

1. Preheat the air fryer to 400°F.
2. Place the edamame in a large bowl and lightly coat them with vegetable oil spray. Toss well, spray again, and toss until they are evenly coated.
3. When the machine is at temperature, pour the edamame into the basket and air-fry, tossing the basket quite often to rearrange the edamame, for 7 minutes, or until warm and aromatic. (Air-fry for 10 minutes if the edamame were frozen and not thawed.)
4. Pour the edamame into a bowl and sprinkle the salt on top. Toss well, then set aside for a couple of minutes before serving with an empty bowl on the side for the pods.

Onion Ring Nachos

Servings: 3
Cooking Time: 8 Minutes

Ingredients:

- ¾ pound Frozen breaded (not battered) onion rings (do not thaw)
- 1½ cups (about 6 ounces) Shredded Cheddar, Monterey Jack, or Swiss cheese, or a purchased Tex-Mex blend
- Up to 12 Pickled jalapeño rings

Directions:

1. Preheat the air fryer to 400°F.
2. When the machine is at temperature, spread the onion rings in the basket in a fairly even layer. Air-fry undisturbed for 6 minutes, or until crisp. Remove the basket from the machine.
3. Cut a circle of parchment paper to line a 6-inch round cake pan for a small air fryer, a 7-inch round cake pan for a medium air fryer, or an 8-inch round cake pan for a large machine.
4. Pour the onion rings into a fairly even layer in the cake pan, then sprinkle the cheese evenly over them. Dot with the jalapeño rings.
5. Set the pan in the basket and air-fry undisturbed for 2 minutes, until the cheese has melted and is bubbling.
6. Remove the pan from the basket. Cool for 5 minutes before serving.

Spiced Nuts

Servings: 3
Cooking Time: 25 Minutes

Ingredients:

- 1 egg white, lightly beaten
- ¼ cup sugar
- 1 teaspoon salt
- ½ teaspoon ground cinnamon
- ¼ teaspoon ground cloves
- ¼ teaspoon ground allspice
- pinch ground cayenne pepper
- 1 cup pecan halves
- 1 cup cashews
- 1 cup almonds

Directions:

1. Combine the egg white with the sugar and spices in a bowl.
2. Preheat the air fryer to 300°F.
3. Spray or brush the air fryer basket with vegetable oil. Toss the nuts together in the spiced egg white and transfer the nuts to the air fryer basket.
4. Air-fry for 25 minutes, stirring the nuts in the basket a few times during the cooking process. Taste the nuts to see if they are crunchy and nicely toasted. Air-fry for a few more minutes if necessary.
5. Serve warm or cool to room temperature and store in an airtight container for up to two weeks.

Grilled Cheese Sandwich

Servings: 2
Cooking Time: 5 Minutes

Ingredients:

- 4 slices bread
- 4 ounces Cheddar cheese slices
- 2 teaspoons butter or oil

Directions:

1. Lay the four cheese slices on two of the bread slices and top with the remaining two slices of bread.
2. Brush both sides with butter or oil and cut the sandwiches in rectangular halves.
3. Place in air fryer basket and cook at 390°F for 5minutes until the outside is crisp and the cheese melts.

Warm Spinach Dip With Pita Chips

Servings: 6
Cooking Time: 40 Minutes

Ingredients:

- Pita Chips:
- 4 pita breads
- 1 tablespoon olive oil
- ½ teaspoon paprika
- salt and freshly ground black pepper
- Spinach Dip:
- 8 ounces cream cheese, softened at room , Temperature: 1 cup ricotta cheese
- 1 cup grated Fontina cheese

- ½ teaspoon Italian seasoning
- ½ teaspoon garlic powder
- ¾ teaspoon salt
- freshly ground black pepper
- 16 ounces frozen chopped spinach, thawed and squeezed dry
- ¼ cup grated Parmesan cheese
- ½ tomato, finely diced
- ¼ teaspoon dried oregano

Directions:

1. Preheat the air fryer to 390°F.
2. Split the pita breads open so you have 2 circles. Cut each circle into 8 wedges. Place all the wedges into a large bowl and toss with the olive oil. Season with the paprika, salt and pepper and toss to coat evenly. Air-fry the pita triangles in two batches for 5 minutes each, shaking the basket once or twice while they cook so they brown and crisp evenly.
3. Combine the cream cheese, ricotta cheese, Fontina cheese, Italian seasoning, garlic powder, salt and pepper in a large bowl. Fold in the spinach and mix well.
4. Transfer the spinach-cheese mixture to a 7-inch ceramic baking dish or cake pan. Sprinkle the Parmesan cheese on top and wrap the dish with aluminum foil. Transfer the dish to the basket of the air fryer, lowering the dish into the basket using a sling made of aluminum foil (fold a piece of aluminum foil into a strip about 2-inches wide by 24-inches long). Fold the ends of the aluminum foil over the top of the dish before returning the basket to the air fryer. Air-fry for 30 minutes at 390°F. With 4 minutes left on the air fryer timer, remove the foil and let the cheese brown on top.
5. Sprinkle the diced tomato and oregano on the warm dip and serve immediately with the pita chips.

Thick-crust Pepperoni Pizza

Servings: 2

Cooking Time: 10 Minutes

Ingredients:

- 10 ounces Purchased fresh pizza dough (not a prebaked crust)
- Olive oil spray
- ¼ cup Purchased pizza sauce
- 10 slices Sliced pepperoni
- ⅓ cup Purchased shredded Italian 3- or 4-cheese blend

Directions:

1. Preheat the air fryer to 400°F.
2. Generously coat the inside of a 6-inch round cake pan for a small air fryer, a 7-inch round cake pan for a medium air fryer, or an 8-inch round cake pan for a large model with olive oil spray.
3. Set the dough in the pan and press it to fill the bottom in an even, thick layer. Spread the sauce over the dough, then top with the pepperoni and cheese.
4. When the machine is at temperature, set the pan in the basket and air-fry undisturbed for 10 minutes, or until puffed, brown, and bubbling.
5. Use kitchen tongs to transfer the cake pan to a wire rack. Cool for only a minute or so. Use a spatula to loosen the pizza from the pan and lift it out and onto the rack. Continue cooling for a few minutes before cutting into wedges to serve.

Blooming Onion

Servings: 4

Cooking Time: 25 Minutes

Ingredients:

- 1 large Vidalia onion, peeled
- 2 eggs
- ½ cup milk
- 1 cup flour
- 1 teaspoon salt
- ½ teaspoon freshly ground black pepper
- ¼ teaspoon ground cayenne pepper
- ½ teaspoon paprika
- ½ teaspoon garlic powder
- Dipping Sauce:
- ½ cup mayonnaise
- ½ cup ketchup
- 1 teaspoon Worcestershire sauce
- ½ teaspoon ground cayenne pepper
- ½ teaspoon paprika
- ½ teaspoon onion powder

Directions:

1. Cut off the top inch of the onion, leaving the root end of the onion intact. Place the now flat, stem end of the onion down on a cutting board with the root end facing up. Make 16 slices around the onion, starting with your knife tip ½-inch away from the root so that you never slice through the root. Begin by making slices at 12, 3, 6 and 9 o'clock around the onion. Then make three slices down the onion in between each of the original four slices. Turn the onion over, gently separate the onion petals, and remove the loose pieces of onion in the center.
2. Combine the eggs and milk in a bowl. In a second bowl, combine the flour, salt, black pepper, cayenne pepper, paprika, and garlic powder.
3. Preheat the air fryer to 350°F.
4. Place the onion cut side up into a third empty bowl. Sprinkle the flour mixture all over the onion to cover it and get in between the onion petals. Turn the onion over to carefully shake off the excess flour and then transfer the onion to the empty flour bowl, again cut side up.
5. Pour the egg mixture all over the onion to cover all the flour. Let it soak for a minute in the mixture. Carefully remove the onion, tipping it upside down to drain off any excess egg, and transfer it to the empty egg bowl, again cut side up.
6. Finally, sprinkle the flour mixture over the onion a second time, making sure the onion is well coated and all the petals have the seasoned flour mixture on them. Carefully turn the onion over, shake off any excess flour and transfer it to a plate or baking sheet. Spray the onion generously with vegetable oil.
7. Transfer the onion, cut side up to the air fryer basket and air-fry for 25 minutes. The onion petals will open more fully as it cooks, so spray with more vegetable oil at least twice during the cooking time.
8. While the onion is cooking, make the dipping sauce by combining all the dip ingredients and mixing well. Serve the Blooming Onion as soon as it comes out of the air fryer with dipping sauce on the side.

Cauliflower-crust Pizza

Servings: 3
Cooking Time: 14 Minutes

Ingredients:

- 1 pound 2 ounces Riced cauliflower
- 1 plus 1 large egg yolk Large egg(s)
- 3 tablespoons (a little more than ½ ounce) Finely grated Parmesan cheese
- 1½ tablespoons Potato starch
- ¾ teaspoon Dried oregano
- ¾ teaspoon Table salt
- Vegetable oil spray
- 3 tablespoons Purchased pizza sauce
- 6 tablespoons (about 1½ ounces) Shredded semi-firm mozzarella

Directions:

1. Pour the riced cauliflower into a medium microwave-safe bowl. Microwave on high for 4 minutes. Stir well, then cool for 15 minutes.
2. Preheat the air fryer to 400°F.
3. Pour the riced cauliflower into a clean kitchen towel or a large piece of cheesecloth. Gather the towel or cheesecloth together. Working over the sink, squeeze the moisture out of the cauliflower, getting out as much of the liquid as you can.
4. Pour the squeezed cauliflower back into that same medium bowl and stir in the egg, egg yolk (if using), cheese, potato starch, oregano, and salt to form a loose, uniform "dough."
5. Cut a piece of aluminum foil or parchment paper into a 6-inch circle for a small pizza, a 7-inch circle for a medium one, or an 8-inch circle for a large one. Coat the circle with vegetable oil spray, then place it in the air-fryer basket. Using a small offset spatula or the back of a flatware tablespoon, spread and smooth the cauliflower mixture onto the circle right to the edges. Air-fry undisturbed for 10 minutes.
6. Remove the basket from the air fryer. Reduce the machine's temperature to 350°F .
7. Using a large nonstick-safe spatula, flip over the cauliflower circle along with its foil or parchment paper right in the basket. Peel off and discard the foil or parchment paper. Spread the pizza sauce evenly over the crust and sprinkle with the cheese.
8. Air-fry undisturbed for 4 minutes, or until the cheese has melted and begun to bubble. Remove the

basket from the machine and cool for 5 minutes. Use the same spatula to transfer the pizza to a wire rack to cool for 5 minutes more before cutting the pie into wedges to serve.

Veggie Cheese Bites

Servings: 4

Cooking Time: 8 Minutes

Ingredients:

- 2 cups riced vegetables (see the Note below)
- ½ cup shredded zucchini
- ½ teaspoon garlic powder
- ¼ teaspoon black pepper
- ¼ teaspoon salt
- 1 large egg
- ¾ cup shredded cheddar cheese
- ⅓ cup whole-wheat flour

Directions:

1. Preheat the air fryer to 350°F.
2. In a large bowl, mix together the riced vegetables, zucchini, garlic powder, pepper, and salt. Mix in the egg. Stir in the shredded cheese and whole-wheat flour until a thick, doughlike consistency forms. If you need to, add 1 teaspoon of flour at a time so you can mold the batter into balls.
3. Using a 1-inch scoop, portion the batter out into about 12 balls.
4. Liberally spray the air fryer basket with olive oil spray. Then place the veggie bites inside. Leave enough room between each bite so the air can flow around them.
5. Cook for 8 minutes, or until the outside is slightly browned. Depending on the size of your air fryer, you may need to cook these in batches.
6. Remove and let cool slightly before serving.

Crispy Tofu Bites

Servings: 4

Cooking Time: 20 Minutes

Ingredients:

- 1 pound Extra firm unflavored tofu
- Vegetable oil spray

Directions:

1. Wrap the piece of tofu in a triple layer of paper towels. Place it on a wooden cutting board and set a large pot on top of it to press out excess moisture. Set aside for 10 minutes.
2. Preheat the air fryer to 400°F.
3. Remove the pot and unwrap the tofu. Cut it into 1-inch cubes. Place these in a bowl and coat them generously with vegetable oil spray. Toss gently, then spray generously again before tossing, until all are glistening.
4. Gently pour the tofu pieces into the basket, spread them into as close to one layer as possible, and air-fry for 20 minutes, using kitchen tongs to gently rearrange the pieces at the 7- and 14-minute marks, until light brown and crisp.
5. Gently pour the tofu pieces onto a wire rack. Cool for 5 minutes before serving warm.

Zucchini Chips

Servings: 3

Cooking Time: 17 Minutes

Ingredients:

- 1½ small (about 1½ cups) Zucchini, washed but not peeled, and cut into ¼-inch-thick rounds
- Olive oil spray
- ¼ teaspoon Table salt

Directions:

1. Preheat the air fryer to 375°F .
2. Lay some paper towels on your work surface. Set the zucchini rounds on top, then set more paper towels over the rounds. Press gently to remove some of the moisture. Remove the top layer of paper towels and lightly coat the rounds with olive oil spray on both sides.
3. When the machine is at temperature, set the rounds in the basket, overlapping them a bit as needed. (They'll shrink as they cook.) Air-fry for 15 minutes, tossing and rearranging the rounds at the 5- and 10-minute marks, until browned, soft, yet crisp at the edges. (You'll need to air-fry the rounds 2 minutes more if the temperature is set at 360°F.)
4. Gently pour the contents of the basket onto a wire rack. Cool for at least 10 minutes or up to 2 hours before serving.

Cinnamon Pita Chips

Servings: 4
Cooking Time: 6 Minutes

Ingredients:

- 2 tablespoons sugar
- 2 teaspoons cinnamon
- 2 whole 6-inch pitas, whole grain or white
- oil for misting or cooking spray

Directions:

1. Mix sugar and cinnamon together.
2. Cut each pita in half and each half into 4 wedges. Break apart each wedge at the fold.
3. Mist one side of pita wedges with oil or cooking spray. Sprinkle them all with half of the cinnamon sugar.
4. Turn the wedges over, mist the other side with oil or cooking spray, and sprinkle with the remaining cinnamon sugar.
5. Place pita wedges in air fryer basket and cook at 330°F for 2minutes.
6. Shake basket and cook 2 more minutes. Shake again, and if needed cook 2 more minutes, until crisp. Watch carefully because at this point they will cook very quickly.

Crispy Wontons

Servings: 8
Cooking Time: 10 Minutes

Ingredients:

- ½ cup refried beans
- 3 tablespoons salsa
- ¼ cup canned artichoke hearts, drained and patted dry
- ¼ cup frozen spinach, defrosted and squeezed dry
- 2 ounces cream cheese
- 1½ teaspoons dried oregano, divided
- ¼ teaspoon garlic powder
- ¼ teaspoon onion powder
- ½ teaspoon salt
- ¼ cup chopped pepperoni
- ¼ cup grated mozzarella cheese
- 1 tablespoon grated Parmesan
- 2 ounces cream cheese
- ½ teaspoon dried oregano
- 32 wontons
- 1 cup water

Directions:

1. Preheat the air fryer to 370°F.
2. In a medium bowl, mix together the refried beans and salsa.
3. In a second medium bowl, mix together the artichoke hearts, spinach, cream cheese, oregano, garlic powder, onion powder, and salt.
4. In a third medium bowl, mix together the pepperoni, mozzarella cheese, Parmesan cheese, cream cheese, and the remaining ½ teaspoon of oregano.
5. Get a towel lightly damp with water and ring it out. While working with the wontons, leave the unfilled wontons under the damp towel so they don't dry out.
6. Working with 8 wontons at a time, place 2 teaspoons of one of the fillings into the center of the wonton, rotating among the different fillings (one filling per wonton). Working one at a time, use a pastry brush, dip the pastry brush into the water, and brush the edges of the dough with the water. Fold the dough in half to form a triangle and set aside. Continue until 8 wontons are formed. Spray the wontons with cooking spray and cover with a dry towel. Repeat until all 32 wontons have been filled.
7. Place the wontons into the air fryer basket, leaving space between the wontons, and cook for 5 minutes. Turn over and check for brownness, and then cook for another 5 minutes.

Buffalo Wings

Servings: 2
Cooking Time: 12 Minutes Per Batch

Ingredients:

- 2 pounds chicken wings
- 3 tablespoons butter, melted
- ¼ cup hot sauce (like Crystal® or Frank's®)
- Finishing Sauce:
- 3 tablespoons butter, melted
- ¼ cup hot sauce (like Crystal® or Frank's®)
- 1 teaspoon Worcestershire sauce

Directions:

1. Prepare the chicken wings by cutting off the wing tips and discarding (or freezing for chicken stock). Divide the drumettes from the wingettes by cutting through the joint. Place the chicken wing pieces in a large bowl.
2. Combine the melted butter and the hot sauce and stir to blend well. Pour the marinade over the chicken wings, cover and let the wings marinate for 2 hours or up to overnight in the refrigerator.
3. Preheat the air fryer to 400°F.
4. Air-fry the wings in two batches for 10 minutes per batch, shaking the basket halfway through the cooking process. When both batches are done, toss all the wings back into the basket for another 2 minutes to heat through and finish cooking.
5. While the wings are air-frying, combine the remaining 3 tablespoons of butter, ¼ cup of hot sauce and the Worcestershire sauce. Remove the wings from the air fryer, toss them in the finishing sauce and serve with some cooling blue cheese dip and celery sticks.

Stuffed Baby Bella Caps

Servings: 16
Cooking Time: 12 Minutes

Ingredients:

- 16 fresh, small Baby Bella mushrooms
- 2 green onions
- 4 ounces mozzarella cheese
- ½ cup diced ham
- 2 tablespoons breadcrumbs
- ½ teaspoon garlic powder
- ¼ teaspoon ground oregano
- ¼ teaspoon ground black pepper
- 1 to 2 teaspoons olive oil

Directions:

1. Remove stems and wash mushroom caps.
2. Cut green onions and cheese in small pieces and place in food processor.
3. Add ham, breadcrumbs, garlic powder, oregano, and pepper and mince ingredients.
4. With food processor running, dribble in just enough olive oil to make a thick paste.
5. Divide stuffing among mushroom caps and pack down lightly.
6. Place stuffed mushrooms in air fryer basket in single layer and cook at 390°F for 12minutes or until tops are golden brown and mushrooms are tender.
7. Repeat step 6 to cook remaining mushrooms.

Corn Tortilla Chips

Servings: 4
Cooking Time: 12 Minutes

Ingredients:

- Eight 6-inch corn tortillas
- ½ teaspoon sea salt
- ¼ teaspoon ground cumin
- ¼ teaspoon chili powder
- ¼ teaspoon garlic powder
- ⅛ teaspoon onion powder
- 1 tablespoon avocado oil

Directions:

1. Cut each corn tortilla into quarters, creating 32 chips in total.
2. Preheat the air fryer to 350°F.
3. In a small bowl, mix together the sea salt, cumin, chili powder, garlic powder, and onion powder.
4. Spray or brush one side of the tortillas with avocado oil. Sprinkle the seasoning mixture evenly over the oiled side of the chips.
5. Working in batches, place half the chips in the air fryer basket. Cook for 8 minutes, shake the basket, and cook another 2 to 4 minutes, checking for crispness. When the chips are golden brown, spread them out onto paper towels and allow them to cool for 3 minutes before serving. Repeat with the remaining chips.

Arancini With Sun-dried Tomatoes And Mozzarella

Servings: 6
Cooking Time: 15 Minutes

Ingredients:

- 1 tablespoon olive oil
- ½ small onion, finely chopped
- 1 cup Arborio rice

- ¼ cup white wine or dry vermouth
- 1 cup vegetable or chicken stock
- 1½ cups water
- 1 teaspoon salt
- freshly ground black pepper
- ⅓ cup grated Parmigiano-Reggiano cheese
- 2 to 3 ounces mozzarella cheese
- 2 eggs, lightly beaten
- ¼ cup chopped oil-packed sun-dried tomatoes
- 1½ cups Italian seasoned breadcrumbs, divided
- olive oil
- marinara sauce, for serving

Directions:

1. .Start by cooking the Arborio rice.
2. Stovetop Method: Preheat a medium saucepan over medium heat. Add the olive oil and sauté the onion until it starts to become tender – about 5 minutes. Add the rice and stir well to coat all the grains of rice. Add the white wine or vermouth. Let this simmer and get absorbed by the rice. Then add the stock and water, cover, reduce the heat to low and simmer for 20 minutes.
3. Pressure-Cooker Method: Preheat the pressure cooker using the BROWN setting. Add the oil and cook the onion for a few minutes. Add the rice, wine, stock, water, salt and freshly ground black pepper, give everything one good stir and lock the lid in place. Pressure cook on HIGH for 7 minutes. Reduce the pressure with the QUICK-RELEASE method and carefully remove the lid.
4. Taste the rice to make sure it is tender. Season with salt and freshly ground black pepper and stir in the grated Parmigiano-Reggiano cheese. Spread the rice out onto a baking sheet to cool.
5. While the rice is cooling, cut the mozzarella into ¾-inch cubes.
6. Once the rice has cooled, combine the rice with the eggs, sun-dried tomatoes and ½ cup of the breadcrumbs. Place the remaining breadcrumbs in a shallow dish. Shape the rice mixture into 12 balls. Press a hole in the rice ball with your finger and push one or two cubes of mozzarella cheese into the hole. Mold the rice back into a ball, enclosing the cheese. Roll the finished rice balls in the breadcrumbs and place them on a baking sheet while you make the remaining rice balls. Spray or brush the rice balls with olive oil.
7. Preheat the air fryer to 380°F.
8. Cook 6 arancini at a time. Air-fry for 10 minutes. Gently turn the arancini over, brush or spray with oil again and air-fry for another 5 minutes. Serve warm with the marinara sauce.

Popcorn Chicken Bites

Servings: 2

Cooking Time: 8 Minutes

Ingredients:

- 1 pound chicken breasts, cutlets or tenders
- 1 cup buttermilk
- 3 to 6 dashes hot sauce (optional)
- 8 cups cornflakes (or 2 cups cornflake crumbs)
- ½ teaspoon salt
- 1 tablespoon butter, melted
- 2 tablespoons chopped fresh parsley

Directions:

1. Cut the chicken into bite-sized pieces (about 1-inch) and place them in a bowl with the buttermilk and hot sauce (if using). Cover and let the chicken marinate in the buttermilk for 1 to 3 hours in the refrigerator.
2. Preheat the air fryer to 380°F.
3. Crush the cornflakes into fine crumbs by either crushing them with your hands in a bowl, rolling them with a rolling pin in a plastic bag or processing them in a food processor. Place the crumbs in a bowl, add the salt, melted butter and parsley and mix well. Working in batches, remove the chicken from the buttermilk marinade, letting any excess drip off and transfer the chicken to the cornflakes. Toss the chicken pieces in the cornflake mixture to coat evenly, pressing the crumbs onto the chicken.
4. Air-fry the chicken in two batches for 8 minutes per batch, shaking the basket halfway through the cooking process. Re-heat the first batch with the second batch for a couple of minutes if desired.
5. Serve the popcorn chicken bites warm with BBQ sauce or honey mustard for dipping.

Fried Goat Cheese

Servings: 3

Cooking Time: 4 Minutes

Ingredients:

- 7 ounces 1- to 1½-inch-diameter goat cheese log
- 2 Large egg(s)
- 1¾ cups Plain dried bread crumbs (gluten-free, if a concern)
- Vegetable oil spray

Directions:

1. Slice the goat cheese log into ½-inch-thick rounds. Set these flat on a small cutting board, a small baking sheet, or a large plate. Freeze uncovered for 30 minutes.
2. Preheat the air fryer to 400°F.
3. Set up and fill two shallow soup plates or small pie plates on your counter: one in which you whisk the egg(s) until uniform and the other for the bread crumbs.
4. Take the goat cheese rounds out of the freezer. With clean, dry hands, dip one round in the egg(s) to coat it on all sides. Let the excess egg slip back into the rest, then dredge the round in the bread crumbs, turning it to coat all sides, even the edges. Repeat this process—egg, then bread crumbs—for a second coating. Coat both sides of the round and its edges with vegetable oil spray, then set it aside. Continue double-dipping, double-dredging, and spraying the remaining rounds.
5. Place the rounds in one layer in the basket. Air-fry undisturbed for 4 minutes, or until lightly browned and crunchy. Do not overcook. Some of the goat cheese may break through the crust. A few little breaks are fine but stop the cooking before the coating reaches structural failure.
6. Remove the basket from the machine and set aside for 3 minutes. Use a nonstick-safe spatula, and maybe a flatware fork for balance, to transfer the rounds to a wire rack. Cool for 5 minutes more before serving.

Prosciutto Mozzarella Bites

Servings: 8

Cooking Time: 6 Minutes

Ingredients:

- 8 pieces full-fat mozzarella string cheese
- 8 thin slices prosciutto
- 16 basil leaves

Directions:

1. Preheat the air fryer to 360°F.
2. Cut the string cheese in half across the center, not lengthwise. Do the same with the prosciutto.
3. Place a piece of prosciutto onto a clean workspace. Top the prosciutto with a basil leaf and then a piece of string cheese. Roll up the string cheese inside the prosciutto and secure with a wooden toothpick. Repeat with the remaining cheese sticks.
4. Place the prosciutto mozzarella bites into the air fryer basket and cook for 6 minutes, checking for doneness at 4 minutes.

Potato Chips

Servings: 2

Cooking Time: 15 Minutes

Ingredients:

- 2 medium potatoes
- 2 teaspoons extra-light olive oil
- oil for misting or cooking spray
- salt and pepper

Directions:

1. Peel the potatoes.
2. Using a mandoline or paring knife, shave potatoes into thin slices, dropping them into a bowl of water as you cut them.
3. Dry potatoes as thoroughly as possible with paper towels or a clean dish towel. Toss potato slices with the oil to coat completely.
4. Spray air fryer basket with cooking spray and add potato slices.
5. Stir and separate with a fork.
6. Cook 390°F for 5minutes. Stir and separate potato slices. Cook 5 more minutes. Stir and separate potatoes again. Cook another 5minutes.
7. Season to taste.

Muffuletta Sliders

Servings: 8
Cooking Time: 7 Minutes

Ingredients:

- ¼ pound thin-sliced deli ham
- ¼ pound thin-sliced pastrami
- 4 ounces low-fat mozzarella cheese, grated or sliced thin
- 8 slider buns
- olive oil for misting
- 1 tablespoon sesame seeds
- Olive Mix
- ¼ cup sliced black olives
- ½ cup sliced green olives with pimentos
- ¼ cup chopped kalamata olives
- 1 teaspoon red wine vinegar
- ¼ teaspoon basil
- ⅛ teaspoon garlic powder

Directions:

1. In a small bowl, stir together all the Olive Mix ingredients.
2. Divide the meats and cheese into 8 equal portions. To assemble sliders, stack in this order: bottom bun, ham, pastrami, 2 tablespoons olive mix, cheese, top bun.
3. Mist tops of sliders lightly with oil. Sprinkle with sesame seeds.
4. Cooking 4 at a time, place sliders in air fryer basket and cook at 360°F for 7 minutes to melt cheese and heat through.

Greek Street Tacos

Servings: 8
Cooking Time: 3 Minutes

Ingredients:

- 8 small flour tortillas (4-inch diameter)
- 8 tablespoons hummus
- 4 tablespoons crumbled feta cheese
- 4 tablespoons chopped kalamata or other olives (optional)
- olive oil for misting

Directions:

1. Place 1 tablespoon of hummus or tapenade in the center of each tortilla. Top with 1 teaspoon of feta crumbles and 1 teaspoon of chopped olives, if using.
2. Using your finger or a small spoon, moisten the edges of the tortilla all around with water.
3. Fold tortilla over to make a half-moon shape. Press center gently. Then press the edges firmly to seal in the filling.
4. Mist both sides with olive oil.
5. Place in air fryer basket very close but try not to overlap.
6. Cook at 390°F for 3minutes, just until lightly browned and crispy.

Cuban Sliders

Servings: 8
Cooking Time: 8 Minutes

Ingredients:

- 8 slices ciabatta bread, ¼-inch thick
- cooking spray
- 1 tablespoon brown mustard
- 6-8 ounces thin sliced leftover roast pork
- 4 ounces thin deli turkey
- ⅓ cup bread and butter pickle slices
- 2–3 ounces Pepper Jack cheese slices

Directions:

1. Spray one side of each slice of bread with butter or olive oil cooking spray.
2. Spread brown mustard on other side of each slice.
3. Layer pork roast, turkey, pickles, and cheese on 4 of the slices. Top with remaining slices.
4. Cook at 390°F for approximately 8minutes. The sandwiches should be golden brown.
5. Cut each slider in half to make 8 portions.

Kale Chips

Servings: 2
Cooking Time: 5 Minutes

Ingredients:

- 4 Medium kale leaves, about 1 ounce each
- 2 teaspoons Olive oil
- 2 teaspoons Regular or low-sodium soy sauce or gluten-free tamari sauce

Directions:

1. Preheat the air fryer to 400°F.
2. Cut the stems from the leaves (all the stems, all the way up the leaf). Tear each leaf into three pieces. Put them in a large bowl.
3. Add the olive oil and soy or tamari sauce. Toss well to coat. You can even gently rub the leaves along the side of the bowl to get the liquids to stick to them.
4. When the machine is at temperature, put the leaf pieces in the basket in one layer. Air-fry for 5 minutes, turning and rearranging with kitchen tongs once halfway through, until the chips are dried out and crunchy. Watch carefully so they don't turn dark brown at the edges.
5. Gently pour the contents of the basket onto a wire rack. Cool for at least 5 minutes before serving. The chips can keep for up to 8 hours uncovered on the rack (provided it's not a humid day).

Savory Sausage Balls

Servings: 10
Cooking Time: 8 Minutes

Ingredients:

- 2 cups all-purpose flour
- 1 tablespoon baking powder
- ½ teaspoon garlic powder
- ¼ teaspoon onion powder
- ½ teaspoon salt
- 3 tablespoons milk
- 2½ cups grated pepper jack cheese
- 1 pound fresh sausage, casing removed

Directions:

1. Preheat the air fryer to 370°F.
2. In a large bowl, whisk together the flour, baking powder, garlic powder, onion powder, and salt. Add in the milk, grated cheese, and sausage.
3. Using a tablespoon, scoop out the sausage and roll it between your hands to form a rounded ball. You should end up with approximately 32 balls. Place them in the air fryer basket in a single layer and working in batches as necessary.
4. Cook for 8 minutes, or until the outer coating turns light brown.
5. Carefully remove, repeating with the remaining sausage balls.

Buffalo Bites

Servings: 16
Cooking Time: 12 Minutes

Ingredients:

- 1 pound ground chicken
- 8 tablespoons buffalo wing sauce
- 2 ounces Gruyère cheese, cut into 16 cubes
- 1 tablespoon maple syrup

Directions:

1. Mix 4 tablespoons buffalo wing sauce into all the ground chicken.
2. Shape chicken into a log and divide into 16 equal portions.
3. With slightly damp hands, mold each chicken portion around a cube of cheese and shape into a firm ball. When you have shaped 8 meatballs, place them in air fryer basket.
4. Cook at 390°F for approximately 5minutes. Shake basket, reduce temperature to 360°F, and cook for 5 minutes longer.
5. While the first batch is cooking, shape remaining chicken and cheese into 8 more meatballs.
6. Repeat step 4 to cook second batch of meatballs.
7. In a medium bowl, mix the remaining 4 tablespoons of buffalo wing sauce with the maple syrup. Add all the cooked meatballs and toss to coat.
8. Place meatballs back into air fryer basket and cook at 390°F for 2 minutes to set the glaze. Skewer each with a toothpick and serve.

Meatball Arancini

Servings: 6
Cooking Time: 10 Minutes

Ingredients:

- 1⅓ cups Water
- ⅔ cup Raw white Arborio rice
- 2 teaspoons Butter
- ¼ teaspoon Table salt
- 2 Large egg(s), well beaten
- ¾ cup Seasoned Italian-style dried bread crumbs (gluten-free, if a concern)
- ⅓ cup (about 1 ounce) Finely grated Parmesan cheese
- 6 ½-ounce "bite-size" frozen meatballs (any variety, even vegan and/or gluten-free, if a concern), thawed
- Olive oil spray

Directions:

1. Combine the water, rice, butter, and salt in a small saucepan. Bring to a boil over medium-high heat, stirring occasionally. Cover, reduce the heat to very low, and simmer very slowly for 20 minutes.
2. Take the saucepan off the heat and let it stand, covered, for 10 minutes. Uncover it and fluff the rice. Cool for 20 minutes. (The rice can be made up to 1 hour in advance; keep it covered in its saucepan.)
3. Preheat the air fryer to 375°F .
4. Set up and fill two shallow soup plates or small bowls on your counter: one with the beaten egg(s) and one with the bread crumbs mixed with the grated cheese.
5. With clean but wet hands, scoop up about 3 tablespoons of the cooked rice and form it into a ball around a mini meatball, forming a sealed casing. Dip the ball in the egg(s) to coat completely, letting any excess egg slip back into the rest. Set the ball in the bread-crumb mixture and roll it gently to coat evenly but lightly all over. Set aside and continue making more rice balls.
6. Generously spray the balls with olive oil spray, then set them in the basket in one layer. They must not touch. Air-fry undisturbed for 10 minutes, or until crunchy and golden brown. Use kitchen tongs to gently transfer the balls to a wire rack. Cool for at least 5 minutes before serving.

Spanakopita Spinach, Feta And Pine Nut Phyllo Bites

Servings: 8
Cooking Time: 10 Minutes

Ingredients:

- ½ (10-ounce) package frozen spinach, thawed and squeezed dry (about 1 cup)
- ¾ cup crumbled feta cheese
- ¼ cup grated Parmesan cheese
- ¼ cup pine nuts, toasted
- ⅛ teaspoon ground nutmeg
- 1 egg, lightly beaten
- ½ teaspoon salt
- freshly ground black pepper
- 6 sheets phyllo dough
- ½ cup butter, melted

Directions:

1. Combine the spinach, cheeses, pine nuts, nutmeg and egg in a bowl. Season with salt and freshly ground black pepper.
2. While building the phyllo triangles, always keep the dough sheets you are not working with covered with plastic wrap and a damp clean kitchen towel. Remove one sheet of the phyllo and place it on a flat surface. Brush the phyllo sheet with melted butter and then layer another sheet of phyllo on top. Brush the second sheet of phyllo with butter. Cut the layered phyllo sheets into 6 strips, about 2½- to 3-inches wide.
3. Place a heaping tablespoon of the spinach filling at the end of each strip of dough. Fold the bottom right corner of the strip over the filling towards the left edge of the strip to make a triangle. Continue to fold the phyllo dough around the spinach as you would fold a flag, making triangle after triangle. Brush the outside of the phyllo triangle with more melted butter and set it aside until you've finished the 6 strips of dough, making 6 triangles.
4. Preheat the air fryer to 350°F.
5. Transfer the first six phyllo triangles to the air fryer basket and air-fry for 5 minutes. Turn the triangles over and air-fry for another 5 minutes.

6. While the first batch of triangles is air-frying, build another set of triangles and air-fry in the same manner. You should do three batches total. These can be warmed in the air fryer for a minute or two just before serving if you like.

Loaded Potato Skins

Servings: 8
Cooking Time: 8 Minutes

Ingredients:

- 12 round baby potatoes
- 3 ounces cream cheese
- 4 slices cooked bacon, crumbled or chopped
- 2 green onions, finely chopped
- ½ cup grated cheddar cheese, divided
- ¼ cup sour cream
- 1 tablespoon milk
- 2 teaspoons hot sauce

Directions:

1. Preheat the air fryer to 320°F.
2. Poke holes into the baby potatoes with a fork. Place the potatoes onto a microwave-safe plate and microwave on high for 4 to 5 minutes, or until soft to squeeze. Let the potatoes cool until they're safe to handle, about 5 minutes.
3. Meanwhile, in a medium bowl, mix together the cream cheese, bacon, green onions, and ¼ cup of the cheddar cheese; set aside.
4. Slice the baby potatoes in half. Using a spoon, scoop out the pulp, leaving enough pulp on the inside to retain the shape of the potato half. Place the potato pulp into the cream cheese mixture and mash together with a fork. Using a spoon, refill the potato halves with filling.
5. Place the potato halves into the air fryer basket and top with the remaining ¼ cup of cheddar cheese.
6. Cook the loaded baked potato bites in batches for 8 minutes.
7. Meanwhile, make the sour cream sauce. In a small bowl, whisk together the sour cream, milk, and hot sauce. Add more hot sauce if desired.
8. When the potatoes have all finished cooking, place them onto a serving platter and serve with sour cream sauce drizzled over the top or as a dip.

Fried Green Tomatoes

Servings: 4
Cooking Time: 15 Minutes

Ingredients:

- 2 eggs
- ¼ cup buttermilk
- ½ cup cornmeal
- ½ cup breadcrumbs
- ¼ teaspoon salt
- 1½ pounds firm green tomatoes, cut in ¼-inch slices
- oil for misting or cooking spray
- Horseradish Drizzle
- ¼ cup mayonnaise
- ¼ cup sour cream
- 2 teaspoons prepared horseradish
- ½ teaspoon Worcestershire sauce
- ½ teaspoon lemon juice
- ⅛ teaspoon black pepper

Directions:

1. Mix all ingredients for Horseradish Drizzle together and chill while you prepare the green tomatoes.
2. Preheat air fryer to 390°F.
3. Beat the eggs and buttermilk together in a shallow bowl.
4. Mix cornmeal, breadcrumbs, and salt together in a plate or shallow dish.
5. Dip 4 tomato slices in the egg mixture, then roll in the breadcrumb mixture.
6. Mist one side with oil and place in air fryer basket, oil-side down, in a single layer.
7. Mist the top with oil.
8. Cook for 15minutes, turning once, until brown and crispy.
9. Repeat steps 5 through 8 to cook remaining tomatoes.
10. Drizzle horseradish sauce over tomatoes just before serving.

Crispy Ravioli Bites

Servings: 5
Cooking Time: 7 Minutes

Ingredients:

- ⅓ cup All-purpose flour
- 1 Large egg(s), well beaten
- ⅔ cup Seasoned Italian-style dried bread crumbs
- 10 ounces (about 20) Frozen mini ravioli, meat or cheese, thawed
- Olive oil spray

Directions:

1. Preheat the air fryer to 400°F.
2. Pour the flour into a medium bowl. Set up and fill two shallow soup plates or small pie plates on your counter: one with the beaten egg(s) and one with the bread crumbs.
3. Pour all the ravioli into the flour and toss well to coat. Pick up 1 ravioli, gently shake off any excess flour, and dip the ravioli in the egg(s), coating both sides. Let any excess egg slip back into the rest, then set the ravioli in the bread crumbs, turning it several times until lightly and evenly coated on all sides. Set aside on a cutting board and continue on with the remaining ravioli.
4. Lightly coat the ravioli on both sides with olive oil spray, then set them in the basket in as close to a single layer as you can. Some can lean up against the side of the basket. Air-fry for 7 minutes, tossing the basket at the 4-minute mark to rearrange the pieces, until brown and crisp.
5. Pour the contents of the basket onto a wire rack. Cool for 5 minutes before serving.

Avocado Egg Rolls

Servings: 8
Cooking Time: 8 Minutes

Ingredients:

- 8 full-size egg roll wrappers
- 1 medium avocado, sliced into 8 pieces
- 1 cup cooked black beans, divided
- ½ cup mild salsa, divided
- ½ cup shredded Mexican cheese, divided
- ⅓ cup filtered water, divided
- ½ cup sour cream
- 1 teaspoon chipotle hot sauce

Directions:

1. Preheat the air fryer to 400°F.
2. Place the egg roll wrapper on a flat surface and place 1 strip of avocado down in the center.
3. Top the avocado with 2 tablespoons of black beans, 1 tablespoon of salsa, and 1 tablespoon of shredded cheese.
4. Place two of your fingers into the water, and then moisten the four outside edges of the egg roll wrapper with water (so the outer edges will secure shut).
5. Fold the bottom corner up, covering the filling. Then secure the sides over the top, remembering to lightly moisten them so they stick. Tightly roll the egg roll up and moisten the final flap of the wrapper and firmly press it into the egg roll to secure it shut.
6. Repeat Steps 2–5 until all 8 egg rolls are complete.
7. When ready to cook, spray the air fryer basket with olive oil spray and place the egg rolls into the basket. Depending on the size and type of air fryer you have, you may need to do this in two sets.
8. Cook for 4 minutes, flip, and then cook the remaining 4 minutes.
9. Repeat until all the egg rolls are cooked. Meanwhile, mix the sour cream with the hot sauce to serve as a dipping sauce.
10. Serve warm.

Tempura Fried Veggies

Servings: 4
Cooking Time: 6 Minutes

Ingredients:

- ½ cup all-purpose flour
- ½ teaspoon black pepper
- ¼ teaspoon salt
- 2 large eggs
- 1¼ cups panko breadcrumbs
- 1 tablespoon extra-virgin olive oil
- 1 cup white button mushrooms, cleaned
- 1 medium zucchini, skinned and sliced
- 1 medium carrot, skinned sliced

Directions:

1. Preheat the air fryer to 400°F.
2. In a small bowl, mix the flour, pepper, and salt.
3. In a separate bowl, whisk the eggs.
4. In a third bowl, mix together the breadcrumbs and olive oil.
5. Begin to batter the vegetables by placing them one at a time into the flour, then dipping them in the eggs, and coating them in breadcrumbs. When you've prepared enough to begin air frying, liberally spray the air fryer basket with olive oil and place the vegetables inside.
6. Cook for 6 minutes, or until the breadcrumb coating on the outside appears golden brown. Repeat coating the other vegetables while the first batch is cooking.
7. When the cooking completes, carefully remove the vegetables and keep them warm. Repeat cooking for the remaining vegetables until all are cooked.
8. Serve warm.

Zucchini Fries With Roasted Garlic Aïoli

Servings: 4
Cooking Time: 12 Minutes

Ingredients:

- Roasted Garlic Aïoli:
- 1 teaspoon roasted garlic
- ½ cup mayonnaise
- 2 tablespoons olive oil
- juice of ½ lemon
- salt and pepper
- Zucchini Fries:
- ½ cup flour
- 2 eggs, beaten
- 1 cup seasoned breadcrumbs
- salt and pepper
- 1 large zucchini, cut into ½-inch sticks
- olive oil in a spray bottle, can or mister

Directions:

1. To make the aïoli, combine the roasted garlic, mayonnaise, olive oil and lemon juice in a bowl and whisk well. Season the aïoli with salt and pepper to taste.
2. Prepare the zucchini fries. Create a dredging station with three shallow dishes. Place the flour in the first shallow dish and season well with salt and freshly ground black pepper. Put the beaten eggs in the second shallow dish. In the third shallow dish, combine the breadcrumbs, salt and pepper. Dredge the zucchini sticks, coating with flour first, then dipping them into the eggs to coat, and finally tossing in breadcrumbs. Shake the dish with the breadcrumbs and pat the crumbs onto the zucchini sticks gently with your hands so they stick evenly.
3. Place the zucchini fries on a flat surface and let them sit at least 10 minutes before air-frying to let them dry out a little. Preheat the air fryer to 400°F.
4. Spray the zucchini sticks with olive oil, and place them into the air fryer basket. You can air-fry the zucchini in two layers, placing the second layer in the opposite direction to the first. Air-fry for 12 minutes turning and rotating the fries halfway through the cooking time. Spray with additional oil when you turn them over.
5. Serve zucchini fries warm with the roasted garlic aïoli.

Sweet Potato Chips

Servings: 4
Cooking Time: 10 Minutes

Ingredients:

- 2 medium sweet potatoes, washed
- 2 cups filtered water
- 1 tablespoon avocado oil
- 2 teaspoons brown sugar
- ½ teaspoon salt

Directions:

1. Using a mandolin, slice the potatoes into ⅛-inch pieces.
2. Add the water to a large bowl. Place the potatoes in the bowl, and soak for at least 30 minutes.
3. Preheat the air fryer to 350°F.
4. Drain the water and pat the chips dry with a paper towel or kitchen cloth. Toss the chips with the avocado oil, brown sugar, and salt. Liberally spray the air fryer basket with olive oil mist.
5. Set the chips inside the air fryer, separating them so they're not on top of each other. Cook for 5 minutes, shake the basket, and cook another 5 minutes, or until browned.

6. Remove and let cool a few minutes prior to serving. Repeat until all the chips are cooked.

Roasted Red Pepper Dip

Servings: 2

Cooking Time: 15 Minutes

Ingredients:

- 2 Medium-size red bell pepper(s)
- 1¾ cups (one 15-ounce can) Canned white beans, drained and rinsed
- 1 tablespoon Fresh oregano leaves, packed
- 3 tablespoons Olive oil
- 1 tablespoon Lemon juice
- ½ teaspoon Table salt
- ½ teaspoon Ground black pepper

Directions:

1. Preheat the air fryer to 400°F.
2. Set the pepper(s) in the basket and air-fry undisturbed for 15 minutes, until blistered and even blackened.
3. Use kitchen tongs to transfer the pepper(s) to a zip-closed plastic bag or small bowl. Seal the bag or cover the bowl with plastic wrap. Set aside for 20 minutes.
4. Peel each pepper, then stem it, cut it in half, and remove all its seeds and their white membranes.
5. Set the pieces of the pepper in a food processor. Add the beans, oregano, olive oil, lemon juice, salt, and pepper. Cover and process until smooth, stopping the machine at least once to scrape down the inside of the canister. Scrape the dip into a bowl and serve warm, or cover and refrigerate for up to 3 days (although the dip tastes best if it's allowed to come back to room temperature).

Desserts And Sweets

Molten Chocolate Almond Cakes

Servings: 3

Cooking Time: 13 Minutes

Ingredients:

- butter and flour for the ramekins
- 4 ounces bittersweet chocolate, chopped
- ½ cup (1 stick) unsalted butter
- 2 eggs
- 2 egg yolks
- ¼ cup sugar
- ½ teaspoon pure vanilla extract, or almond extract
- 1 tablespoon all-purpose flour
- 3 tablespoons ground almonds
- 8 to 12 semisweet chocolate discs (or 4 chunks of chocolate)
- cocoa powder or powdered sugar, for dusting
- toasted almonds, coarsely chopped

Directions:

1. Butter and flour three (6-ounce) ramekins. (Butter the ramekins and then coat the butter with flour by shaking it around in the ramekin and dumping out any excess.)
2. Melt the chocolate and butter together, either in the microwave or in a double boiler. In a separate bowl, beat the eggs, egg yolks and sugar together until light and smooth. Add the vanilla extract. Whisk the chocolate mixture into the egg mixture. Stir in the flour and ground almonds.
3. Preheat the air fryer to 330°F.
4. Transfer the batter carefully to the buttered ramekins, filling halfway. Place two or three chocolate discs in the center of the batter and then fill the ramekins to ½-inch below the top with the remaining batter. Place the ramekins into the air fryer basket and air-fry at 330°F for 13 minutes. The sides of the cake should be set, but the centers should be slightly soft. Remove the ramekins from the air fryer and let the cakes sit for 5 minutes. (If you'd like the cake a little less molten, air-fry for 14 minutes and let the cakes sit for 4 minutes.)
5. Run a butter knife around the edge of the ramekins and invert the cakes onto a plate. Lift the ramekin off the plate slowly and carefully so that the cake doesn't break. Dust with cocoa powder or powdered sugar and serve with a scoop of ice cream and some coarsely chopped toasted almonds.

Giant Buttery Chocolate Chip Cookie

Servings: 4

Cooking Time: 16 Minutes

Ingredients:

- ⅔ cup plus 1 tablespoon All-purpose flour
- ¼ teaspoon Baking soda
- ¼ teaspoon Table salt
- Baking spray (see the headnote)
- 4 tablespoons (¼ cup/½ stick) plus 1 teaspoon Butter, at room temperature
- ¼ cup plus 1 teaspoon Packed dark brown sugar
- 3 tablespoons plus 1 teaspoon Granulated white sugar
- 2½ tablespoons Pasteurized egg substitute, such as Egg Beaters
- ½ teaspoon Vanilla extract
- ¾ cup plus 1 tablespoon Semisweet or bittersweet chocolate chips

Directions:

1. Preheat the air fryer to 350°F .
2. Whisk the flour, baking soda, and salt in a bowl until well combined.
3. For a small air fryer, coat the inside of a 6-inch round cake pan with baking spray. For a medium air fryer, coat the inside of a 7-inch round cake pan with baking spray. And for a large air fryer, coat the inside of an 8-inch round cake pan with baking spray.
4. Using a hand electric mixer at medium speed, beat the butter, brown sugar, and granulated white sugar in a bowl until smooth and thick, about 3 minutes, scraping down the inside of the bowl several times.
5. Beat in the pasteurized egg substitute or egg (as applicable) and vanilla until uniform. Scrape down and remove the beaters. Fold in the flour mixture and

chocolate chips with a rubber spatula, just until combined. Scrape and gently press this dough into the prepared pan, getting it even across the pan to the perimeter.

6. Set the pan in the basket and air-fry undisturbed for 16 minutes, or until the cookie is puffed, browned, and feels set to the touch.

7. Transfer the pan to a wire rack and cool for 10 minutes. Loosen the cookie from the perimeter with a spatula, then invert the pan onto a cutting board and let the cookie come free. Remove the pan and reinvert the cookie onto the wire rack. Cool for 5 minutes more before slicing into wedges to serve.

Chewy Coconut Cake

Servings: 6

Cooking Time: 18-22 Minutes

Ingredients:

- ¾ cup plus 2½ tablespoons All-purpose flour
- ¾ teaspoon Baking powder
- ⅛ teaspoon Table salt
- 7½ tablespoons (1 stick minus ½ tablespoon) Butter, at room temperature
- ⅓ cup plus 1 tablespoon Granulated white sugar
- 5 tablespoons Packed light brown sugar
- 5 tablespoons Pasteurized egg substitute, such as Egg Beaters
- 2 teaspoons Vanilla extract
- ½ cup Unsweetened shredded coconut (see here)
- Baking spray

Directions:

1. Preheat the air fryer to 325°F (or 330°F, if that's the closest setting).
2. Mix the flour, baking powder, and salt in a small bowl until well combined.
3. Using an electric hand mixer at medium speed , beat the butter, granulated white sugar, and brown sugar in a medium bowl until creamy and smooth, about 3 minutes, occasionally scraping down the inside of the bowl. Beat in the egg substitute or egg and vanilla until smooth.
4. Scrape down and remove the beaters. Fold in the flour mixture with a rubber spatula just until all the flour is moistened. Fold in the coconut until the mixture is a uniform color.
5. Use the baking spray to generously coat the inside of a 6-inch round cake pan for a small batch, a 7-inch round cake pan for a medium batch, or an 8-inch round cake pan for a large batch. Scrape and spread the batter into the pan, smoothing the batter out to an even layer.
6. Set the pan in the basket and air-fry for 18 minutes for a 6-inch layer, 20 minutes for a 7-inch layer, or 22 minutes for an 8-inch layer, or until the cake is well browned and set even if there's a little soft give right at the center. Start checking it at the 16-minute mark to know where you are.
7. Use hot pads or silicone baking mitts to transfer the cake pan to a wire rack. Cool for at least 1 hour or up to 4 hours. Use a nonstick-safe knife to slice the cake into wedges right in the pan, lifting them out one by one.

Coconut-custard Pie

Servings: 4

Cooking Time: 20 Minutes

Ingredients:

- 1 cup milk
- ¼ cup plus 2 tablespoons sugar
- ¼ cup biscuit baking mix
- 1 teaspoon vanilla
- 2 eggs
- 2 tablespoons melted butter
- cooking spray
- ½ cup shredded, sweetened coconut

Directions:

1. Place all ingredients except coconut in a medium bowl.
2. Using a hand mixer, beat on high speed for 3minutes.
3. Let sit for 5minutes.
4. Preheat air fryer to 330°F.
5. Spray a 6-inch round or 6 x 6-inch square baking pan with cooking spray and place pan in air fryer basket.
6. Pour filling into pan and sprinkle coconut over top.
7. Cook pie at 330°F for 20 minutes or until center sets.

Fudgy Brownie Cake

Servings: 6

Cooking Time: 25-35 Minutes

Ingredients:

- 6½ tablespoons All-purpose flour
- ¼ cup plus 1 teaspoon Unsweetened cocoa powder
- ½ teaspoon Baking powder
- ¼ teaspoon Table salt
- 6½ tablespoons Butter, at room temperature
- 9½ tablespoons Granulated white sugar
- 1 egg plus 1 large egg white Large egg(s)
- ¾ teaspoon Vanilla extract
- Baking spray (see here)

Directions:

1. Preheat the air fryer to 325°F (or 330°F, if that's the closest setting).
2. Mix the flour, cocoa powder, baking powder, and salt in a small bowl until well combined.
3. Using an electric hand mixer at medium speed, beat the butter and sugar in a medium bowl until creamy and smooth, about 3 minutes, occasionally scraping down the inside of the bowl.
4. Beat in the egg(s) and the white or yolk (as necessary), as well as the vanilla, until smooth. Turn off the beaters and add the flour mixture. Beat at low speed until thick and smooth.
5. Use the baking spray to generously coat the inside of a 6-inch round cake pan for a small batch, a 7-inch round cake pan for a medium batch, or an 8-inch round cake pan for a large batch. Scrape and spread the batter into the pan, smoothing the batter out to an even layer.
6. Set the pan in the basket and air-fry for 25 minutes for a 6-inch layer, 30 minutes for a 7-inch layer, or 35 minutes for an 8-inch layer, or until the cake is set but soft to the touch. Start checking it at the 20-minute mark to know where you are.
7. Use hot pads or silicone baking mitts to transfer the cake pan to a wire rack. Cool for at least 1 hour or up to 4 hours. Using a nonstick-safe knife, slice the cake into wedges right in the pan and lift them out one by one.

Honey-pecan Yogurt Cake

Servings: 6

Cooking Time: 18-24 Minutes

Ingredients:

- 1 cup plus 3½ tablespoons All-purpose flour
- ¼ teaspoon Baking powder
- ¼ teaspoon Baking soda
- ¼ teaspoon Table salt
- 5 tablespoons Plain full-fat, low-fat, or fat-free Greek yogurt
- 5 tablespoons Honey
- 5 tablespoons Pasteurized egg substitute, such as Egg Beaters
- 2 teaspoons Vanilla extract
- ⅔ cup Chopped pecans
- Baking spray (see here)

Directions:

1. Preheat the air fryer to 325°F (or 330°F, if the closest setting).
2. Mix the flour, baking powder, baking soda, and salt in a small bowl until well combined.
3. Using an electric hand mixer at medium speed , beat the yogurt, honey, egg substitute or egg, and vanilla in a medium bowl until smooth, about 2 minutes, scraping down the inside of the bowl once or twice.
4. Turn off the mixer; scrape down and remove the beaters. Fold in the flour mixture with a rubber spatula, just until all of the flour has been moistened. Fold in the pecans until they are evenly distributed in the mixture.
5. Use the baking spray to generously coat the inside of a 6-inch round cake pan for a small batch, a 7-inch round cake pan for a medium batch, or an 8-inch round cake pan for a large batch. Scrape and spread the batter into the pan, smoothing the batter out to an even layer.
6. Set the pan in the basket and air-fry for 18 minutes for a 6-inch layer, 22 minutes for a 7-inch layer, or 24 minutes for an 8-inch layer, or until a toothpick or cake tester inserted into the center of the cake comes out clean. Start checking it at the 15-minute mark to know where you are.
7. Use hot pads or silicone baking mitts to transfer the cake pan to a wire rack. Cool for 5 minutes. To unmold,

set a cutting board over the baking pan and invert both the board and the pan. Lift the still-warm pan off the cake layer. Set the wire rack on top of that layer and invert all of it with the cutting board so that the cake layer is now right side up on the wire rack. Remove the cutting board and continue cooling the cake for at least 10 minutes or to room temperature, about 30 minutes, before slicing into wedges.

Gingerbread

Servings: 6

Cooking Time: 20 Minutes

Ingredients:

- cooking spray
- 1 cup flour
- 2 tablespoons sugar
- ¾ teaspoon ground ginger
- ¼ teaspoon cinnamon
- 1 teaspoon baking powder
- ½ teaspoon baking soda
- ⅛ teaspoon salt
- 1 egg
- ¼ cup molasses
- ½ cup buttermilk
- 2 tablespoons oil
- 1 teaspoon pure vanilla extract

Directions:

1. Preheat air fryer to 330°F.
2. Spray 6 x 6-inch baking dish lightly with cooking spray.
3. In a medium bowl, mix together all the dry ingredients.
4. In a separate bowl, beat the egg. Add molasses, buttermilk, oil, and vanilla and stir until well mixed.
5. Pour liquid mixture into dry ingredients and stir until well blended.
6. Pour batter into baking dish and cook at 330°F for 20minutes or until toothpick inserted in center of loaf comes out clean.

Peanut Butter S'mores

Servings:10

Cooking Time: 1 Minute

Ingredients:

- 10 Graham crackers (full, double-square cookies as they come out of the package)
- 5 tablespoons Natural-style creamy or crunchy peanut butter
- ½ cup Milk chocolate chips
- 10 Standard-size marshmallows (not minis and not jumbo campfire ones)

Directions:

1. Preheat the air fryer to 350°F .
2. Break the graham crackers in half widthwise at the marked place, so the rectangle is now in two squares. Set half of the squares flat side up on your work surface. Spread each with about 1½ teaspoons peanut butter, then set 10 to 12 chocolate chips point side up into the peanut butter on each, pressing gently so the chips stick.
3. Flatten a marshmallow between your clean, dry hands and set it atop the chips. Do the same with the remaining marshmallows on the other coated graham crackers. Do not set the other half of the graham crackers on top of these coated graham crackers.
4. When the machine is at temperature, set the treats graham cracker side down in a single layer in the basket. They may touch, but even a fraction of an inch between them will provide better air flow. Air-fry undisturbed for 45 seconds.
5. Use a nonstick-safe spatula to transfer the topped graham crackers to a wire rack. Set the other graham cracker squares flat side down over the marshmallows. Cool for a couple of minutes before serving.

Coconut Macaroons

Servings: 12

Cooking Time: 8 Minutes

Ingredients:

- 1⅓ cups shredded, sweetened coconut
- 4½ teaspoons flour
- 2 tablespoons sugar
- 1 egg white
- ½ teaspoon almond extract

Directions:

1. Preheat air fryer to 330°F.
2. Mix all ingredients together.
3. Shape coconut mixture into 12 balls.
4. Place all 12 macaroons in air fryer basket. They won't expand, so you can place them close together, but they shouldn't touch.
5. Cook at 330°F for 8 minutes, until golden.

Sweet Potato Donut Holes

Servings: 18

Cooking Time: 4 Minutes Per Batch

Ingredients:

- 1 cup flour
- ⅓ cup sugar
- ¼ teaspoon baking soda
- 1 teaspoon baking powder
- ⅛ teaspoon salt
- ½ cup cooked mashed purple sweet potatoes
- 1 egg, beaten
- 2 tablespoons butter, melted
- 1 teaspoon pure vanilla extract
- oil for misting or cooking spray

Directions:

1. Preheat air fryer to 390°F.
2. In a large bowl, stir together the flour, sugar, baking soda, baking powder, and salt.
3. In a separate bowl, combine the potatoes, egg, butter, and vanilla and mix well.
4. Add potato mixture to dry ingredients and stir into a soft dough.
5. Shape dough into 1½-inch balls. Mist lightly with oil or cooking spray.
6. Place 9 donut holes in air fryer basket, leaving a little space in between. Cook for 4 minutes, until done in center and lightly browned outside.
7. Repeat step 6 to cook remaining donut holes.

Nutella® Torte

Servings: 6

Cooking Time: 55 Minutes

Ingredients:

- ¼ cup unsalted butter, softened
- ½ cup sugar
- 2 eggs
- 1 teaspoon vanilla
- 1¼ cups Nutella® (or other chocolate hazelnut spread), divided
- ¼ cup flour
- 1 teaspoon baking powder
- ¼ teaspoon salt
- dark chocolate fudge topping
- coarsely chopped toasted hazelnuts

Directions:

1. Cream the butter and sugar together with an electric hand mixer until light and fluffy. Add the eggs, vanilla, and ¾ cup of the Nutella® and mix until combined. Combine the flour, baking powder and salt together, and add these dry ingredients to the butter mixture, beating for 1 minute.
2. Preheat the air fryer to 350°F.
3. Grease a 7-inch cake pan with butter and then line the bottom of the pan with a circle of parchment paper. Grease the parchment paper circle as well. Pour the batter into the prepared cake pan and wrap the pan completely with aluminum foil. Lower the pan into the air fryer basket with an aluminum sling (fold a piece of aluminum foil into a strip about 2-inches wide by 24-inches long). Fold the ends of the aluminum foil over the top of the dish before returning the basket to the air fryer. Air-fry for 30 minutes. Remove the foil and air-fry for another 25 minutes.
4. Remove the cake from air fryer and let it cool for 10 minutes. Invert the cake onto a plate, remove the parchment paper and invert the cake back onto a serving platter. While the cake is still warm, spread the remaining ½ cup of Nutella® over the top of the cake. Melt the dark chocolate fudge in the microwave for about 10 seconds so it melts enough to be pourable. Drizzle the sauce on top of the cake in a zigzag motion. Turn the cake 90 degrees and drizzle more sauce in zigzags perpendicular to the first zigzags. Garnish the edges of the torte with the toasted hazelnuts and serve.

Carrot Cake With Cream Cheese Icing

Servings: 6

Cooking Time: 55 Minutes

Ingredients:

- 1¼ cups all-purpose flour
- 1 teaspoon baking powder
- ½ teaspoon baking soda
- 1 teaspoon ground cinnamon
- ¼ teaspoon ground nutmeg
- ¼ teaspoon salt
- 2 cups grated carrot (about 3 to 4 medium carrots or 2 large)
- ¾ cup granulated sugar
- ¼ cup brown sugar
- 2 eggs
- ¾ cup canola or vegetable oil
- For the icing:
- 8 ounces cream cheese, softened at room , Temperature: 8 tablespoons butter (4 ounces or 1 stick), softened at room , Temperature: 1 cup powdered sugar
- 1 teaspoon pure vanilla extract

Directions:

1. Grease a 7-inch cake pan.
2. Combine the flour, baking powder, baking soda, cinnamon, nutmeg and salt in a bowl. Add the grated carrots and toss well. In a separate bowl, beat the sugars and eggs together until light and frothy. Drizzle in the oil, beating constantly. Fold the egg mixture into the dry ingredients until everything is just combined and you no longer see any traces of flour. Pour the batter into the cake pan and wrap the pan completely in greased aluminum foil.
3. Preheat the air fryer to 350°F.
4. Lower the cake pan into the air fryer basket using a sling made of aluminum foil (fold a piece of aluminum foil into a strip about 2-inches wide by 24-inches long). Fold the ends of the aluminum foil into the air fryer, letting them rest on top of the cake. Air-fry for 40 minutes. Remove the aluminum foil cover and air-fry for an additional 15 minutes or until a skewer inserted into the center of the cake comes out clean and the top is nicely browned.
5. While the cake is cooking, beat the cream cheese, butter, powdered sugar and vanilla extract together using a hand mixer, stand mixer or food processor (or a lot of elbow grease!).
6. Remove the cake pan from the air fryer and let the cake cool in the cake pan for 10 minutes or so. Then remove the cake from the pan and let it continue to cool completely. Frost the cake with the cream cheese icing and serve.

Orange Gooey Butter Cake

Servings: 6

Cooking Time: 85 Minutes

Ingredients:

- Crust Layer:
- ½ cup flour
- ¼ cup sugar
- ½ teaspoon baking powder
- ⅛ teaspoon salt
- 2 ounces (½ stick) unsalted European style butter, melted
- 1 egg
- 1 teaspoon orange extract
- 2 tablespoons orange zest
- Gooey Butter Layer:
- 8 ounces cream cheese, softened
- 4 ounces (1 stick) unsalted European style butter, melted
- 2 eggs
- 2 teaspoons orange extract
- 2 tablespoons orange zest
- 4 cups powdered sugar
- Garnish:
- powdered sugar
- orange slices

Directions:

1. Preheat the air fryer to 350°F.
2. Grease a 7-inch cake pan and line the bottom with parchment paper. Combine the flour, sugar, baking powder and salt in a bowl. Add the melted butter, egg, orange extract and orange zest. Mix well and press this mixture into the bottom of the greased cake pan. Lower the pan into the basket using an aluminum foil sling

(fold a piece of aluminum foil into a strip about 2-inches wide by 24-inches long). Fold the ends of the aluminum foil over the top of the dish before returning the basket to the air fryer. Air-fry uncovered for 8 minutes.

3. To make the gooey butter layer, beat the cream cheese, melted butter, eggs, orange extract and orange zest in a large bowl using an electric hand mixer. Add the powdered sugar in stages, beat until smooth with each addition. Pour this mixture on top of the baked crust in the cake pan. Wrap the pan with a piece of greased aluminum foil, tenting the top of the foil to leave a little room for the cake to rise.

4. Air-fry for 60 minutes at 350°F. Remove the aluminum foil and air-fry for an additional 17 minutes.

5. Let the cake cool inside the pan for at least 10 minutes. Then, run a butter knife around the cake and let the cake cool completely in the pan. When cooled, run the butter knife around the edges of the cake again and invert it onto a plate and then back onto a serving platter. Sprinkle the powdered sugar over the top of the cake and garnish with orange slices.

Giant Oatmeal–peanut Butter Cookie

Servings: 4

Cooking Time: 18 Minutes

Ingredients:

- 1 cup Rolled oats (not quick-cooking or steel-cut oats)
- ½ cup All-purpose flour
- ½ teaspoon Ground cinnamon
- ½ teaspoon Baking soda
- ⅓ cup Packed light brown sugar
- ¼ cup Solid vegetable shortening
- 2 tablespoons Natural-style creamy peanut butter
- 3 tablespoons Granulated white sugar
- 2 tablespoons (or 1 small egg, well beaten) Pasteurized egg substitute, such as Egg Beaters
- ⅓ cup Roasted, salted peanuts, chopped
- Baking spray

Directions:

1. Preheat the air fryer to 350°F .

2. Stir the oats, flour, cinnamon, and baking soda in a bowl until well combined.

3. Using an electric hand mixer at medium speed, beat the brown sugar, shortening, peanut butter, granulated white sugar, and egg substitute or egg (as applicable) until smooth and creamy, about 3 minutes, scraping down the inside of the bowl occasionally.

4. Scrape down and remove the beaters. Fold in the flour mixture and peanuts with a rubber spatula just until all the flour is moistened and the peanut bits are evenly distributed in the dough.

5. For a small air fryer, coat the inside of a 6-inch round cake pan with baking spray. For a medium air fryer, coat the inside of a 7-inch round cake pan with baking spray. And for a large air fryer, coat the inside of an 8-inch round cake pan with baking spray. Scrape and gently press the dough into the prepared pan, spreading it into an even layer to the perimeter.

6. Set the pan in the basket and air-fry undisturbed for 18 minutes, or until well browned.

7. Transfer the pan to a wire rack and cool for 15 minutes. Loosen the cookie from the perimeter with a spatula, then invert the pan onto a cutting board and let the cookie come free. Remove the pan and reinvert the cookie onto the wire rack. Cool for 5 minutes more before slicing into wedges to serve.

Giant Vegan Chocolate Chip Cookie

Servings: 4

Cooking Time: 16 Minutes

Ingredients:

- ⅔ cup All-purpose flour
- 5 tablespoons Rolled oats (not quick-cooking or steel-cut oats)
- ¼ teaspoon Baking soda
- ¼ teaspoon Table salt
- 5 tablespoons Granulated white sugar
- ¼ cup Vegetable oil
- 2½ tablespoons Tahini (see here)
- 2½ tablespoons Maple syrup
- 2 teaspoons Vanilla extract
- ⅔ cup Vegan semisweet or bittersweet chocolate chips
- Baking spray

Directions:

1. Preheat the air fryer to 325°F (or 330°F, if that's the closest setting).

2. Whisk the flour, oats, baking soda, and salt in a bowl until well combined.

3. Using an electric hand mixer at medium speed, beat the sugar, oil, tahini, maple syrup, and vanilla until rich and creamy, about 3 minutes, scraping down the inside of the bowl occasionally.

4. Scrape down and remove the beaters. Fold in the flour mixture and chocolate chips with a rubber spatula just until all the flour is moistened and the chocolate chips are even throughout the dough.

5. For a small air fryer, coat the inside of a 6-inch round cake pan with baking spray. For a medium air fryer, coat the inside of a 7-inch round cake pan with baking spray. And for a large air fryer, coat the inside of an 8-inch round cake pan with baking spray. Scrape and gently press the dough into the prepared pan, spreading it into an even layer to the perimeter.

6. Set the pan in the basket and air-fry undisturbed for 16 minutes, or until puffed, browned, and firm to the touch.

7. Transfer the pan to a wire rack and cool for 10 minutes. Loosen the cookie from the perimeter with a spatula, then invert the pan onto a cutting board and let the cookie come free. Remove the pan and reinvert the cookie onto the wire rack. Cool for 5 minutes more before slicing into wedges to serve.

Black And Blue Clafoutis

Servings: 2

Cooking Time: 15minutes

Ingredients:

- 6-inch pie pan
- 3 large eggs
- ½ cup sugar
- 1 teaspoon vanilla extract
- 2 tablespoons butter, melted 1 cup milk
- ½ cup all-purpose flour*
- 1 cup blackberries
- 1 cup blueberries
- 2 tablespoons confectioners' sugar

Directions:

1. Preheat the air fryer to 320°F.

2. Combine the eggs and sugar in a bowl and whisk vigorously until smooth, lighter in color and well combined. Add the vanilla extract, butter and milk and whisk together well. Add the flour and whisk just until no lumps or streaks of white remain.

3. Scatter half the blueberries and blackberries in a greased (6-inch) pie pan or cake pan. Pour half of the batter (about 1¼ cups) on top of the berries and transfer the tart pan to the air fryer basket. You can use an aluminum foil sling to help with this by taking a long piece of aluminum foil, folding it in half lengthwise twice until it is roughly 26-inches by 3-inches. Place this under the pie dish and hold the ends of the foil to move the pie dish in and out of the air fryer basket. Tuck the ends of the foil beside the pie dish while it cooks in the air fryer.

4. Air-fry at 320°F for 15 minutes or until the clafoutis has puffed up and is still a little jiggly in the center. Remove the clafoutis from the air fryer, invert it onto a plate and let it cool while you bake the second batch. Serve the clafoutis warm, dusted with confectioners' sugar on top.

Baked Apple Crisp

Servings: 4

Cooking Time: 23 Minutes

Ingredients:

- 2 large Granny Smith apples, peeled, cored, and chopped
- ¼ cup granulated sugar
- ¼ cup plus 2 teaspoons flour, divided
- 2 teaspoons milk
- ¼ teaspoon cinnamon
- ¼ cup oats
- ¼ cup brown sugar
- 2 tablespoons unsalted butter
- ⅛ teaspoon baking powder
- ⅛ teaspoon salt

Directions:

1. Preheat the air fryer to 350°F.

2. In a medium bowl, mix the apples, the granulated sugar, 2 teaspoons of the flour, the milk, and the cinnamon.
3. Spray 4 oven-safe ramekins with cooking spray. Divide the filling among the four ramekins.
4. In a small bowl, mix the oats, the brown sugar, the remaining ¼ cup of flour, the butter, the baking powder, and the salt. Use your fingers or a pastry blender to crumble the butter into pea-size pieces. Divide the topping over the top of the apple filling. Cover the apple crisps with foil.
5. Place the covered apple crisps in the air fryer basket and cook for 20 minutes. Uncover and continue cooking for 3 minutes or until the surface is golden and crunchy.

Blueberry Cheesecake Tartlets

Servings: 9
Cooking Time: 6 Minutes

Ingredients:

- 8 ounces cream cheese, softened
- ¼ cup sugar
- 1 egg
- ½ teaspoon vanilla extract
- zest of 2 lemons, divided
- 9 mini graham cracker tartlet shells*
- 2 cups blueberries
- ½ teaspoon ground cinnamon
- juice of ½ lemon
- ¼ cup apricot preserves

Directions:

1. Preheat the air fryer to 330°F.
2. Combine the cream cheese, sugar, egg, vanilla and the zest of one lemon in a medium bowl and blend until smooth by hand or with an electric hand mixer. Pour the cream cheese mixture into the tartlet shells.
3. Air-fry 3 tartlets at a time at 330°F for 6 minutes, rotating them in the air fryer basket halfway through the cooking time.
4. Combine the blueberries, cinnamon, zest of one lemon and juice of half a lemon in a bowl. Melt the apricot preserves in the microwave or over low heat in a saucepan. Pour the apricot preserves over the blueberries and gently toss to coat.
5. Allow the cheesecakes to cool completely and then top each one with some of the blueberry mixture. Garnish the tartlets with a little sugared lemon peel and refrigerate until you are ready to serve.

Midnight Nutella® Banana Sandwich

Servings: 2
Cooking Time: 8 Minutes

Ingredients:

- butter, softened
- 4 slices white bread*
- ¼ cup chocolate hazelnut spread (Nutella®)
- 1 banana

Directions:

1. Preheat the air fryer to 370°F.
2. Spread the softened butter on one side of all the slices of bread and place the slices buttered side down on the counter. Spread the chocolate hazelnut spread on the other side of the bread slices. Cut the banana in half and then slice each half into three slices lengthwise. Place the banana slices on two slices of bread and top with the remaining slices of bread (buttered side up) to make two sandwiches. Cut the sandwiches in half (triangles or rectangles) – this will help them all fit in the air fryer at once. Transfer the sandwiches to the air fryer.
3. Air-fry at 370°F for 5 minutes. Flip the sandwiches over and air-fry for another 2 to 3 minutes, or until the top bread slices are nicely browned. Pour yourself a glass of milk or a midnight nightcap while the sandwiches cool slightly and enjoy!

Fried Pineapple Chunks

Servings: 3
Cooking Time: 10 Minutes

Ingredients:

- 3 tablespoons Cornstarch
- 1 Large egg white, beaten until foamy
- 1 cup (4 ounces) Ground vanilla wafer cookies (not low-fat cookies)
- ¼ teaspoon Ground dried ginger
- 18 (about 2¼ cups) Fresh 1-inch chunks peeled and cored pineapple

Directions:

1. Preheat the air fryer to 400°F.
2. Put the cornstarch in a medium or large bowl. Put the beaten egg white in a small bowl. Pour the cookie crumbs and ground dried ginger into a large zip-closed plastic bag, shaking it a bit to combine them.
3. Dump the pineapple chunks into the bowl with the cornstarch. Toss and stir until well coated. Use your cleaned fingers or a large fork like a shovel to pick up a few pineapple chunks, shake off any excess cornstarch, and put them in the bowl with the egg white. Stir gently, then pick them up and let any excess egg white slip back into the rest. Put them in the bag with the crumb mixture. Repeat the cornstarch-then-egg process until all the pineapple chunks are in the bag. Seal the bag and shake gently, turning the bag this way and that, to coat the pieces well.
4. Set the coated pineapple chunks in the basket with as much air space between them as possible. Even a fraction of an inch will work, but they should not touch. Air-fry undisturbed for 10 minutes, or until golden brown and crisp.
5. Gently dump the contents of the basket onto a wire rack. Cool for at least 5 minutes or up to 15 minutes before serving.

Hasselback Apple Crisp

Servings: 4

Cooking Time: 20 Minutes

Ingredients:

- 2 large Gala apples, peeled, cored and cut in half
- ¼ cup butter, melted
- ½ teaspoon ground cinnamon
- 2 tablespoons sugar
- Topping
- 3 tablespoons butter, melted
- 2 tablespoons brown sugar
- ¼ cup chopped pecans
- 2 tablespoons rolled oats*
- 1 tablespoon flour*
- vanilla ice cream
- caramel sauce

Directions:

1. Place the apples cut side down on a cutting board. Slicing from stem end to blossom end, make 8 to 10 slits down the apple halves but only slice three quarters of the way through the apple, not all the way through to the cutting board.
2. Preheat the air fryer to 330°F and pour a little water into the bottom of the air fryer drawer. (This will help prevent the grease that drips into the bottom drawer from burning and smoking.)
3. Transfer the apples to the air fryer basket, flat side down. Combine ¼ cup of melted butter, cinnamon and sugar in a small bowl. Brush this butter mixture onto the apples and air-fry at 330°F for 15 minutes. Baste the apples several times with the butter mixture during the cooking process.
4. While the apples are air-frying, make the filling. Combine 3 tablespoons of melted butter with the brown sugar, pecans, rolled oats and flour in a bowl. Stir with a fork until the mixture resembles small crumbles.
5. When the timer on the air fryer is up, spoon the topping down the center of the apples. Air-fry at 330°F for an additional 5 minutes.
6. Transfer the apples to a serving plate and serve with vanilla ice cream and caramel sauce.

Chocolate Cake

Servings: 8

Cooking Time: 20 Minutes

Ingredients:

- ½ cup sugar
- ¼ cup flour, plus 3 tablespoons
- 3 tablespoons cocoa
- ½ teaspoon baking powder
- ½ teaspoon baking soda
- ¼ teaspoon salt
- 1 egg
- 2 tablespoons oil
- ½ cup milk
- ½ teaspoon vanilla extract

Directions:

1. Preheat air fryer to 330°F.
2. Grease and flour a 6 x 6-inch baking pan.

3. In a medium bowl, stir together the sugar, flour, cocoa, baking powder, baking soda, and salt.
4. Add all other ingredients and beat with a wire whisk until smooth.
5. Pour batter into prepared pan and bake at 330°F for 20 minutes, until toothpick inserted in center comes out clean or with crumbs clinging to it.

Air-fried Strawberry Hand Tarts

Servings: 9
Cooking Time: 9 Minutes

Ingredients:

- ½ cup butter, softened
- ½ cup sugar
- 2 eggs
- 1 teaspoon vanilla extract
- 2 tablespoons lemon zest
- 2½ cups all-purpose flour
- 1 teaspoon baking powder
- ¼ teaspoon salt
- 1¼ cups strawberry jam, divided
- 1 egg white, beaten
- 1 cup powdered sugar
- 2 teaspoons milk

Directions:

1. Combine the butter and sugar in a bowl and beat with an electric mixer until the mixture is light and fluffy. Add the eggs one at a time. Add the vanilla extract and lemon zest and mix well. In a separate bowl, combine the flour, baking powder and salt. Add the dry ingredients to the wet ingredients, mixing just until the dough comes together. Transfer the dough to a floured surface and knead by hand for 10 minutes. Cover with a clean kitchen towel and let the dough rest for 30 minutes. (Alternatively, dough can be mixed and kneaded in a stand mixer.)
2. Divide the dough in half and roll each half out into a ¼-inch thick rectangle that measures 12-inches x 9-inches. Cut each rectangle of dough into nine 4-inch x 3-inch rectangles (a pizza cutter is very helpful for this task). You should have 18 rectangles. Spread two teaspoons of strawberry jam in the center of nine of the rectangles leaving a ¼-inch border around the edges. Brush the egg white around the edges of each rectangle and top with the remaining nine rectangles of dough. Press the back of a fork around the edges to seal the tarts shut. Brush the top of the tarts with the beaten egg white and pierce the dough three or four times down the center of the tart with a fork.
3. Preheat the air fryer to 350°F.
4. Air-fry the tarts in batches at 350°F for 6 minutes. Flip the tarts over and air-fry for an additional 3 minutes.
5. While the tarts are air-frying, make the icing. Combine the powdered sugar, ¼ cup strawberry preserves and milk in a bowl, whisking until the icing is smooth. Spread the icing over the top of each tart, leaving an empty border around the edges. Decorate with sprinkles if desired.

Brownies After Dark

Servings: 4
Cooking Time: 13 Minutes

Ingredients:

- 1 egg
- ½ cup granulated sugar
- ¼ teaspoon salt
- ½ teaspoon vanilla
- ¼ cup butter, melted
- ¼ cup flour, plus 2 tablespoons
- ¼ cup cocoa
- cooking spray
- Optional
- vanilla ice cream
- caramel sauce
- whipped cream

Directions:

1. Beat together egg, sugar, salt, and vanilla until light.
2. Add melted butter and mix well.
3. Stir in flour and cocoa.
4. Spray 6 x 6-inch baking pan lightly with cooking spray.
5. Spread batter in pan and cook at 330°F for 13 minutes. Cool and cut into 4 large squares or 16 small brownie bites.

Sweet Potato Pie Rolls

Servings:3
Cooking Time: 8 Minutes

Ingredients:

- 6 Spring roll wrappers
- 1½ cups Canned yams in syrup, drained
- 2 tablespoons Light brown sugar
- ¼ teaspoon Ground cinnamon
- 1 Large egg(s), well beaten
- Vegetable oil spray

Directions:

1. Preheat the air fryer to 400°F.
2. Set a spring roll wrapper on a clean, dry work surface. Scoop up ¼ cup of the pulpy yams and set along one edge of the wrapper, leaving 2 inches on each side of the yams. Top the yams with about 1 teaspoon brown sugar and a pinch of ground cinnamon. Fold the sides of the wrapper perpendicular to the yam filling up and over the filling, partially covering it. Brush beaten egg(s) over the side of the wrapper farthest from the yam. Starting with the yam end, roll the wrapper closed, ending at the part with the beaten egg that you can press gently to seal. Lightly coat the roll on all sides with vegetable oil spray. Set it aside seam side down and continue filling, rolling, and spraying the remaining wrappers in the same way.
3. Set the rolls seam side down in the basket with as much air space between them as possible. Air-fry undisturbed for 8 minutes, or until crisp and golden brown.
4. Use a nonstick-safe spatula and perhaps kitchen tongs for balance to gently transfer the rolls to a wire rack. Cool for at least 5 minutes or up to 30 minutes before serving.

Mixed Berry Hand Pies

Servings: 4
Cooking Time: 15 Minutes

Ingredients:

- ¾ cup sugar
- ½ teaspoon ground cinnamon
- 1 tablespoon cornstarch
- 1 cup blueberries
- 1 cup blackberries
- 1 cup raspberries, divided
- 1 teaspoon water
- 1 package refrigerated pie dough (or your own homemade pie dough)
- 1 egg, beaten

Directions:

1. Combine the sugar, cinnamon, and cornstarch in a small saucepan. Add the blueberries, blackberries, and ½ cup of the raspberries. Toss the berries gently to coat them evenly. Add the teaspoon of water to the saucepan and turn the stovetop on to medium-high heat, stirring occasionally. Once the berries break down, release their juice and start to simmer (about 5 minutes), simmer for another couple of minutes and then transfer the mixture to a bowl, stir in the remaining ½ cup of raspberries and let it cool.
2. Preheat the air fryer to 370°F.
3. Cut the pie dough into four 5-inch circles and four 6-inch circles.
4. Spread the 6-inch circles on a flat surface. Divide the berry filling between all four circles. Brush the perimeter of the dough circles with a little water. Place the 5-inch circles on top of the filling and press the perimeter of the dough circles together to seal. Roll the edges of the bottom circle up over the top circle to make a crust around the filling. Press a fork around the crust to make decorative indentations and to seal the crust shut. Brush the pies with egg wash and sprinkle a little sugar on top. Poke a small hole in the center of each pie with a paring knife to vent the dough.
5. Air-fry two pies at a time. Brush or spray the air fryer basket with oil and place the pies into the basket. Air-fry for 9 minutes. Turn the pies over and air-fry for another 6 minutes. Serve warm or at room temperature.

Apple Crisp

Servings: 4

Cooking Time: 16 Minutes

Ingredients:

- Filling
- 3 Granny Smith apples, thinly sliced (about 4 cups)
- ¼ teaspoon ground cinnamon
- ⅛ teaspoon salt
- 1½ teaspoons lemon juice
- 2 tablespoons honey
- 1 tablespoon brown sugar
- cooking spray
- Crumb Topping
- 2 tablespoons oats
- 2 tablespoons oat bran
- 2 tablespoons cooked quinoa
- 2 tablespoons chopped walnuts
- 2 tablespoons brown sugar
- 2 teaspoons coconut oil

Directions:

1. Combine all filling ingredients and stir well so that apples are evenly coated.
2. Spray air fryer baking pan with nonstick cooking spray and spoon in the apple mixture.
3. Cook at 360°F for 5minutes. Stir well, scooping up from the bottom to mix apples and sauce.
4. At this point, the apples should be crisp-tender. Continue cooking in 3-minute intervals until apples are as soft as you like.
5. While apples are cooking, combine all topping ingredients in a small bowl. Stir until coconut oil mixes in well and distributes evenly. If your coconut oil is cold, it may be easier to mix in by hand.
6. When apples are cooked to your liking, sprinkle crumb mixture on top. Cook at 360°F for 8 minutes or until crumb topping is golden brown and crispy.

Puff Pastry Apples

Servings: 4

Cooking Time: 10 Minutes

Ingredients:

- 3 Rome or Gala apples, peeled
- 2 tablespoons sugar
- 1 teaspoon all-purpose flour
- 1 teaspoon ground cinnamon
- ⅛ teaspoon ground ginger
- pinch ground nutmeg
- 1 sheet puff pastry
- 1 tablespoon butter, cut into 4 pieces
- 1 egg, beaten
- vegetable oil
- vanilla ice cream (optional)
- caramel sauce (optional)

Directions:

1. Remove the core from the apple by cutting the four sides off the apple around the core. Slice the pieces of apple into thin half-moons, about ¼-inch thick. Combine the sugar, flour, cinnamon, ginger, and nutmeg in a large bowl. Add the apples to the bowl and gently toss until the apples are evenly coated with the spice mixture. Set aside.
2. Cut the puff pastry sheet into a 12-inch by 12-inch square. Then quarter the sheet into four 6-inch squares. Save any remaining pastry for decorating the apples at the end.
3. Divide the spiced apples between the four puff pastry squares, stacking the apples in the center of each square and placing them flat on top of each other in a circle. Top the apples with a piece of the butter.
4. Brush the four edges of the pastry with the egg wash. Bring the four corners of the pastry together, wrapping them around the apple slices and pinching them together at the top in the style of a "beggars purse" appetizer. Fold the ends of the pastry corners down onto the apple making them look like leaves. Brush the entire apple with the egg wash.
5. Using the leftover dough, make leaves to decorate the apples. Cut out 8 leaf shapes, about 1½-inches long, "drawing" the leaf veins on the pastry leaves with a paring knife. Place 2 leaves on the top of each apple, tucking the ends of the leaves under the pastry in the center of the apples. Brush the top of the leaves with additional egg wash. Sprinkle the entire apple with some granulated sugar.
6. Preheat the air fryer to 350°F.

7. Spray or brush the inside of the air fryer basket with oil. Place the apples in the basket and air-fry for 6 minutes. Carefully turn the apples over – it's easiest to remove one apple, then flip the others over and finally return the last apple to the air fryer. Air-fry for an additional 4 minutes.
8. Serve the puff pastry apples warm with vanilla ice cream and drizzle with some caramel sauce.

Thumbprint Sugar Cookies

Servings: 10
Cooking Time: 8 Minutes

Ingredients:

- 2½ tablespoons butter
- ⅓ cup cane sugar
- 1 teaspoon pure vanilla extract
- 1 large egg
- 1 cup all-purpose flour
- ½ teaspoon baking soda
- ¼ teaspoon salt
- 10 chocolate kisses

Directions:

1. Preheat the air fryer to 350°F.
2. In a large bowl, cream the butter with the sugar and vanilla. Whisk in the egg and set aside.
3. In a separate bowl, mix the flour, baking soda, and salt. Then gently mix the dry ingredients into the wet. Portion the dough into 10 balls; then press down on each with the bottom of a cup to create a flat cookie.
4. Liberally spray the metal trivet of an air fryer basket with olive oil mist.
5. Place the cookies in the air fryer basket on the trivet and cook for 8 minutes or until the tops begin to lightly brown.
6. Remove and immediately press the chocolate kisses into the tops of the cookies while still warm.
7. Let cool 5 minutes and then enjoy.

Vanilla Butter Cake

Servings: 6
Cooking Time: 20-24 Minutes

Ingredients:

- ¾ cup plus 1 tablespoon All-purpose flour
- 1 teaspoon Baking powder
- ¼ teaspoon Table salt
- 8 tablespoons (½ cup/1 stick) Butter, at room temperature
- ½ cup Granulated white sugar
- 2 Large egg(s)
- 2 tablespoons Whole or low-fat milk (not fat-free)
- ¾ teaspoon Vanilla extract
- Baking spray (see here)

Directions:

1. Preheat the air fryer to 325°F (or 330°F, if that's the closest setting).
2. Mix the flour, baking powder, and salt in a small bowl until well combined.
3. Using an electric hand mixer at medium speed, beat the butter and sugar in a medium bowl until creamy and smooth, about 3 minutes, occasionally scraping down the inside of the bowl.
4. Beat in the egg or eggs, as well as the white or a yolk as necessary. Beat in the milk and vanilla until smooth. Turn off the beaters and add the flour mixture. Beat at low speed until thick and smooth.
5. Use the baking spray to generously coat the inside of a 6-inch round cake pan for a small batch, a 7-inch round cake pan for a medium batch, or an 8-inch round cake pan for a large batch. Scrape and spread the batter into the pan, smoothing the batter out to an even layer.
6. Set the pan in the basket and air-fry undisturbed for 20 minutes for a 6-inch layer, 22 minutes for a 7-inch layer, or 24 minutes for an 8-inch layer, or until a toothpick or cake tester inserted into the center of the cake comes out clean. Start checking it at the 15-minute mark to know where you are.
7. Use hot pads or silicone baking mitts to transfer the cake pan to a wire rack. Cool for 5 minutes. To unmold, set a cutting board over the baking pan and invert both the board and the pan. Lift the still-warm pan off the cake layer. Set the wire rack on top of the cake layer and invert all of it with the cutting board so that the cake layer is now right side up on the wire rack. Remove the cutting board and continue cooling the cake for at least 10 minutes or to room temperature, about 30 minutes, before slicing into wedges.

Struffoli

Servings: X
Cooking Time: 20 Minutes

Ingredients:

- ¼ cup butter, softened
- ⅔ cup sugar
- 5 eggs
- 2 teaspoons vanilla extract
- zest of 1 lemon
- 4 cups all-purpose flour
- 2 teaspoons baking soda
- ¼ teaspoon salt
- 16 ounces honey
- 1 teaspoon ground cinnamon
- zest of 1 orange
- 2 tablespoons water
- nonpareils candy sprinkles

Directions:

1. Cream the butter and sugar together in a bowl until light and fluffy using a hand mixer (or a stand mixer). Add the eggs, vanilla and lemon zest and mix. In a separate bowl, combine the flour, baking soda and salt. Add the dry ingredients to the wet ingredients and mix until you have a soft dough. Shape the dough into a ball, wrap it in plastic and let it rest for 30 minutes.
2. Divide the dough ball into four pieces. Roll each piece into a long rope. Cut each rope into about 25 (½-inch) pieces. Roll each piece into a tight ball. You should have 100 little balls when finished.
3. Preheat the air fryer to 370°F.
4. In batches of about 20, transfer the dough balls to the air fryer basket, leaving a small space in between them. Air-fry the dough balls at 370°F for 3 to 4 minutes, shaking the basket when one minute of cooking time remains.
5. After all the dough balls are air-fried, make the honey topping. Melt the honey in a small saucepan on the stovetop. Add the cinnamon, orange zest, and water. Simmer for one minute. Place the air-fried dough balls in a large bowl and drizzle the honey mixture over top. Gently toss to coat all the dough balls evenly. Transfer the coated struffoli to a platter and sprinkle the nonpareil candy sprinkles over top. You can dress the presentation up by piling the balls into the shape of a wreath or pile them high in a cone shape to resemble a Christmas tree.
6. Struffoli can be made ahead. Store covered tightly.

Peach Cobbler

Servings: 4
Cooking Time: 12 Minutes

Ingredients:

- 16 ounces frozen peaches, thawed, with juice (do not drain)
- 6 tablespoons sugar
- 1 tablespoon cornstarch
- 1 tablespoon water
- Crust
- ½ cup flour
- ¼ teaspoon salt
- 3 tablespoons butter
- 1½ tablespoons cold water
- ¼ teaspoon sugar

Directions:

1. Place peaches, including juice, and sugar in air fryer baking pan. Stir to mix well.
2. In a small cup, dissolve cornstarch in the water. Stir into peaches.
3. In a medium bowl, combine the flour and salt. Cut in butter using knives or a pastry blender. Stir in the cold water to make a stiff dough.
4. On a floured board or wax paper, pat dough into a square or circle slightly smaller than your air fryer baking pan. Cut diagonally into 4 pieces.
5. Place dough pieces on top of peaches, leaving a tiny bit of space between the edges. Sprinkle very lightly with sugar, no more than about ¼ teaspoon.
6. Cook at 360°F for 12 minutes, until fruit bubbles and crust browns.

Custard

Servings: 4
Cooking Time: 45 Minutes

Ingredients:

- 2 cups whole milk
- 2 eggs
- ¼ cup sugar
- ⅛ teaspoon salt
- ¼ teaspoon vanilla
- cooking spray
- ⅛ teaspoon nutmeg

Directions:

1. In a blender, process milk, egg, sugar, salt, and vanilla until smooth.
2. Spray a 6 x 6-inch baking pan with nonstick spray and pour the custard into it.
3. Cook at 300°F for 45 minutes. Custard is done when the center sets.
4. Sprinkle top with the nutmeg.
5. Allow custard to cool slightly.
6. Serve it warm, at room temperature, or chilled.

Cinnamon Sugar Banana Rolls

Servings: 6
Cooking Time: 8 Minutes

Ingredients:

- ¼ cup Granulated white sugar
- 2 teaspoons Ground cinnamon
- 2 tablespoons Peach or apricot jam or orange marmalade
- 6 Spring roll wrappers, thawed if necessary
- 2 Ripe banana(s), peeled and cut into 3-inch-long sections
- 1 Large egg, well beaten
- Vegetable oil spray

Directions:

1. Preheat the air fryer to 400°F.
2. Stir the sugar and cinnamon in a small bowl until well combined. Stir the jam or marmalade with a fork to loosen it up.
3. Set a spring roll wrapper on a clean, dry work surface. Roll a banana section in the sugar mixture until evenly and well coated. Set the coated banana along one edge of the wrapper. Top it with about 1 teaspoon of the jam or marmalade. Fold the sides of the wrapper perpendicular to the banana up and over the banana, partially covering it. Brush beaten egg over the side of the wrapper farthest from the banana. Starting with the banana, roll the wrapper closed, ending at the part with the beaten egg. Press gently to seal. Set the roll aside seam side down and continue filling and rolling the remaining wrappers in the same way.
4. Lightly coat the wrappers with vegetable oil spray. Set them seam side down in the basket with as much air space between them as possible. Air-fry undisturbed for 8 minutes, or until crisp and golden brown.
5. Use kitchen tongs to gently transfer the rolls to a wire rack. Cool for at least 5 minutes or up to 30 minutes before serving.

Cherry Hand Pies

Servings: 8
Cooking Time: 8 Minutes

Ingredients:

- 4 cups frozen or canned pitted tart cherries (if using canned, drain and pat dry)
- 2 teaspoons lemon juice
- ½ cup sugar
- ¼ cup cornstarch
- 1 teaspoon vanilla extract
- 1 Basic Pie Dough (see the preceding recipe) or store-bought pie dough

Directions:

1. In a medium saucepan, place the cherries and lemon juice and cook over medium heat for 10 minutes, or until the cherries begin to break down.
2. In a small bowl, stir together the sugar and cornstarch. Pour the sugar mixture into the cherries, stirring constantly. Cook the cherry mixture over low heat for 2 to 3 minutes, or until thickened. Remove from the heat and stir in the vanilla extract. Allow the cherry mixture to cool to room temperature, about 30 minutes.
3. Meanwhile, bring the pie dough to room temperature. Divide the dough into 8 equal pieces. Roll out the dough to ¼-inch thickness in circles. Place ¼ cup

filling in the center of each rolled dough. Fold the dough to create a half-circle. Using a fork, press around the edges to seal the hand pies. Pierce the top of the pie with a fork for steam release while cooking. Continue until 8 hand pies are formed.

4. Preheat the air fryer to 350°F.
5. Place a single layer of hand pies in the air fryer basket and spray with cooking spray. Cook for 8 to 10 minutes or until golden brown and cooked through.

Wild Blueberry Sweet Empanadas

Servings: 12

Cooking Time: 8 Minutes

Ingredients:

- 2 cups frozen wild blueberries
- 5 tablespoons chia seeds
- ¼ cup honey
- 1 tablespoon lemon or lime juice
- ¼ cup water
- 1½ cups all-purpose flour
- 1 cup whole-wheat flour
- ½ teaspoon salt
- 1 tablespoon sugar
- ½ cup cold unsalted butter
- 1 egg
- ½ cup plus 2 tablespoons milk, divided
- 1 cup powdered sugar
- 1 teaspoon vanilla extract

Directions:

1. To make the wild blueberry chia jam, place the blueberries, chia seeds, honey, lemon or lime juice, and water into a blender and pulse for 2 minutes. Pour the chia jam into a glass jar or bowl and cover. Store in the refrigerator at least 4 to 8 hours or until the jam is thickened.
2. In a food processor, place the all-purpose flour, whole-wheat flour, salt, sugar, and butter and process for 2 minutes, scraping down the sides of the food processor every 30 seconds. Add in the egg and blend for 30 seconds. Using the pulse button, add in ½ cup of the milk 1 tablespoon at a time or until the dough is moist enough to handle and be rolled into a ball. Let the dough rest at room temperature for 30 minutes.
3. On a floured surface, cut the dough in half; then form a ball and cut each ball into 6 equal pieces, totaling 12 equal pieces. Work with one piece at a time, and cover the remaining dough with a towel. Roll out the dough into a 6-inch round, much like a tortilla, with ¼ inch thickness. Place 4 tablespoons of filling in the center of round, fold over to form a half-circle. Using a fork, crimp the edges together and pierce the top with a fork for air holes. Repeat with the remaining dough and filling.
4. Preheat the air fryer to 350°F.
5. Working in batches, place 3 to 4 empanadas in the air fryer basket and spray with cooking spray. Cook for 8 minutes. Repeat in batches, as needed. Allow the sweet empanadas to cool for 15 minutes. Meanwhile, in a small bowl, whisk together the powdered sugar, the remaining 2 tablespoons of milk, and the vanilla extract. Then drizzle the glaze over the surface and serve.

Brown Sugar Baked Apples

Servings: 4

Cooking Time: 15 Minutes

Ingredients:

- 3 Small tart apples, preferably McIntosh
- 4 tablespoons (¼ cup/½ stick) Butter
- 6 tablespoons Light brown sugar
- Ground cinnamon
- Table salt

Directions:

1. Preheat the air fryer to 400°F.
2. Stem the apples, then cut them in half through their "equators" (that is, not the stem ends). Use a melon baller to core the apples, taking care not to break through the flesh and skin at any point but creating a little well in the center of each half.
3. When the machine is at temperature, remove the basket and set it on a heat-safe work surface. Set the apple halves cut side up in the basket with as much air space between them as possible. Even a fraction of an inch will work. Drop 2 teaspoons of butter into the well in the center of each apple half. Sprinkle each half with 1 tablespoon brown sugar and a pinch each ground cinnamon and table salt.

4. Return the basket to the machine. Air-fry undisturbed for 15 minutes, or until the apple halves have softened and the brown sugar has caramelized.

5. Use a nonstick-safe spatula to transfer the apple halves cut side up to a wire rack. Cool for at least 10 minutes before serving, or serve at room temperature.

Cheesecake Wontons

Servings:16

Cooking Time: 6 Minutes

Ingredients:

- ¼ cup Regular or low-fat cream cheese (not fat-free)
- 2 tablespoons Granulated white sugar
- 1½ tablespoons Egg yolk
- ¼ teaspoon Vanilla extract
- ⅛ teaspoon Table salt
- 1½ tablespoons All-purpose flour
- 16 Wonton wrappers (vegetarian, if a concern)
- Vegetable oil spray

Directions:

1. Preheat the air fryer to 400°F.
2. Using a flatware fork, mash the cream cheese, sugar, egg yolk, and vanilla in a small bowl until smooth. Add the salt and flour and continue mashing until evenly combined.
3. Set a wonton wrapper on a clean, dry work surface so that one corner faces you (so that it looks like a diamond on your work surface). Set 1 teaspoon of the cream cheese mixture in the middle of the wrapper but just above a horizontal line that would divide the wrapper in half. Dip your clean finger in water and run it along the edges of the wrapper. Fold the corner closest to you up and over the filling, lining it up with the corner farthest from you, thereby making a stuffed triangle. Press gently to seal. Wet the two triangle tips nearest you, then fold them up and together over the filling. Gently press together to seal and fuse. Set aside and continue making more stuffed wontons, 11 more for the small batch, 15 more for the medium batch, or 23 more for the large one.
4. Lightly coat the stuffed wrappers on all sides with vegetable oil spray. Set them with the fused corners up in the basket with as much air space between them as possible. Air-fry undisturbed for 6 minutes, or until golden brown and crisp.
5. Gently dump the contents of the basket onto a wire rack. Cool for at least 5 minutes before serving.

Vegan Brownie Bites

Servings: 10

Cooking Time: 8 Minutes

Ingredients:

- ⅔ cup walnuts
- ⅓ cup all-purpose flour
- ¼ cup dark cocoa powder
- ⅓ cup cane sugar
- ¼ teaspoon salt
- 2 tablespoons vegetable oil
- 1 teaspoon pure vanilla extract
- 1 tablespoon almond milk
- 1 tablespoon powdered sugar

Directions:

1. Preheat the air fryer to 350°F.
2. To a blender or food processor fitted with a metal blade, add the walnuts, flour, cocoa powder, sugar, and salt. Pulse until smooth, about 30 seconds. Add in the oil, vanilla, and milk and pulse until a dough is formed.
3. Remove the dough and place in a bowl. Form into 10 equal-size bites.
4. Liberally spray the metal trivet in the air fryer basket with olive oil mist. Place the brownie bites into the basket and cook for 8 minutes, or until the outer edges begin to slightly crack.
5. Remove the basket from the air fryer and let cool. Sprinkle the brownie bites with powdered sugar and serve.

S'mores Pockets

Servings: 6

Cooking Time: 5 Minutes

Ingredients:

- 12 sheets phyllo dough, thawed
- 1½ cups butter, melted
- ¾ cup graham cracker crumbs
- 1 (7-ounce) Giant Hershey's® milk chocolate bar

- 12 marshmallows, cut in half

Directions:

1. Place one sheet of the phyllo on a large cutting board. Keep the rest of the phyllo sheets covered with a slightly damp, clean kitchen towel. Brush the phyllo sheet generously with some melted butter. Place a second phyllo sheet on top of the first and brush it with more butter. Repeat with one more phyllo sheet until you have a stack of 3 phyllo sheets with butter brushed between the layers. Cover the phyllo sheets with one quarter of the graham cracker crumbs leaving a 1-inch border on one of the short ends of the rectangle. Cut the phyllo sheets lengthwise into 3 strips.
2. Take 2 of the strips and crisscross them to form a cross with the empty borders at the top and to the left. Place 2 of the chocolate rectangles in the center of the cross. Place 4 of the marshmallow halves on top of the chocolate. Now fold the pocket together by folding the bottom phyllo strip up over the chocolate and marshmallows. Then fold the right side over, then the top strip down and finally the left side over. Brush all the edges generously with melted butter to seal shut. Repeat with the next three sheets of phyllo, until all the sheets have been used. You will be able to make 2 pockets with every second batch because you will have an extra graham cracker crumb strip from the previous set of sheets.
3. Preheat the air fryer to 350°F.
4. Transfer 3 pockets at a time to the air fryer basket. Air-fry at 350°F for 4 to 5 minutes, until the phyllo dough is light brown in color. Flip the pockets over halfway through the cooking process. Repeat with the remaining 3 pockets.
5. Serve warm.

One-bowl Chocolate Buttermilk Cake

Servings: 6

Cooking Time: 16-20 Minutes

Ingredients:

- ¾ cup All-purpose flour
- ½ cup Granulated white sugar
- 3 tablespoons Unsweetened cocoa powder
- ½ teaspoon Baking soda
- ¼ teaspoon Table salt
- ½ cup Buttermilk
- 2 tablespoons Vegetable oil
- ¾ teaspoon Vanilla extract
- Baking spray (see here)

Directions:

1. Preheat the air fryer to 325°F (or 330°F, if that's the closest setting).
2. Stir the flour, sugar, cocoa powder, baking soda, and salt in a large bowl until well combined. Add the buttermilk, oil, and vanilla. Stir just until a thick, grainy batter forms.
3. Use the baking spray to generously coat the inside of a 6-inch round cake pan for a small batch, a 7-inch round cake pan for a medium batch, or an 8-inch round cake pan for a large batch. Scrape and spread the chocolate batter into this pan, smoothing the batter out to an even layer.
4. Set the pan in the basket and air-fry undisturbed for 16 minutes for a 6-inch layer, 18 minutes for a 7-inch layer, or 20 minutes for an 8-inch layer, or until a toothpick or cake tester inserted into the center of the cake comes out clean. Start checking it at the 14-minute mark to know where you are.
5. Use hot pads or silicone baking mitts to transfer the cake pan to a wire rack. Cool for 5 minutes. To unmold, set a cutting board over the baking pan and invert both the board and the pan. Lift the still-warm pan off the cake layer. Set the wire rack on top of the cake layer and invert all of it with the cutting board so that the cake layer is now right side up on the wire rack. Remove the cutting board and continue cooling the cake for at least 10 minutes or to room temperature, about 30 minutes, before slicing into wedges.

Donut Holes

Servings: 13

Cooking Time: 12 Minutes

Ingredients:

- 6 tablespoons Granulated white sugar
- 1½ tablespoons Butter, melted and cooled
- 2 tablespoons (or 1 small egg, well beaten) Pasteurized egg substitute, such as Egg Beaters

- 6 tablespoons Regular or low-fat sour cream (not fat-free)
- ¾ teaspoon Vanilla extract
- 1⅔ cups All-purpose flour
- ¾ teaspoon Baking powder
- ¼ teaspoon Table salt
- Vegetable oil spray

Directions:

1. Preheat the air fryer to 350°F .
2. Whisk the sugar and melted butter in a medium bowl until well combined. Whisk in the egg substitute or egg , then the sour cream and vanilla until smooth. Remove the whisk and stir in the flour, baking powder, and salt with a wooden spoon just until a soft dough forms.
3. Use 2 tablespoons of this dough to create a ball between your clean palms. Set it aside and continue making balls: 8 more for the small batch, 12 more for the medium batch, or 17 more for the large one.
4. Coat the balls in the vegetable oil spray, then set them in the basket with as much air space between them as possible. Even a fraction of an inch will be enough, but they should not touch. Air-fry undisturbed for 12 minutes, or until browned and cooked through. A toothpick inserted into the center of a ball should come out clean.
5. Pour the contents of the basket onto a wire rack. Cool for at least 5 minutes before serving.

Strawberry Pastry Rolls

Servings: 4

Cooking Time: 6 Minutes

Ingredients:

- 3 ounces low-fat cream cheese
- 2 tablespoons plain yogurt
- 2 teaspoons sugar
- ¼ teaspoon pure vanilla extract
- 8 ounces fresh strawberries
- 8 sheets phyllo dough
- butter-flavored cooking spray
- ¼–½ cup dark chocolate chips (optional)

Directions:

1. In a medium bowl, combine the cream cheese, yogurt, sugar, and vanilla. Beat with hand mixer at high speed until smooth, about 1 minute.
2. Wash strawberries and destem. Chop enough of them to measure ½ cup. Stir into cheese mixture.
3. Preheat air fryer to 330°F.
4. Phyllo dough dries out quickly, so cover your stack of phyllo sheets with waxed paper and then place a damp dish towel on top of that. Remove only one sheet at a time as you work.
5. To create one pastry roll, lay out a single sheet of phyllo. Spray lightly with butter-flavored spray, top with a second sheet of phyllo, and spray the second sheet lightly.
6. Place a quarter of the filling (about 3 tablespoons) about ½ inch from the edge of one short side. Fold the end of the phyllo over the filling and keep rolling a turn or two. Fold in both the left and right sides so that the edges meet in the middle of your roll. Then roll up completely. Spray outside of pastry roll with butter spray.
7. When you have 4 rolls, place them in the air fryer basket, seam side down, leaving some space in between each. Cook at 330°F for 6 minutes, until they turn a delicate golden brown.
8. Repeat step 7 for remaining rolls.
9. Allow pastries to cool to room temperature.
10. When ready to serve, slice the remaining strawberries. If desired, melt the chocolate chips in microwave or double boiler. Place 1 pastry on each dessert plate, and top with sliced strawberries. Drizzle melted chocolate over strawberries and onto plate.

Fried Cannoli Wontons

Servings: 10

Cooking Time: 8 Minutes

Ingredients:

- 8 ounces Neufchâtel cream cheese
- ¼ cup powdered sugar
- 1 teaspoon vanilla extract
- ¼ teaspoon salt
- ¼ cup mini chocolate chips
- 2 tablespoons chopped pecans (optional)
- 20 wonton wrappers

- ¼ cup filtered water

Directions:

1. Preheat the air fryer to 370°F.
2. In a large bowl, use a hand mixer to combine the cream cheese with the powdered sugar, vanilla, and salt. Fold in the chocolate chips and pecans. Set aside.
3. Lay the wonton wrappers out on a flat, smooth surface and place a bowl with the filtered water next to them.
4. Use a teaspoon to evenly divide the cream cheese mixture among the 20 wonton wrappers, placing the batter in the center of the wontons.
5. Wet the tip of your index finger, and gently moisten the outer edges of the wrapper. Then fold each wrapper until it creates a secure pocket.
6. Liberally spray the air fryer basket with olive oil mist.
7. Place the wontons into the basket, and cook for 5 to 8 minutes. When the outer edges begin to brown, remove the wontons from the air fryer basket. Repeat cooking with remaining wontons.
8. Serve warm.

Glazed Cherry Turnovers

Servings: 8

Cooking Time: 14 Minutes

Ingredients:

- 2 sheets frozen puff pastry, thawed
- 1 (21-ounce) can premium cherry pie filling
- 2 teaspoons ground cinnamon
- 1 egg, beaten
- 1 cup sliced almonds
- 1 cup powdered sugar
- 2 tablespoons milk

Directions:

1. Roll a sheet of puff pastry out into a square that is approximately 10-inches by 10-inches. Cut this large square into quarters.
2. Mix the cherry pie filling and cinnamon together in a bowl. Spoon ¼ cup of the cherry filling into the center of each puff pastry square. Brush the perimeter of the pastry square with the egg wash. Fold one corner of the puff pastry over the cherry pie filling towards the opposite corner, forming a triangle. Seal the two edges of the pastry together with the tip of a fork, making a design with the tines. Brush the top of the turnovers with the egg wash and sprinkle sliced almonds over each one. Repeat these steps with the second sheet of puff pastry. You should have eight turnovers at the end.
3. Preheat the air fryer to 370°F.
4. Air-fry two turnovers at a time for 14 minutes, carefully turning them over halfway through the cooking time.
5. While the turnovers are cooking, make the glaze by whisking the powdered sugar and milk together in a small bowl until smooth. Let the glaze sit for a minute so the sugar can absorb the milk. If the consistency is still too thick to drizzle, add a little more milk, a drop at a time, and stir until smooth.
6. Let the cooked cherry turnovers sit for at least 10 minutes. Then drizzle the glaze over each turnover in a zigzag motion. Serve warm or at room temperature.

Chocolate Macaroons

Servings: 16

Cooking Time: 8 Minutes

Ingredients:

- 2 Large egg white(s), at room temperature
- ⅛ teaspoon Table salt
- ½ cup Granulated white sugar
- 1½ cups Unsweetened shredded coconut
- 3 tablespoons Unsweetened cocoa powder

Directions:

1. Preheat the air fryer to 375°F .
2. Using an electric mixer at high speed, beat the egg white(s) and salt in a medium or large bowl until stiff peaks can be formed when the turned-off beaters are dipped into the mixture.
3. Still working with the mixer at high speed, beat in the sugar in a slow stream until the meringue is shiny and thick.
4. Scrape down and remove the beaters. Fold in the coconut and cocoa with a rubber spatula until well combined, working carefully to deflate the meringue as little as possible.
5. Scoop up 2 tablespoons of the mixture. Wet your clean hands and roll that little bit of coconut bliss into a

ball. Set it aside and continue making more balls: 7 more for a small batch, 15 more for a medium batch, or 23 more for a large one.

6. Line the bottom of the machine's basket or the basket attachment with parchment paper. Set the balls on the parchment with as much air space between them as possible. Air-fry undisturbed for 8 minutes, or until dry, set, and lightly browned.

7. Use a nonstick-safe spatula to transfer the macaroons to a wire rack. Cool for at least 10 minutes before serving. Or cool to room temperature, about 30 minutes, then store in a sealed container at room temperature for up to 3 days.

Apple Dumplings

Servings: 4

Cooking Time: 25 Minutes

Ingredients:

- 1 Basic Pie Dough (see the following recipe)
- 4 medium Granny Smith or Pink Lady apples, peeled and cored
- 4 tablespoons sugar
- 4 teaspoons cinnamon
- ½ teaspoon ground nutmeg
- 4 tablespoons unsalted butter, melted
- 4 scoops ice cream, for serving

Directions:

1. Preheat the air fryer to 330°F.
2. Bring the pie crust recipe to room temperature.
3. Place the pie crust on a floured surface. Divide the dough into 4 equal pieces. Roll out each piece to ¼-inch-thick rounds. Place an apple onto each dough round. Sprinkle 1 tablespoon of sugar in the core part of each apple; sprinkle 1 teaspoon cinnamon and ⅛ teaspoon nutmeg over each. Place 1 tablespoon of butter into the center of each. Fold up the sides and fully cover the cored apples.
4. Place the dumplings into the air fryer basket and spray with cooking spray. Cook for 25 minutes. Check after 14 minutes cooking; if they're getting too brown, reduce the heat to 320°F and complete the cooking.
5. Serve hot apple dumplings with a scoop of ice cream.

Peanut Butter Cup Doughnut Holes

Servings: 24

Cooking Time: 4 Minutes

Ingredients:

- 1½ cups bread flour
- 1 teaspoon active dry yeast
- 1 tablespoon sugar
- ¼ teaspoon salt
- ½ cup warm milk
- ½ teaspoon vanilla extract
- 2 egg yolks
- 2 tablespoons melted butter
- 24 miniature peanut butter cups, plus a few more for garnish
- vegetable oil, in a spray bottle
- Doughnut Topping
- 1 cup chocolate chips
- 2 tablespoons milk

Directions:

1. Combine the flour, yeast, sugar and salt in a bowl. Add the milk, vanilla, egg yolks and butter. Mix well until the dough starts to come together. Transfer the dough to a floured surface and knead by hand for 2 minutes. Shape the dough into a ball and transfer it to a large oiled bowl. Cover the bowl with a towel and let the dough rise in a warm place for 1 to 1½ hours, until the dough has doubled in size.
2. When the dough has risen, punch it down and roll it into a 24-inch long log. Cut the dough into 24 pieces. Push a peanut butter cup into the center of each piece of dough, pinch the dough shut and roll it into a ball. Place the dough balls on a cookie sheet and let them rise in a warm place for 30 minutes.
3. Preheat the air fryer to 400°F.
4. Spray or brush the dough balls lightly with vegetable oil. Air-fry eight at a time, at 400°F for 4 minutes, turning them over halfway through the cooking process.
5. While the doughnuts are air frying, prepare the topping. Place the chocolate chips and milk in a microwave safe bowl. Microwave on high for 1 minute. Stir and microwave for an additional 30 seconds if

necessary to get all the chips to melt. Stir until the chips are melted and smooth.

6. Dip the top half of the doughnut holes into the melted chocolate. Place them on a rack to set up for just a few minutes and watch them disappear.

Chocolate Soufflés

Servings: 2
Cooking Time: 14 Minutes

Ingredients:

- butter and sugar for greasing the ramekins
- 3 ounces semi-sweet chocolate, chopped
- ¼ cup unsalted butter
- 2 eggs, yolks and white separated
- 3 tablespoons sugar
- ½ teaspoon pure vanilla extract
- 2 tablespoons all-purpose flour
- powdered sugar, for dusting the finished soufflés
- heavy cream, for serving

Directions:

1. Butter and sugar two 6-ounce ramekins. (Butter the ramekins and then coat the butter with sugar by shaking it around in the ramekin and dumping out any excess.)
2. Melt the chocolate and butter together, either in the microwave or in a double boiler. In a separate bowl, beat the egg yolks vigorously. Add the sugar and the vanilla extract and beat well again. Drizzle in the chocolate and butter, mixing well. Stir in the flour, combining until there are no lumps.
3. Preheat the air fryer to 330°F.
4. In a separate bowl, whisk the egg whites to soft peak stage (the point at which the whites can almost stand up on the end of your whisk). Fold the whipped egg whites into the chocolate mixture gently and in stages.
5. Transfer the batter carefully to the buttered ramekins, leaving about ½-inch at the top. (You may have a little extra batter, depending on how airy the batter is, so you might be able to squeeze out a third soufflé if you want to.) Place the ramekins into the air fryer basket and air-fry for 14 minutes. The soufflés should have risen nicely and be brown on top. (Don't worry if the top gets a little dark – you'll be covering it with powdered sugar in the next step.)
6. Dust with powdered sugar and serve immediately with heavy cream to pour over the top at the table.

Honey-roasted Mixed Nuts

Servings: 8
Cooking Time: 15 Minutes

Ingredients:

- ½ cup raw, shelled pistachios
- ½ cup raw almonds
- 1 cup raw walnuts
- 2 tablespoons filtered water
- 2 tablespoons honey
- 1 tablespoon vegetable oil
- 2 tablespoons sugar
- ½ teaspoon salt

Directions:

1. Preheat the air fryer to 300°F.
2. Lightly spray an air-fryer-safe pan with olive oil; then place the pistachios, almonds, and walnuts inside the pan and place the pan inside the air fryer basket.
3. Cook for 15 minutes, shaking the basket every 5 minutes to rotate the nuts.
4. While the nuts are roasting, boil the water in a small pan and stir in the honey and oil. Continue to stir while cooking until the water begins to evaporate and a thick sauce is formed. Note: The sauce should stick to the back of a wooden spoon when mixed. Turn off the heat.
5. Remove the nuts from the air fryer (cooking should have just completed) and spoon the nuts into the stovetop pan. Use a spatula to coat the nuts with the honey syrup.
6. Line a baking sheet with parchment paper and spoon the nuts onto the sheet. Lightly sprinkle the sugar and salt over the nuts and let cool in the refrigerator for at least 2 hours.
7. When the honey and sugar have hardened, store the nuts in an airtight container in the refrigerator.

Boston Cream Donut Holes

Servings: 24
Cooking Time: 12 Minutes

Ingredients:

- 1½ cups bread flour
- 1 teaspoon active dry yeast
- 1 tablespoon sugar
- ¼ teaspoon salt
- ½ cup warm milk
- ½ teaspoon pure vanilla extract
- 2 egg yolks
- 2 tablespoons butter, melted
- vegetable oil
- Custard Filling:
- 1 (3.4-ounce) box French vanilla instant pudding mix
- ¾ cup whole milk
- ¼ cup heavy cream
- Chocolate Glaze:
- 1 cup chocolate chips
- ⅓ cup heavy cream

Directions:

1. Combine the flour, yeast, sugar and salt in the bowl of a stand mixer. Add the milk, vanilla, egg yolks and butter. Mix until the dough starts to come together in a ball. Transfer the dough to a floured surface and knead the dough by hand for 2 minutes. Shape the dough into a ball, place it in a large oiled bowl, cover the bowl with a clean kitchen towel and let the dough rise for 1 to 1½ hours or until the dough has doubled in size.
2. When the dough has risen, punch it down and roll it into a 24-inch log. Cut the dough into 24 pieces and roll each piece into a ball. Place the dough balls on a baking sheet and let them rise for another 30 minutes.
3. Preheat the air fryer to 400°F.
4. Spray or brush the dough balls lightly with vegetable oil and air-fry eight at a time for 4 minutes, turning them over halfway through the cooking time.
5. While donut holes are cooking, make the filling and chocolate glaze. To make the filling, use an electric hand mixer to beat the French vanilla pudding, milk and ¼ cup of heavy cream together for 2 minutes.
6. To make the chocolate glaze, place the chocolate chips in a medium-sized bowl. Bring the heavy cream to a boil on the stovetop and pour it over the chocolate chips. Stir until the chips are melted and the glaze is smooth.
7. To fill the donut holes, place the custard filling in a pastry bag with a long tip. Poke a hole into the side of the donut hole with a small knife. Wiggle the knife around to make room for the filling. Place the pastry bag tip into the hole and slowly squeeze the custard into the center of the donut. Dip the top half of the donut into the chocolate glaze, letting any excess glaze drip back into the bowl. Let the glazed donut holes sit for a few minutes before serving.

Caramel Apple Crumble

Servings: 6
Cooking Time: 50 Minutes

Ingredients:

- 4 apples, peeled and thinly sliced
- 2 tablespoons sugar
- 1 tablespoon flour
- 1 teaspoon ground cinnamon
- ¼ teaspoon ground allspice
- healthy pinch ground nutmeg
- 10 caramel squares, cut into small pieces
- Crumble Topping:
- ¾ cup rolled oats
- ¼ cup sugar
- ⅓ cup flour
- ¼ teaspoon ground cinnamon
- 6 tablespoons butter, melted

Directions:

1. Preheat the air fryer to 330°F.
2. Combine the apples, sugar, flour, and spices in a large bowl and toss to coat. Add the caramel pieces and mix well. Pour the apple mixture into a 1-quart round baking dish that will fit in your air fryer basket (6-inch diameter).
3. To make the crumble topping, combine the rolled oats, sugar, flour and cinnamon in a small bowl. Add the melted butter and mix well. Top the apples with the crumble mixture. Cover the entire dish with aluminum

foil and transfer the dish to the air fryer basket, lowering the dish into the basket using a sling made of aluminum foil (fold a piece of aluminum foil into a strip about 2-inches wide by 24-inches long). Fold the ends of the aluminum foil over the top of the dish before returning the basket to the air fryer.

4. Air-fry at 330°F for 25 minutes. Remove the aluminum foil and continue to air-fry for another 25 minutes. Serve the crumble warm with whipped cream or vanilla ice cream, if desired.

White Chocolate Cranberry Blondies

Servings: 6

Cooking Time: 18 Minutes

Ingredients:

- ⅓ cup butter
- ½ cup sugar
- 1 teaspoon vanilla extract
- 1 large egg
- 1 cup all-purpose flour
- ½ teaspoon baking powder
- ⅛ teaspoon salt
- ¼ cup dried cranberries
- ¼ cup white chocolate chips

Directions:

1. Preheat the air fryer to 320°F.
2. In a large bowl, cream the butter with the sugar and vanilla extract. Whisk in the egg and set aside.
3. In a separate bowl, mix the flour with the baking powder and salt. Then gently mix the dry ingredients into the wet. Fold in the cranberries and chocolate chips.
4. Liberally spray an oven-safe 7-inch springform pan with olive oil and pour the batter into the pan.
5. Cook for 17 minutes or until a toothpick inserted in the center comes out clean.
6. Remove and let cool 5 minutes before serving.

Almond-roasted Pears

Servings: 4

Cooking Time: 15 Minutes

Ingredients:

- Yogurt Topping
- 1 container vanilla Greek yogurt (5–6 ounces)
- ¼ teaspoon almond flavoring
- 2 whole pears
- ¼ cup crushed Biscoff cookies (approx. 4 cookies)
- 1 tablespoon sliced almonds
- 1 tablespoon butter

Directions:

1. Stir almond flavoring into yogurt and set aside while preparing pears.
2. Halve each pear and spoon out the core.
3. Place pear halves in air fryer basket.
4. Stir together the cookie crumbs and almonds. Place a quarter of this mixture into the hollow of each pear half.
5. Cut butter into 4 pieces and place one piece on top of crumb mixture in each pear.
6. Cook at 360°F for 15 minutes or until pears have cooked through but are still slightly firm.
7. Serve pears warm with a dollop of yogurt topping.

Baked Apple

Servings: 6

Cooking Time: 20 Minutes

Ingredients:

- 3 small Honey Crisp or other baking apples
- 3 tablespoons maple syrup
- 3 tablespoons chopped pecans
- 1 tablespoon firm butter, cut into 6 pieces

Directions:

1. Put ½ cup water in the drawer of the air fryer.
2. Wash apples well and dry them.
3. Split apples in half. Remove core and a little of the flesh to make a cavity for the pecans.
4. Place apple halves in air fryer basket, cut side up.
5. Spoon 1½ teaspoons pecans into each cavity.
6. Spoon ½ tablespoon maple syrup over pecans in each apple.
7. Top each apple with ½ teaspoon butter.
8. Cook at 360°F for 20 minutes, until apples are tender.

Coconut Crusted Bananas With Pineapple Sauce

Servings: 4
Cooking Time: 5 Minutes

Ingredients:

- Pineapple Sauce
- 1½ cups puréed fresh pineapple
- 2 tablespoons sugar
- juice of 1 lemon
- ¼ teaspoon ground cinnamon
- 3 firm bananas
- ¼ cup sweetened condensed milk
- 1¼ cups shredded coconut
- ⅓ cup crushed graham crackers (crumbs)*
- vegetable or canola oil, in a spray bottle
- vanilla frozen yogurt or ice cream

Directions:

1. Make the pineapple sauce by combining the pineapple, sugar, lemon juice and cinnamon in a saucepan. Simmer the mixture on the stovetop for 20 minutes, and then set it aside.
2. Slice the bananas diagonally into ½-inch thick slices and place them in a bowl. Pour the sweetened condensed milk into the bowl and toss the bananas gently to coat. Combine the coconut and graham cracker crumbs together in a shallow dish. Remove the banana slices from the condensed milk and let any excess milk drip off. Dip the banana slices in the coconut and crumb mixture to coat both sides. Spray the coated slices with oil.
3. Preheat the air fryer to 400°F.
4. Grease the bottom of the air fryer basket with a little oil. Air-fry the bananas in batches at 400°F for 5 minutes, turning them over halfway through the cooking time. Air-fry until the bananas are golden brown on both sides.
5. Serve warm over vanilla frozen yogurt with some of the pineapple sauce spooned over top.

Sea-salted Caramel Cookie Cups

Servings: 12
Cooking Time: 12 Minutes

Ingredients:

- ⅓ cup butter
- ¼ cup brown sugar
- 1 teaspoon vanilla extract
- 1 large egg
- 1 cup all-purpose flour
- ½ cup old-fashioned oats
- ½ teaspoon baking soda
- ¼ teaspoon salt
- ⅓ cup sea-salted caramel chips

Directions:

1. Preheat the air fryer to 300°F.
2. In a large bowl, cream the butter with the brown sugar and vanilla. Whisk in the egg and set aside.
3. In a separate bowl, mix the flour, oats, baking soda, and salt. Then gently mix the dry ingredients into the wet. Fold in the caramel chips.
4. Divide the batter into 12 silicon muffin liners. Place the cookie cups into the air fryer basket and cook for 12 minutes or until a toothpick inserted in the center comes out clean.
5. Remove and let cool 5 minutes before serving.

Coconut Rice Cake

Servings: 8
Cooking Time: 30 Minutes

Ingredients:

- 1 cup all-natural coconut water
- 1 cup unsweetened coconut milk
- 1 teaspoon almond extract
- ¼ teaspoon salt
- 4 tablespoons honey
- cooking spray
- ¾ cup raw jasmine rice
- 2 cups sliced or cubed fruit

Directions:

1. In a medium bowl, mix together the coconut water, coconut milk, almond extract, salt, and honey.
2. Spray air fryer baking pan with cooking spray and add the rice.
3. Pour liquid mixture over rice.
4. Cook at 360°F for 15minutes. Stir and cook for 15 minutes longer or until rice grains are tender.

5. Allow cake to cool slightly. Run a dull knife around edge of cake, inside the pan. Turn the cake out onto a platter and garnish with fruit.

Pear And Almond Biscotti Crumble

Servings: 6

Cooking Time: 65 Minutes

Ingredients:

- 7-inch cake pan or ceramic dish
- 3 pears, peeled, cored and sliced
- ½ cup brown sugar
- ¼ teaspoon ground ginger
- 1 teaspoon ground cinnamon
- ⅛ teaspoon ground nutmeg
- 2 tablespoons cornstarch
- 1¼ cups (4 to 5) almond biscotti, coarsely crushed
- ¼ cup all-purpose flour
- ¼ cup sliced almonds
- ¼ cup butter, melted

Directions:

1. Combine the pears, brown sugar, ginger, cinnamon, nutmeg and cornstarch in a bowl. Toss to combine and then pour the pear mixture into a greased 7-inch cake pan or ceramic dish.
2. Combine the crushed biscotti, flour, almonds and melted butter in a medium bowl. Toss with a fork until the mixture resembles large crumbles. Sprinkle the biscotti crumble over the pears and cover the pan with aluminum foil.
3. Preheat the air fryer to 350°F.
4. Air-fry at 350°F for 60 minutes. Remove the aluminum foil and air-fry for an additional 5 minutes to brown the crumble layer.
5. Serve warm.

Roasted Pears

Servings: 4

Cooking Time: 10 Minutes

Ingredients:

- 2 Ripe pears, preferably Anjou, stemmed, peeled, halved lengthwise, and cored
- 2 tablespoons Butter, melted
- 2 teaspoons Granulated white sugar
- Grated nutmeg
- ¼ cup Honey
- ½ cup (about 1½ ounces) Shaved Parmesan cheese

Directions:

1. Preheat the air fryer to 400°F.
2. Brush each pear half with about 1½ teaspoons of the melted butter, then sprinkle their cut sides with ½ teaspoon sugar. Grate a pinch of nutmeg over each pear.
3. When the machine is at temperature, set the pear halves cut side up in the basket with as much air space between them as possible. Air-fry undisturbed for 10 minutes, or until hot and softened.
4. Use a nonstick-safe spatula, and perhaps a flatware tablespoon for balance, to transfer the pear halves to a serving platter or plates. Cool for a minute or two, then drizzle each pear half with 1 tablespoon of the honey. Lay about 2 tablespoons of shaved Parmesan over each half just before serving.

Fried Twinkies

Servings:6

Cooking Time: 5 Minutes

Ingredients:

- 2 Large egg white(s)
- 2 tablespoons Water
- 1½ cups (about 9 ounces) Ground gingersnap cookie crumbs
- 6 Twinkies
- Vegetable oil spray

Directions:

1. Preheat the air fryer to 400°F.
2. Set up and fill two shallow soup plates or small pie plates on your counter: one for the egg white(s), whisked with the water until foamy; and one for the gingersnap crumbs.
3. Dip a Twinkie in the egg white(s), turning it to coat on all sides, even the ends. Let the excess egg white mixture slip back into the rest, then set the Twinkie in the crumbs. Roll it to coat on all sides, even the ends, pressing gently to get an even coating. Then repeat this process: egg white(s), followed by crumbs. Lightly coat the prepared Twinkie on all sides with vegetable oil spray.

Set aside and coat each of the remaining Twinkies with the same double-dipping technique, followed by spraying.
4. Set the Twinkies flat side up in the basket with as much air space between them as possible. Air-fry for 5 minutes, or until browned and crunchy.
5. Use a nonstick-safe spatula to gently transfer the Twinkies to a wire rack. Cool for at least 10 minutes before serving.

Oreo-coated Peanut Butter Cups

Servings:8
Cooking Time: 4 Minutes

Ingredients:

- 8 Standard ¾-ounce peanut butter cups, frozen
- ⅓ cup All-purpose flour
- 2 Large egg white(s), beaten until foamy
- 16 Oreos or other creme-filled chocolate sandwich cookies, ground to crumbs in a food processor
- Vegetable oil spray

Directions:

1. Set up and fill three shallow soup plates or small pie plates on your counter: one for the flour, one for the beaten egg white(s), and one for the cookie crumbs.
2. Dip a frozen peanut butter cup in the flour, turning it to coat all sides. Shake off any excess, then set it in the beaten egg white(s). Turn it to coat all sides, then let any excess egg white slip back into the rest. Set the candy bar in the cookie crumbs. Turn to coat on all parts, even the sides. Dip the peanut butter cup back in the egg white(s) as before, then into the cookie crumbs as before, making sure you have a solid, even coating all around the cup. Set aside while you dip and coat the remaining cups.
3. When all the peanut butter cups are dipped and coated, lightly coat them on all sides with the vegetable oil spray. Set them on a plate and freeze while the air fryer heats.
4. Preheat the air fryer to 400°F.
5. Set the dipped cups wider side up in the basket with as much air space between them as possible. Air-fry undisturbed for 4 minutes, or until they feel soft but the coating is set.
6. Turn off the machine and remove the basket from it. Set aside the basket with the fried cups for 10 minutes. Use a nonstick-safe spatula to transfer the fried cups to a wire rack. Cool for at least another 5 minutes before serving.

Easy Churros

Servings: 12
Cooking Time: 10 Minutes

Ingredients:

- ½ cup Water
- 4 tablespoons (¼ cup/½ stick) Butter
- ¼ teaspoon Table salt
- ½ cup All-purpose flour
- 2 Large egg(s)
- ¼ cup Granulated white sugar
- 2 teaspoons Ground cinnamon

Directions:

1. Bring the water, butter, and salt to a boil in a small saucepan set over high heat, stirring occasionally.
2. When the butter has fully melted, reduce the heat to medium and stir in the flour to form a dough. Continue cooking, stirring constantly, to dry out the dough until it coats the bottom and sides of the pan with a film, even a crust. Remove the pan from the heat, scrape the dough into a bowl, and cool for 15 minutes.
3. Using an electric hand mixer at medium speed, beat in the egg, or eggs one at a time, until the dough is smooth and firm enough to hold its shape.
4. Mix the sugar and cinnamon in a small bowl. Scoop up 1 tablespoon of the dough and roll it in the sugar mixture to form a small, coated tube about ½ inch in diameter and 2 inches long. Set it aside and make 5 more tubes for the small batch or 11 more for the large one.
5. Set the tubes on a plate and freeze for 20 minutes. Meanwhile, Preheat the air fryer to 375°F .
6. Set 3 frozen tubes in the basket for a small batch or 6 for a large one with as much air space between them as possible. Air-fry undisturbed for 10 minutes, or until puffed, brown, and set.
7. Use kitchen tongs to transfer the churros to a wire rack to cool for at least 5 minutes. Meanwhile, air-fry and cool the second batch of churros in the same way.

Dark Chocolate Peanut Butter S'mores

Servings: 4

Cooking Time: 6 Minutes

Ingredients:

- 4 graham cracker sheets
- 4 marshmallows
- 4 teaspoons chunky peanut butter
- 4 ounces dark chocolate
- ½ teaspoon ground cinnamon

Directions:

1. Preheat the air fryer to 390°F. Break the graham crackers in half so you have 8 pieces.
2. Place 4 pieces of graham cracker on the bottom of the air fryer. Top each with one of the marshmallows and bake for 6 or 7 minutes, or until the marshmallows have a golden brown center.
3. While cooking, slather each of the remaining graham crackers with 1 teaspoon peanut butter.
4. When baking completes, carefully remove each of the graham crackers, add 1 ounce of dark chocolate on top of the marshmallow, and lightly sprinkle with cinnamon. Top with the remaining peanut butter graham cracker to make the sandwich. Serve immediately.

Fried Banana S'mores

Servings: 4

Cooking Time: 6 Minutes

Ingredients:

- 4 bananas
- 3 tablespoons mini semi-sweet chocolate chips
- 3 tablespoons mini peanut butter chips
- 3 tablespoons mini marshmallows
- 3 tablespoons graham cracker cereal

Directions:

1. Preheat the air fryer to 400°F.
2. Slice into the un-peeled bananas lengthwise along the inside of the curve, but do not slice through the bottom of the peel. Open the banana slightly to form a pocket.
3. Fill each pocket with chocolate chips, peanut butter chips and marshmallows. Poke the graham cracker cereal into the filling.
4. Place the bananas in the air fryer basket, resting them on the side of the basket and each other to keep them upright with the filling facing up. Air-fry for 6 minutes, or until the bananas are soft to the touch, the peels have blackened and the chocolate and marshmallows have melted and toasted.
5. Let them cool for a couple of minutes and then simply serve with a spoon to scoop out the filling.

Beef，Pork & Lamb Recipes

Crunchy Veal Cutlets

Servings: 2

Cooking Time: 5 Minutes

Ingredients:

- ½ cup All-purpose flour or tapioca flour
- 1 Large egg(s), well beaten
- ¾ cup Seasoned Italian-style dried bread crumbs (gluten-free, if a concern)
- 2 tablespoons Yellow cornmeal
- 4 Thinly pounded 2-ounce veal leg cutlets (less than ¼ inch thick)
- Olive oil spray

Directions:

1. Preheat the air fryer to 400°F.
2. Set up and fill three shallow soup plates or small pie plates on your counter: one for the flour; one for the egg(s); and one for the bread crumbs, whisked with the cornmeal until well combined.
3. Dredge a veal cutlet in the flour, coating it on both sides. Gently shake off any excess flour, then gently dip it in the beaten egg(s), coating both sides. Let the excess egg slip back into the rest. Dip the cutlet in the bread-crumb mixture, turning it several times and pressing gently to make an even coating on both sides. Coat it on both sides with olive oil spray, then set it aside and continue dredging and coating more cutlets.
4. When the machine is at temperature, set the cutlets in the basket so that they don't touch each other. Air-fry undisturbed for 5 minutes, or until crisp and brown. (If only some of the veal cutlets will fit in one layer for any selected batch—the sizes of air fryer baskets vary dramatically—work in batches as necessary.)
5. Use kitchen tongs to transfer the cutlets to a wire rack. Cool for only 1 to 2 minutes before serving.

City "chicken"

Servings: 3

Cooking Time: 10 Minutes

Ingredients:

- 1 pound Pork tenderloin, cut into 2-inch cubes
- ½ cup All-purpose flour or tapioca flour
- 1 Large egg(s)
- 1 teaspoon Dried poultry seasoning blend
- 1¼ cups Plain panko bread crumbs (gluten-free, if a concern)
- Vegetable oil spray

Directions:

1. Preheat the air fryer to 350°F .
2. Thread 3 or 4 pieces of pork on a 4-inch bamboo skewer. You'll need 2 or 3 skewers for a small batch, 3 or 4 for a medium, and up to 6 for a large batch.
3. Set up and fill three shallow soup plates or small pie plates on your counter: one for the flour; one for the egg(s), beaten with the poultry seasoning until foamy; and one for the bread crumbs.
4. Dip and roll one skewer into the flour, coating all sides of the meat. Gently shake off any excess flour, then dip and roll the skewer in the egg mixture. Let any excess egg mixture slip back into the rest, then set the skewer in the bread crumbs and roll it around, pressing gently, until the exterior surfaces of the meat are evenly coated. Generously coat the meat on the skewer with vegetable oil spray. Set aside and continue dredging, dipping, coating, and spraying the remaining skewers.
5. Set the skewers in the basket in one layer and air-fry undisturbed for 10 minutes, or until brown and crunchy.
6. Use kitchen tongs to transfer the skewers to a wire rack. Cool for a minute or two before serving.

Pepper Steak

Servings: 4

Cooking Time: 30 Minutes

Ingredients:

- 2 tablespoons cornstarch
- 1 tablespoon sugar
- ¾ cup beef broth
- ¼ cup hoisin sauce
- 3 tablespoons soy sauce
- 1 teaspoon sesame oil
- ½ teaspoon freshly ground black pepper

- 1½ pounds boneless New York strip steaks, sliced into ½-inch strips
- 1 onion, sliced
- 3 small bell peppers, red, yellow and green, sliced

Directions:

1. Whisk the cornstarch and sugar together in a large bowl to break up any lumps in the cornstarch. Add the beef broth and whisk until combined and smooth. Stir in the hoisin sauce, soy sauce, sesame oil and freshly ground black pepper. Add the beef, onion and peppers, and toss to coat. Marinate the beef and vegetables at room temperature for 30 minutes, stirring a few times to keep meat and vegetables coated.
2. Preheat the air fryer to 350°F.
3. Transfer the beef, onion, and peppers to the air fryer basket with tongs, reserving the marinade. Air-fry the beef and vegetables for 30 minutes, stirring well two or three times during the cooking process.
4. While the beef is air-frying, bring the reserved marinade to a simmer in a small saucepan over medium heat on the stovetop. Simmer for 5 minutes until the sauce thickens.
5. When the steak and vegetables have finished cooking, transfer them to a serving platter. Pour the hot sauce over the pepper steak and serve with white rice.

Tuscan Veal Chops

Servings: 2

Cooking Time: 12-15 Minutes

Ingredients:

- 4 teaspoons Olive oil
- 2 teaspoons Finely minced garlic
- 2 teaspoons Finely minced fresh rosemary leaves
- 1 teaspoon Finely grated lemon zest
- 1 teaspoon Crushed fennel seeds
- 1 teaspoon Table salt
- Up to ¼ teaspoon Red pepper flakes
- 2 10-ounce bone-in veal loin or rib chop(s), about ½ inch thick

Directions:

1. Preheat the air fryer to 400°F.
2. Mix the oil, garlic, rosemary, lemon zest, fennel seeds, salt, and red pepper flakes in a small bowl. Rub this mixture onto both sides of the veal chop(s). Set aside at room temperature as the machine comes to temperature.
3. Set the chop(s) in the basket. If you're cooking more than one chop, leave as much air space between them as possible. Air-fry undisturbed for 12 minutes for medium-rare, or until an instant-read meat thermometer inserted into the center of a chop (without touching bone) registers 135°F (not USDA-approved). Or air-fry undisturbed for 15 minutes for medium-well, or until an instant-read meat thermometer registers 145°F (USDA-approved).
4. Use kitchen tongs to transfer the chops to a cutting board or a wire rack. Cool for 5 minutes before serving.

Pork Cutlets With Almond-lemon Crust

Servings: 3

Cooking Time: 14 Minutes

Ingredients:

- ¾ cup Almond flour
- ¾ cup Plain dried bread crumbs (gluten-free, if a concern)
- 1½ teaspoons Finely grated lemon zest
- 1¼ teaspoons Table salt
- ¾ teaspoon Garlic powder
- ¾ teaspoon Dried oregano
- 1 Large egg white(s)
- 2 tablespoons Water
- 3 6-ounce center-cut boneless pork loin chops (about ¾ inch thick)
- Olive oil spray

Directions:

1. Preheat the air fryer to 375°F .
2. Mix the almond flour, bread crumbs, lemon zest, salt, garlic powder, and dried oregano in a large bowl until well combined.
3. Whisk the egg white(s) and water in a shallow soup plate or small pie plate until uniform.
4. Dip a chop in the egg white mixture, turning it to coat all sides, even the ends. Let any excess egg white mixture slip back into the rest, then set it in the almond flour mixture. Turn it several times, pressing gently to coat it evenly. Generously coat the chop with olive oil

spray, then set aside to dip and coat the remaining chop(s).

5. Set the chops in the basket with as much air space between them as possible. Air-fry undisturbed for 12 minutes, or until browned and crunchy. You may need to add 2 minutes to the cooking time if the machine is at 360°F.

6. Use kitchen tongs to transfer the chops to a wire rack. Cool for a few minutes before serving.

Better-than-chinese-take-out Pork Ribs

Servings: 3

Cooking Time: 35 Minutes

Ingredients:

- 1½ tablespoons Hoisin sauce (see here; gluten-free, if a concern)
- 1½ tablespoons Regular or low-sodium soy sauce or gluten-free tamari sauce
- 1½ tablespoons Shaoxing (Chinese cooking rice wine), dry sherry, or white grape juice
- 1½ teaspoons Minced garlic
- ¾ teaspoon Ground dried ginger
- ¾ teaspoon Ground white pepper
- 1½ pounds Pork baby back rib rack(s), cut into 2-bone pieces

Directions:

1. Mix the hoisin sauce, soy or tamari sauce, Shaoxing or its substitute, garlic, ginger, and white pepper in a large bowl. Add the rib sections and stir well to coat. Cover and refrigerate for at least 2 hours or up to 24 hours, stirring the rib sections in the marinade occasionally.
2. Preheat the air fryer to 350°F . Set the ribs in their bowl on the counter as the machine heats.
3. When the machine is at temperature, set the rib pieces on their sides in a single layer in the basket with as much air space between them as possible. Air-fry for 35 minutes, turning and rearranging the pieces once, until deeply browned and sizzling.
4. Use kitchen tongs to transfer the rib pieces to a large serving bowl or platter. Wait a minute or two before serving them so the meat can reabsorb some of its own juices.

Fried Spam

Servings: 2

Cooking Time: 12 Minutes

Ingredients:

- ½ cup All-purpose flour or gluten-free all-purpose flour
- 1 Large egg(s)
- 1 tablespoon Wasabi paste
- 1⅓ cups Plain panko bread crumbs (gluten-free, if a concern)
- 4 ½-inch-thick Spam slices
- Vegetable oil spray

Directions:

1. Preheat the air fryer to 400°F.
2. Set up and fill three shallow soup plates or small pie plates on your counter: one for the flour; one for the egg(s), whisked with the wasabi paste until uniform; and one for the bread crumbs.
3. Dip a slice of Spam in the flour, coating both sides. Slip it into the egg mixture and turn to coat on both sides, even along the edges. Let any excess egg mixture slip back into the rest, then set the slice in the bread crumbs. Turn it several times, pressing gently to make an even coating on both sides. Generously coat both sides of the slice with vegetable oil spray. Set aside so you can dip, coat, and spray the remaining slice(s).
4. Set the slices in the basket in a single layer so that they don't touch (even if they're close together). Air-fry undisturbed for 12 minutes, or until very brown and quite crunchy.
5. Use kitchen tongs to transfer the slices to a wire rack. Cool for a minute or two before serving.

Garlic And Oregano Lamb Chops

Servings: 4

Cooking Time: 17 Minutes

Ingredients:

- 1½ tablespoons Olive oil
- 1 tablespoon Minced garlic
- 1 teaspoon Dried oregano
- 1 teaspoon Finely minced orange zest
- ¾ teaspoon Fennel seeds
- ¾ teaspoon Table salt
- ¾ teaspoon Ground black pepper
- 6 4-ounce, 1-inch-thick lamb loin chops

Directions:

1. Mix the olive oil, garlic, oregano, orange zest, fennel seeds, salt, and pepper in a large bowl. Add the chops and toss well to coat. Set aside as the air fryer heats, tossing one more time.
2. Preheat the air fryer to 400°F.
3. Set the chops bone side down in the basket (that is, so they stand up on their bony edge) with as much air space between them as possible. Air-fry undisturbed for 14 minutes for medium-rare, or until an instant-read meat thermometer inserted into the thickest part of a chop (without touching bone) registers 132°F (not USDA-approved). Or air-fry undisturbed for 17 minutes for well done, or until an instant-read meat thermometer registers 145°F (USDA-approved).
4. Use kitchen tongs to transfer the chops to a wire rack. Cool for 5 minutes before serving.

Kielbasa Sausage With Pierogies And Caramelized Onions

Servings: 3

Cooking Time: 30 Minutes

Ingredients:

- 1 Vidalia or sweet onion, sliced
- olive oil
- salt and freshly ground black pepper
- 2 tablespoons butter, cut into small cubes
- 1 teaspoon sugar
- 1 pound light Polish kielbasa sausage, cut into 2-inch chunks
- 1 (13-ounce) package frozen mini pierogies
- 2 teaspoons vegetable or olive oil
- chopped scallions

Directions:

1. Preheat the air fryer to 400°F.
2. Toss the sliced onions with a little olive oil, salt and pepper and transfer them to the air fryer basket. Dot the onions with pieces of butter and air-fry at 400°F for 2 minutes. Then sprinkle the sugar over the onions and stir. Pour any melted butter from the bottom of the air fryer drawer over the onions (do this over the sink – some of the butter will spill through the basket). Continue to air-fry for another 13 minutes, stirring or shaking the basket every few minutes to cook the onions evenly.
3. Add the kielbasa chunks to the onions and toss. Air-fry for another 5 minutes, shaking the basket halfway through the cooking time. Transfer the kielbasa and onions to a bowl and cover with aluminum foil to keep warm.
4. Toss the frozen pierogies with the vegetable or olive oil and transfer them to the air fryer basket. Air-fry at 400°F for 8 minutes, shaking the basket twice during the cooking time.
5. When the pierogies have finished cooking, return the kielbasa and onions to the air fryer and gently toss with the pierogies. Air-fry for 2 more minutes and then transfer everything to a serving platter. Garnish with the chopped scallions and serve hot with the spicy sour cream sauce below.
6. Kielbasa Sausage with Pierogies and Caramelized Onions

Blackberry Bbq Glazed Country-style Ribs

Servings: 2

Cooking Time: 40 Minutes

Ingredients:

- ½ cup + 2 tablespoons sherry or Madeira wine, divided
- 1 pound boneless country-style pork ribs
- salt and freshly ground black pepper
- 1 tablespoon Chinese 5-spice powder

- ¼ cup blackberry preserves
- ¼ cup hoisin sauce*
- 1 clove garlic, minced
- 1 generous tablespoon grated fresh ginger
- 2 scallions, chopped
- 1 tablespoon sesame seeds, toasted

Directions:

1. Preheat the air fryer to 330°F and pour ½ cup of the sherry into the bottom of the air fryer drawer.
2. Season the ribs with salt, pepper and the 5-spice powder.
3. Air-fry the ribs at 330°F for 20 minutes, turning them over halfway through the cooking time.
4. While the ribs are cooking, make the sauce. Combine the remaining sherry, blackberry preserves, hoisin sauce, garlic and ginger in a small saucepan. Bring to a simmer on the stovetop for a few minutes, until the sauce thickens.
5. When the time is up on the air fryer, turn the ribs over, pour a little sauce on the ribs and air-fry for another 10 minutes at 330°F. Turn the ribs over again, pour on more of the sauce and air-fry at 330°F for a final 10 minutes.
6. Let the ribs rest for at least 5 minutes before serving them warm with a little more glaze brushed on and the scallions and sesame seeds sprinkled on top.

Red Curry Flank Steak

Servings: 4

Cooking Time: 18 Minutes

Ingredients:

- 3 tablespoons red curry paste
- ¼ cup olive oil
- 2 teaspoons grated fresh ginger
- 2 tablespoons soy sauce
- 2 tablespoons rice wine vinegar
- 3 scallions, minced
- 1½ pounds flank steak
- fresh cilantro (or parsley) leaves

Directions:

1. Mix the red curry paste, olive oil, ginger, soy sauce, rice vinegar and scallions together in a bowl. Place the flank steak in a shallow glass dish and pour half the marinade over the steak. Pierce the steak several times with a fork or meat tenderizer to let the marinade penetrate the meat. Turn the steak over, pour the remaining marinade over the top and pierce the steak several times again. Cover and marinate the steak in the refrigerator for 6 to 8 hours.
2. When you are ready to cook, remove the steak from the refrigerator and let it sit at room temperature for 30 minutes.
3. Preheat the air fryer to 400°F.
4. Cut the flank steak in half so that it fits more easily into the air fryer and transfer both pieces to the air fryer basket. Pour the marinade over the steak. Air-fry for 18 minutes, depending on your preferred degree of doneness of the steak (12 minutes = medium rare). Flip the steak over halfway through the cooking time.
5. When your desired degree of doneness has been reached, remove the steak to a cutting board and let it rest for 5 minutes before slicing. Thinly slice the flank steak against the grain of the meat. Transfer the slices to a serving platter, pour any juice from the bottom of the air fryer over the sliced flank steak and sprinkle the fresh cilantro on top.

Kielbasa Chunks With Pineapple & Peppers

Servings: 2

Cooking Time: 10 Minutes

Ingredients:

- ¾ pound kielbasa sausage
- 1 cup bell pepper chunks (any color)
- 1 8-ounce can pineapple chunks in juice, drained
- 1 tablespoon barbeque seasoning
- 1 tablespoon soy sauce
- cooking spray

Directions:

1. Cut sausage into ½-inch slices.
2. In a medium bowl, toss all ingredients together.
3. Spray air fryer basket with nonstick cooking spray.
4. Pour sausage mixture into the basket.
5. Cook at 390°F for approximately 5minutes. Shake basket and cook an additional 5minutes.

Pork Schnitzel

Servings: 4

Cooking Time: 14 Minutes

Ingredients:

- 4 boneless pork chops, pounded to ¼-inch thickness
- 1 teaspoon salt, divided
- 1 teaspoon black pepper, divided
- ½ cup all-purpose flour
- 2 eggs
- 1 cup breadcrumbs
- ¼ teaspoon paprika
- 1 lemon, cut into wedges

Directions:

1. Season both sides of the pork chops with ½ teaspoon of the salt and ½ teaspoon of the pepper.
2. On a plate, place the flour.
3. In a large bowl, whisk the eggs.
4. In another large bowl, place the breadcrumbs.
5. Season the flour with the paprika and season the breadcrumbs with the remaining ½ teaspoon of salt and ½ teaspoon of pepper.
6. To bread the pork, place a pork chop in the flour, then into the whisked eggs, and then into the breadcrumbs. Place the breaded pork onto a plate and finish breading the remaining pork chops.
7. Preheat the air fryer to 390°F.
8. Place the pork chops into the air fryer, not overlapping and working in batches as needed. Spray the pork chops with cooking spray and cook for 8 minutes; flip the pork and cook for another 4 to 6 minutes or until cooked to an internal temperature of 145°F.
9. Serve with lemon wedges.

Sweet Potato–crusted Pork Rib Chops

Servings: 2

Cooking Time: 14 Minutes

Ingredients:

- 2 Large egg white(s), well beaten
- 1½ cups (about 6 ounces) Crushed sweet potato chips (certified gluten-free, if a concern)
- 1 teaspoon Ground cinnamon
- 1 teaspoon Ground dried ginger
- 1 teaspoon Table salt (optional)
- 2 10-ounce, 1-inch-thick bone-in pork rib chop(s)

Directions:

1. Preheat the air fryer to 375°F .
2. Set up and fill two shallow soup plates or small pie plates on your counter: one for the beaten egg white(s); and one for the crushed chips, mixed with the cinnamon, ginger, and salt (if using).
3. Dip a chop in the egg white(s), coating it on both sides as well as the edges. Let the excess egg white slip back into the rest, then set it in the crushed chip mixture. Turn it several times, pressing gently, until evenly coated on both sides and the edges. If necessary, set the chop aside and coat the remaining chop(s).
4. Set the chop(s) in the basket with as much air space between them as possible. Air-fry undisturbed for 12 minutes, or until crunchy and browned and an instant-read meat thermometer inserted into the center of a chop (without touching bone) registers 145°F. If the machine is at 360°F, you may need to add 2 minutes to the cooking time.
5. Use kitchen tongs to transfer the chop(s) to a wire rack. Cool for 2 or 3 minutes before serving.

Crispy Ham And Eggs

Servings: 3

Cooking Time: 9 Minutes

Ingredients:

- 2 cups Rice-puff cereal, such as Rice Krispies
- ¼ cup Maple syrup
- ½ pound ¼- to ½-inch-thick ham steak (gluten-free, if a concern)
- 1 tablespoon Unsalted butter
- 3 Large eggs
- ⅛ teaspoon Table salt
- ⅛ teaspoon Ground black pepper

Directions:

1. Preheat the air fryer to 400°F.
2. Pour the cereal into a food processor, cover, and process until finely ground. Pour the ground cereal into a shallow soup plate or a small pie plate.

3. Smear the maple syrup on both sides of the ham, then set the ham into the ground cereal. Turn a few times, pressing gently, until evenly coated.
4. Set the ham steak in the basket and air-fry undisturbed for 5 minutes, or until browned.
5. Meanwhile, melt the butter in a medium or large nonstick skillet set over medium heat. Crack the eggs into the skillet and cook until the whites are set and the yolks are hot, about 3 minutes (or 4 minutes for a more set yolk.) Season with the salt and pepper.
6. When the ham is ready, transfer it to a serving platter, then slip the eggs from the skillet on top of it. Divide into portions to serve.

Stuffed Pork Chops

Servings: 4
Cooking Time: 12 Minutes

Ingredients:

- 4 boneless pork chops
- ½ teaspoon salt
- ½ teaspoon black pepper
- ¼ teaspoon paprika
- 1 cup frozen spinach, defrosted and squeezed dry
- 2 cloves garlic, minced
- 2 ounces cream cheese
- ¼ cup grated Parmesan cheese
- 1 tablespoon extra-virgin olive oil

Directions:

1. Pat the pork chops with a paper towel. Make a slit in the side of each pork chop to create a pouch.
2. Season the pork chops with the salt, pepper, and paprika.
3. In a small bowl, mix together the spinach, garlic, cream cheese, and Parmesan cheese.
4. Divide the mixture into fourths and stuff the pork chop pouches. Secure the pouches with toothpicks.
5. Preheat the air fryer to 400°F.
6. Place the stuffed pork chops in the air fryer basket and spray liberally with cooking spray. Cook for 6 minutes, flip and coat with more cooking spray, and cook another 6 minutes. Check to make sure the meat is cooked to an internal temperature of 145°F. Cook the pork chops in batches, as needed.

Marinated Rib-eye Steak With Herb Roasted Mushrooms

Servings: 2
Cooking Time: 10-15 Minutes

Ingredients:

- 2 tablespoons Worcestershire sauce
- ¼ cup red wine
- 2 (8-ounce) boneless rib-eye steaks
- coarsely ground black pepper
- 8 ounces baby bella (cremini) mushrooms, stems trimmed and caps halved
- 2 tablespoons olive oil
- 1 teaspoon dried parsley
- 1 teaspoon fresh thyme leaves
- salt and freshly ground black pepper
- chopped fresh chives or parsley

Directions:

1. Combine the Worcestershire sauce and red wine in a shallow baking dish. Add the steaks to the marinade, pierce them several times with the tines of a fork or a meat tenderizer and season them generously with the coarsely ground black pepper. Flip the steaks over and pierce the other side in a similar fashion, seasoning again with the coarsely ground black pepper. Marinate the steaks for 2 hours.
2. Preheat the air fryer to 400°F.
3. Toss the mushrooms in a bowl with the olive oil, dried parsley, thyme, salt and freshly ground black pepper. Transfer the steaks from the marinade to the air fryer basket, season with salt and scatter the mushrooms on top.
4. Air-fry the steaks for 10 minutes for medium-rare, 12 minutes for medium, or 15 minutes for well-done, flipping the steaks once halfway through the cooking time.
5. Serve the steaks and mushrooms together with the chives or parsley sprinkled on top. A good steak sauce or some horseradish would be a nice accompaniment.

Indian Fry Bread Tacos

Servings: 4
Cooking Time: 20 Minutes

Ingredients:

- 1 cup all-purpose flour
- 1½ teaspoons salt, divided
- 1½ teaspoons baking powder
- ¼ cup milk
- ¼ cup warm water
- ½ pound lean ground beef
- One 14.5-ounce can pinto beans, drained and rinsed
- 1 tablespoon taco seasoning
- ½ cup shredded cheddar cheese
- 2 cups shredded lettuce
- ¼ cup black olives, chopped
- 1 Roma tomato, diced
- 1 avocado, diced
- 1 lime

Directions:

1. In a large bowl, whisk together the flour, 1 teaspoon of the salt, and baking powder. Make a well in the center and add in the milk and water. Form a ball and gently knead the dough four times. Cover the bowl with a damp towel, and set aside.
2. Preheat the air fryer to 380°F.
3. In a medium bowl, mix together the ground beef, beans, and taco seasoning. Crumble the meat mixture into the air fryer basket and cook for 5 minutes; toss the meat and cook an additional 2 to 3 minutes, or until cooked fully. Place the cooked meat in a bowl for taco assembly; season with the remaining ½ teaspoon salt as desired.
4. On a floured surface, place the dough. Cut the dough into 4 equal parts. Using a rolling pin, roll out each piece of dough to 5 inches in diameter. Spray the dough with cooking spray and place in the air fryer basket, working in batches as needed. Cook for 3 minutes, flip over, spray with cooking spray, and cook for an additional 1 to 3 minutes, until golden and puffy.
5. To assemble, place the fry breads on a serving platter. Equally divide the meat and bean mixture on top of the fry bread. Divide the cheese, lettuce, olives, tomatoes, and avocado among the four tacos. Squeeze lime over the top prior to serving.

Wasabi-coated Pork Loin Chops

Servings: 3
Cooking Time: 14 Minutes

Ingredients:

- 1½ cups Wasabi peas
- ¼ cup Plain panko bread crumbs
- 1 Large egg white(s)
- 2 tablespoons Water
- 3 5- to 6-ounce boneless center-cut pork loin chops (about ½ inch thick)

Directions:

1. Preheat the air fryer to 375°F .
2. Put the wasabi peas in a food processor. Cover and process until finely ground, about like panko bread crumbs. Add the bread crumbs and pulse a few times to blend.
3. Set up and fill two shallow soup plates or small pie plates on your counter: one for the egg white(s), whisked with the water until uniform; and one for the wasabi pea mixture.
4. Dip a pork chop in the egg white mixture, coating the chop on both sides as well as around the edge. Allow any excess egg white mixture to slip back into the rest, then set the chop in the wasabi pea mixture. Press gently and turn it several times to coat evenly on both sides and around the edge. Set aside, then dip and coat the remaining chop(s).
5. Set the chops in the basket with as much air space between them as possible. Air-fry, turning once at the 6-minute mark, for 12 minutes, or until the chops are crisp and browned and an instant-read meat thermometer inserted into the center of a chop registers 145°F. If the machine is at 360°F, you may need to add 2 minutes to the cooking time.
6. Use kitchen tongs to transfer the chops to a wire rack. Cool for a couple of minutes before serving.

Pesto-rubbed Veal Chops

Servings: 2
Cooking Time: 12-15 Minutes

Ingredients:

- ¼ cup Purchased pesto
- 2 10-ounce bone-in veal loin or rib chop(s)
- ½ teaspoon Ground black pepper

Directions:

1. Preheat the air fryer to 400°F.
2. Rub the pesto onto both sides of the veal chop(s). Sprinkle one side of the chop(s) with the ground black pepper. Set aside at room temperature as the machine comes up to temperature.
3. Set the chop(s) in the basket. If you're cooking more than one chop, leave as much air space between them as possible. Air-fry undisturbed for 12 minutes for medium-rare, or until an instant-read meat thermometer inserted into the center of a chop (without touching bone) registers 135°F (not USDA-approved). Or air-fry undisturbed for 15 minutes for medium-well, or until an instant-read meat thermometer registers 145°F (USDA-approved).
4. Use kitchen tongs to transfer the chops to a cutting board or a wire rack. Cool for 5 minutes before serving.

Steakhouse Burgers With Red Onion Compote

Servings: 4
Cooking Time: 22 Minutes

Ingredients:

- 1½ pounds lean ground beef
- 2 cloves garlic, minced and divided
- 1 teaspoon Worcestershire sauce
- 1 teaspoon sea salt, divided
- ½ teaspoon black pepper
- 1 tablespoon extra-virgin olive oil
- 1 red onion, thinly sliced
- ¼ cup balsamic vinegar
- 1 teaspoon sugar
- 1 tablespoon tomato paste
- 2 tablespoons mayonnaise
- 2 tablespoons sour cream
- 4 brioche hamburger buns
- 1 cup arugula

Directions:

1. In a large bowl, mix together the ground beef, 1 of the minced garlic cloves, the Worcestershire sauce, ½ teaspoon of the salt, and the black pepper. Form the meat into 1-inch-thick patties. Make a dent in the center (this helps the center cook evenly). Let the meat sit for 15 minutes.
2. Meanwhile, in a small saucepan over medium heat, cook the olive oil and red onion for 4 minutes, stirring frequently to avoid burning. Add in the balsamic vinegar, sugar, and tomato paste, and cook for an additional 3 minutes, stirring frequently. Transfer the onion compote to a small bowl.
3. Preheat the air fryer to 350°F.
4. In another small bowl, mix together the remaining minced garlic, the mayonnaise, and the sour cream. Spread the mayo mixture on the insides of the brioche buns.
5. Cook the hamburgers for 6 minutes, flip the burgers, and cook an additional 2 to 6 minutes. Check the internal temperature to avoid under- or overcooking. Hamburgers should be cooked to at least 160°F. After cooking, cover with foil and let the meat rest for 5 minutes.
6. Meanwhile, place the buns inside the air fryer and toast them for 3 minutes.
7. To assemble the burgers, place the hamburger on one side of the bun, top with onion compote and ¼ cup arugula, and then place the other half of the bun on top.

Rosemary Lamb Chops

Servings: 4
Cooking Time: 6 Minutes

Ingredients:

- 8 lamb chops
- 1 tablespoon extra-virgin olive oil
- 1 teaspoon dried rosemary, crushed
- 2 cloves garlic, minced
- 1 teaspoon sea salt
- ¼ teaspoon black pepper

Directions:

1. In a large bowl, mix together the lamb chops, olive oil, rosemary, garlic, salt, and pepper. Let sit at room temperature for 10 minutes.
2. Meanwhile, preheat the air fryer to 380°F.
3. Cook the lamb chops for 3 minutes, flip them over, and cook for another 3 minutes.

Glazed Meatloaf

Servings: 4
Cooking Time: 35-55 Minutes

Ingredients:

- ½ cup Seasoned Italian-style panko bread crumbs (gluten-free, if a concern)
- ¼ cup Whole or low-fat milk
- 1 pound Lean ground beef
- 1 pound Bulk mild Italian sausage meat (gluten-free, if a concern)
- 1 Large egg(s), well beaten
- 1 teaspoon Dried thyme
- 1 teaspoon Onion powder
- 1 teaspoon Garlic powder
- Vegetable oil spray
- 1 tablespoon Ketchup (gluten-free, if a concern)
- 1 tablespoon Hoisin sauce (see here; gluten-free, if a concern)
- 2 teaspoons Pickle brine, preferably from a jar of jalapeño rings (gluten-free, if a concern)

Directions:

1. Pour the bread crumbs into a large bowl, add the milk, stir gently, and soak for 10 minutes.
2. Preheat the air fryer to 350°F .
3. Add the ground beef, Italian sausage meat, egg(s), thyme, onion powder, and garlic powder to the bowl with the bread crumbs. Blend gently until well combined. (Clean, dry hands work best!) Form this mixture into an oval loaf about 2 inches tall (its length will vary depending on the amount of ingredients) but with a flat bottom. Generously coat the top, bottom, and all sides of the loaf with vegetable oil spray.
4. Use a large, nonstick-safe spatula or perhaps silicone baking mitts to transfer the loaf to the basket. Air-fry undisturbed for 30 minutes for a small meatloaf, 40 minutes for a medium one, or 50 minutes for a large, until an instant-read meat thermometer inserted into the center of the loaf registers 165°F.
5. Whisk the ketchup, hoisin, and pickle brine in a small bowl until smooth. Brush this over the top and sides of the meatloaf and continue air-frying undisturbed for 5 minutes, or until the glaze has browned a bit. Use that same spatula or those same baking mitts to transfer the meatloaf to a cutting board. Cool for 10 minutes before slicing.

Sausage-cheese Calzone

Servings: 8
Cooking Time: 8 Minutes

Ingredients:

- Crust
- 2 cups white wheat flour, plus more for kneading and rolling
- 1 package (¼ ounce) RapidRise yeast
- 1 teaspoon salt
- ½ teaspoon dried basil
- 1 cup warm water (115°F to 125°F)
- 2 teaspoons olive oil
- Filling
- ¼ pound Italian sausage
- ½ cup ricotta cheese
- 4 ounces mozzarella cheese, shredded
- ¼ cup grated Parmesan cheese
- oil for misting or cooking spray
- marinara sauce for serving

Directions:

1. Crumble Italian sausage into air fryer baking pan and cook at 390°F for 5minutes. Stir, breaking apart, and cook for 3 to 4minutes, until well done. Remove and set aside on paper towels to drain.
2. To make dough, combine flour, yeast, salt, and basil. Add warm water and oil and stir until a soft dough forms. Turn out onto lightly floured board and knead for 3 or 4minutes. Let dough rest for 10minutes.
3. To make filling, combine the three cheeses in a medium bowl and mix well. Stir in the cooked sausage.
4. Cut dough into 8 pieces.
5. Working with 4 pieces of the dough, press each into a circle about 5 inches in diameter. Top each dough

circle with 2 heaping tablespoons of filling. Fold over to create a half-moon shape and press edges firmly together. Be sure that edges are firmly sealed to prevent leakage. Spray both sides with oil or cooking spray.

6. Place 4 calzones in air fryer basket and cook at 360°F for 5minutes. Mist with oil and cook for 3 minutes, until crust is done and nicely browned.

7. While the first batch is cooking, press out the remaining dough, fill, and shape into calzones.

8. Spray both sides with oil and cook for 5minutes. If needed, mist with oil and continue cooking for 3 minutes longer. This second batch will cook a little faster than the first because your air fryer is already hot.

9. Serve with marinara sauce on the side for dipping.

Barbecue Country-style Pork Ribs

Servings: 3

Cooking Time: 30 Minutes

Ingredients:

- 3 8-ounce boneless country-style pork ribs
- 1½ teaspoons Mild smoked paprika
- 1½ teaspoons Light brown sugar
- ¾ teaspoon Onion powder
- ¾ teaspoon Ground black pepper
- ¼ teaspoon Table salt
- Vegetable oil spray

Directions:

1. Preheat the air fryer to 350°F . Set the ribs in a bowl on the counter as the machine heats.

2. Mix the smoked paprika, brown sugar, onion powder, pepper, and salt in a small bowl until well combined. Rub this mixture over all the surfaces of the country-style ribs. Generously coat the country-style ribs with vegetable oil spray.

3. Set the ribs in the basket with as much air space between them as possible. Air-fry undisturbed for 30 minutes, or until browned and sizzling and an instant-read meat thermometer inserted into one rib registers at least 145°F.

4. Use kitchen tongs to transfer the country-style ribs to a wire rack. Cool for 5 minutes before serving.

Almond And Sun-dried Tomato Crusted Pork Chops

Servings: 4

Cooking Time: 10 Minutes

Ingredients:

- ½ cup oil-packed sun-dried tomatoes
- ½ cup toasted almonds
- ¼ cup grated Parmesan cheese
- ½ cup olive oil
- 2 tablespoons water
- ½ teaspoon salt
- freshly ground black pepper
- 4 center-cut boneless pork chops (about 1¼ pounds)

Directions:

1. Place the sun-dried tomatoes into a food processor and pulse them until they are coarsely chopped. Add the almonds, Parmesan cheese, olive oil, water, salt and pepper. Process all the ingredients into a smooth paste. Spread most of the paste (leave a little in reserve) onto both sides of the pork chops and then pierce the meat several times with a needle-style meat tenderizer or a fork. Let the pork chops sit and marinate for at least 1 hour (refrigerate if marinating for longer than 1 hour).

2. Preheat the air fryer to 370°F.

3. Brush a little olive oil on the bottom of the air fryer basket. Transfer the pork chops into the air fryer basket, spooning a little more of the sun-dried tomato paste onto the pork chops if there are any gaps where the paste may have been rubbed off. Air-fry the pork chops at 370°F for 10 minutes, turning the chops over halfway through the cooking process.

4. When the pork chops have finished cooking, transfer them to a serving plate and serve with mashed potatoes and vegetables for a hearty meal.

Honey Mesquite Pork Chops

Servings: 2

Cooking Time: 10 Minutes

Ingredients:

- 2 tablespoons mesquite seasoning
- ¼ cup honey
- 1 tablespoon olive oil
- 1 tablespoon water
- freshly ground black pepper
- 2 bone-in center cut pork chops (about 1 pound)

Directions:

1. Whisk the mesquite seasoning, honey, olive oil, water and freshly ground black pepper together in a shallow glass dish. Pierce the chops all over and on both sides with a fork or meat tenderizer. Add the pork chops to the marinade and massage the marinade into the chops. Cover and marinate for 30 minutes.
2. Preheat the air fryer to 330°F.
3. Transfer the pork chops to the air fryer basket and pour half of the marinade over the chops, reserving the remaining marinade. Air-fry the pork chops for 6 minutes. Flip the pork chops over and pour the remaining marinade on top. Air-fry for an additional 3 minutes at 330°F. Then, increase the air fryer temperature to 400°F and air-fry the pork chops for an additional minute.
4. Transfer the pork chops to a serving plate, and let them rest for 5 minutes before serving. If you'd like a sauce for these chops, pour the cooked marinade from the bottom of the air fryer over the top.

Vietnamese Beef Lettuce Wraps

Servings: 4

Cooking Time: 12 Minutes

Ingredients:

- ⅓ cup low-sodium soy sauce*
- 2 teaspoons fish sauce*
- 2 teaspoons brown sugar
- 1 tablespoon chili paste
- juice of 1 lime
- 2 cloves garlic, minced
- 2 teaspoons fresh ginger, minced
- 1 pound beef sirloin
- Sauce
- ⅓ cup low-sodium soy sauce*
- juice of 2 limes
- 1 tablespoon mirin wine
- 2 teaspoons chili paste
- Serving
- 1 head butter lettuce
- ½ cup julienned carrots
- ½ cup julienned cucumber
- ½ cup sliced radishes, sliced into half moons
- 2 cups cooked rice noodles
- ⅓ cup chopped peanuts

Directions:

1. Combine the soy sauce, fish sauce, brown sugar, chili paste, lime juice, garlic and ginger in a bowl. Slice the beef into thin slices, then cut those slices in half. Add the beef to the marinade and marinate for 1 to 3 hours in the refrigerator. When you are ready to cook, remove the steak from the refrigerator and let it sit at room temperature for 30 minutes.
2. Preheat the air fryer to 400°F.
3. Transfer the beef and marinade to the air fryer basket. Air-fry at 400°F for 12 minutes, shaking the basket a few times during the cooking process.
4. While the beef is cooking, prepare a wrap-building station. Combine the soy sauce, lime juice, mirin wine and chili paste in a bowl and transfer to a little pouring vessel. Separate the lettuce leaves from the head of lettuce and put them in a serving bowl. Place the carrots, cucumber, radish, rice noodles and chopped peanuts all in separate serving bowls.
5. When the beef has finished cooking, transfer it to another serving bowl and invite your guests to build their wraps. To build the wraps, place some beef in a lettuce leaf and top with carrots, cucumbers, some rice noodles and chopped peanuts. Drizzle a little sauce over top, fold the lettuce around the ingredients and enjoy!

Flank Steak With Roasted Peppers And Chimichurri

Servings: 4
Cooking Time: 22 Minutes

Ingredients:

- 2 cups flat-leaf parsley leaves
- ¼ cup fresh oregano leaves
- 3 cloves garlic
- ½ cup olive oil
- ¼ cup red wine vinegar
- ½ teaspoon salt
- freshly ground black pepper
- ¼ teaspoon crushed red pepper flakes
- ½ teaspoon ground cumin
- 1 pound flank steak
- 1 red bell pepper, cut into strips
- 1 yellow bell pepper, cut into strips

Directions:

1. Make the chimichurri sauce by chopping the parsley, oregano and garlic in a food processor. Add the olive oil, vinegar and seasonings and process again. Pour half of the sauce into a shallow dish with the flank steak and set the remaining sauce aside. Pierce the flank steak with a needle-style meat tenderizer or a paring knife and marinate the steak for 2 to 24 hours in the refrigerator. When you are ready to cook, remove the steak from the refrigerator and let it sit at room temperature for 30 minutes.
2. Preheat the air fryer to 400°F.
3. Cut the flank steak in half so that it fits more easily into the air fryer and transfer both pieces to the air fryer basket. Air-fry for 14 minutes, depending on how you like your steak cooked (10 minutes will give you medium for a 1-inch thick flank steak). Flip the steak over halfway through the cooking time.
4. When the flank steak is cooked to your liking, transfer it to a cutting board, loosely tent with foil and let it rest while you cook the peppers.
5. Toss the peppers in a little olive oil, salt and freshly ground black pepper and transfer them to the air fryer basket. Air-fry at 400°F for 8 minutes, shaking the basket once or twice throughout the cooking process. To serve, slice the flank steak against the grain of the meat and top with the roasted peppers. Drizzle the reserved chimichurri sauce on top, thinning the sauce with another tablespoon of olive oil if desired.

Cinnamon-stick Kofta Skewers

Servings: 8
Cooking Time: 15 Minutes

Ingredients:

- 1 pound Lean ground beef
- ½ teaspoon Ground cumin
- ½ teaspoon Onion powder
- ½ teaspoon Ground dried turmeric
- ½ teaspoon Ground cinnamon
- ½ teaspoon Table salt
- Up to a ⅛ teaspoon Cayenne
- 8 3½- to 4-inch-long cinnamon sticks (see the headnote)
- Vegetable oil spray

Directions:

1. Preheat the air fryer to 375°F .
2. Gently mix the ground beef, cumin, onion powder, turmeric, cinnamon, salt, and cayenne in a bowl until the meat is evenly mixed with the spices. (Clean, dry hands work best!) Divide this mixture into 2-ounce portions, each about the size of a golf ball.
3. Wrap one portion of the meat mixture around a cinnamon stick, using about three-quarters of the length of the stick, covering one end but leaving a little "handle" of cinnamon stick protruding from the other end. Set aside and continue making more kofta skewers.
4. Generously coat the formed kofta skewers on all sides with vegetable oil spray. Set them in the basket with as much air space between them as possible. Air-fry undisturbed for 13 minutes, or until browned and cooked through. If the machine is at 360°F, you may need to add 2 minutes to the cooking time.
5. Use a nonstick-safe spatula, and perhaps kitchen tongs for balance, to gently transfer the kofta skewers to a wire rack. Cool for at least 5 minutes or up to 20 minutes before serving.

Mongolian Beef

Servings: 4

Cooking Time: 15 Minutes

Ingredients:

- 1½ pounds flank steak, thinly sliced
- on the bias into ¼-inch strips
- Marinade
- 2 tablespoons soy sauce*
- 1 clove garlic, smashed
- big pinch crushed red pepper flakes
- Sauce
- 1 tablespoon vegetable oil
- 2 cloves garlic, minced
- 1 tablespoon finely grated fresh ginger
- 3 dried red chili peppers
- ¾ cup soy sauce*
- ¾ cup chicken stock
- 5 to 6 tablespoons brown sugar (depending on how sweet you want the sauce)
- ½ cup cornstarch, divided
- 1 bunch scallions, sliced into 2-inch pieces

Directions:

1. Marinate the beef in the soy sauce, garlic and red pepper flakes for one hour.
2. In the meantime, make the sauce. Preheat a small saucepan over medium heat on the stovetop. Add the oil, garlic, ginger and dried chili peppers and sauté for just a minute or two. Add the soy sauce, chicken stock and brown sugar and continue to simmer for a few minutes. Dissolve 3 tablespoons of cornstarch in 3 tablespoons of water and stir this into the saucepan. Stir the sauce over medium heat until it thickens. Set this aside.
3. Preheat the air fryer to 400°F.
4. Remove the beef from the marinade and transfer it to a zipper sealable plastic bag with the remaining cornstarch. Shake it around to completely coat the beef and transfer the coated strips of beef to a baking sheet or plate, shaking off any excess cornstarch. Spray the strips with vegetable oil on all sides and transfer them to the air fryer basket.
5. Air-fry at 400°F for 15 minutes, shaking the basket to toss and rotate the beef strips throughout the cooking process. Add the scallions for the last 4 minutes of the cooking. Transfer the hot beef strips and scallions to a bowl and toss with the sauce (warmed on the stovetop if necessary), coating all the beef strips with the sauce. Serve warm over white rice.

Chicken Fried Steak

Servings: 4

Cooking Time: 15 Minutes

Ingredients:

- 2 eggs
- ½ cup buttermilk
- 1½ cups flour
- ¾ teaspoon salt
- ½ teaspoon pepper
- 1 pound beef cube steaks
- salt and pepper
- oil for misting or cooking spray

Directions:

1. Beat together eggs and buttermilk in a shallow dish.
2. In another shallow dish, stir together the flour, ½ teaspoon salt, and ¼ teaspoon pepper.
3. Season cube steaks with remaining salt and pepper to taste. Dip in flour, buttermilk egg wash, and then flour again.
4. Spray both sides of steaks with oil or cooking spray.
5. Cooking in 2 batches, place steaks in air fryer basket in single layer. Cook at 360°F for 10minutes. Spray tops of steaks with oil and cook 5minutes or until meat is well done.
6. Repeat to cook remaining steaks.

Lamb Burger With Feta And Olives

Servings: 3

Cooking Time: 16 Minutes

Ingredients:

- 2 teaspoons olive oil
- ⅓ onion, finely chopped
- 1 clove garlic, minced
- 1 pound ground lamb
- 2 tablespoons fresh parsley, finely chopped
- 1½ teaspoons fresh oregano, finely chopped

- ½ cup black olives, finely chopped
- ⅓ cup crumbled feta cheese
- ½ teaspoon salt
- freshly ground black pepper
- 4 thick pita breads
- toppings and condiments

Directions:

1. Preheat a medium skillet over medium-high heat on the stovetop. Add the olive oil and cook the onion until tender, but not browned – about 4 to 5 minutes. Add the garlic and cook for another minute. Transfer the onion and garlic to a mixing bowl and add the ground lamb, parsley, oregano, olives, feta cheese, salt and pepper. Gently mix the ingredients together.
2. Divide the mixture into 3 or 4 equal portions and then form the hamburgers, being careful not to over-handle the meat. One good way to do this is to throw the meat back and forth between your hands like a baseball, packing the meat each time you catch it. Flatten the balls into patties, making an indentation in the center of each patty. Flatten the sides of the patties as well to make it easier to fit them into the air fryer basket.
3. Preheat the air fryer to 370°F.
4. If you don't have room for all four burgers, air-fry two or three burgers at a time for 8 minutes at 370°F. Flip the burgers over and air-fry for another 8 minutes. If you cooked your burgers in batches, return the first batch of burgers to the air fryer for the last two minutes of cooking to re-heat. This should give you a medium-well burger. If you'd prefer a medium-rare burger, shorten the cooking time to about 13 minutes. Remove the burgers to a resting plate and let the burgers rest for a few minutes before dressing and serving.
5. While the burgers are resting, toast the pita breads in the air fryer for 2 minutes. Tuck the burgers into the toasted pita breads, or wrap the pitas around the burgers and serve with a tzatziki sauce or some mayonnaise.

T-bone Steak With Roasted Tomato, Corn And Asparagus Salsa

Servings: 2

Cooking Time: 15-20 Minutes

Ingredients:

- 1 (20-ounce) T-bone steak
- salt and freshly ground black pepper
- Salsa
- 1½ cups cherry tomatoes
- ¾ cup corn kernels (fresh, or frozen and thawed)
- 1½ cups sliced asparagus (1-inch slices) (about ½ bunch)
- 1 tablespoon + 1 teaspoon olive oil, divided
- salt and freshly ground black pepper
- 1½ teaspoons red wine vinegar
- 3 tablespoons chopped fresh basil
- 1 tablespoon chopped fresh chives

Directions:

1. Preheat the air fryer to 400°F.
2. Season the steak with salt and pepper and air-fry at 400°F for 10 minutes (medium-rare), 12 minutes (medium), or 15 minutes (well-done), flipping the steak once halfway through the cooking time.
3. In the meantime, toss the tomatoes, corn and asparagus in a bowl with a teaspoon or so of olive oil, salt and freshly ground black pepper.
4. When the steak has finished cooking, remove it to a cutting board, tent loosely with foil and let it rest. Transfer the vegetables to the air fryer and air-fry at 400°F for 5 minutes, shaking the basket once or twice during the cooking process. Transfer the cooked vegetables back into the bowl and toss with the red wine vinegar, remaining olive oil and fresh herbs.
5. To serve, slice the steak on the bias and serve with some of the salsa on top.

Smokehouse-style Beef Ribs

Servings: 3

Cooking Time: 25 Minutes

Ingredients:

- ¼ teaspoon Mild smoked paprika
- ¼ teaspoon Garlic powder
- ¼ teaspoon Onion powder
- ¼ teaspoon Table salt
- ¼ teaspoon Ground black pepper
- 3 10- to 12-ounce beef back ribs (not beef short ribs)

Directions:

1. Preheat the air fryer to 350°F .
2. Mix the smoked paprika, garlic powder, onion powder, salt, and pepper in a small bowl until uniform. Massage and pat this mixture onto the ribs.
3. When the machine is at temperature, set the ribs in the basket in one layer, turning them on their sides if necessary, sort of like they're spooning but with at least ¼ inch air space between them. Air-fry for 25 minutes, turning once, until deep brown and sizzling.
4. Use kitchen tongs to transfer the ribs to a wire rack. Cool for 5 minutes before serving.

Spicy Hoisin Bbq Pork Chops

Servings: 2
Cooking Time: 12 Minutes

Ingredients:

- 3 tablespoons hoisin sauce
- ¼ cup honey
- 1 tablespoon soy sauce
- 3 tablespoons rice vinegar
- 2 tablespoons brown sugar
- 1½ teaspoons grated fresh ginger
- 1 to 2 teaspoons Sriracha sauce, to taste
- 2 to 3 bone-in center cut pork chops, 1-inch thick (about 1¼ pounds)
- chopped scallions, for garnish

Directions:

1. Combine the hoisin sauce, honey, soy sauce, rice vinegar, brown sugar, ginger, and Sriracha sauce in a small saucepan. Whisk the ingredients together and bring the mixture to a boil over medium-high heat on the stovetop. Reduce the heat and simmer the sauce until it has reduced in volume and thickened slightly – about 10 minutes.
2. Preheat the air fryer to 400°F.
3. Place the pork chops into the air fryer basket and pour half the hoisin BBQ sauce over the top. Air-fry for 6 minutes. Then, flip the chops over, pour the remaining hoisin BBQ sauce on top and air-fry for 6 more minutes, depending on the thickness of the pork chops. The internal temperature of the pork chops should be 155°F when tested with an instant read thermometer.
4. Let the pork chops rest for 5 minutes before serving. You can spoon a little of the sauce from the bottom drawer of the air fryer over the top if desired. Sprinkle with chopped scallions and serve.

Wiener Schnitzel

Servings: 4
Cooking Time: 14 Minutes

Ingredients:

- 4 thin boneless pork loin chops
- 2 tablespoons lemon juice
- ½ cup flour
- 1 teaspoon salt
- ¼ teaspoon marjoram
- 1 cup plain breadcrumbs
- 2 eggs, beaten
- oil for misting or cooking spray

Directions:

1. Rub the lemon juice into all sides of pork chops.
2. Mix together the flour, salt, and marjoram.
3. Place flour mixture on a sheet of wax paper.
4. Place breadcrumbs on another sheet of wax paper.
5. Roll pork chops in flour, dip in beaten eggs, then roll in breadcrumbs. Mist all sides with oil or cooking spray.
6. Spray air fryer basket with nonstick cooking spray and place pork chops in basket.
7. Cook at 390°F for 7minutes. Turn, mist again, and cook for another 7 minutes, until well done. Serve with lemon wedges.

Stuffed Bell Peppers

Servings: 4
Cooking Time: 10 Minutes

Ingredients:

- ¼ pound lean ground pork
- ¾ pound lean ground beef
- ¼ cup onion, minced
- 1 15-ounce can Red Gold crushed tomatoes
- 1 teaspoon Worcestershire sauce
- 1 teaspoon barbeque seasoning
- 1 teaspoon honey

- ½ teaspoon dried basil
- ½ cup cooked brown rice
- ½ teaspoon garlic powder
- ½ teaspoon oregano
- ½ teaspoon salt
- 2 small bell peppers

Directions:

1. Place pork, beef, and onion in air fryer baking pan and cook at 360°F for 5minutes.
2. Stir to break apart chunks and cook 3 more minutes. Continue cooking and stirring in 2-minute intervals until meat is well done. Remove from pan and drain.
3. In a small saucepan, combine the tomatoes, Worcestershire, barbeque seasoning, honey, and basil. Stir well to mix in honey and seasonings.
4. In a large bowl, combine the cooked meat mixture, rice, garlic powder, oregano, and salt. Add ¼ cup of the seasoned crushed tomatoes. Stir until well mixed.
5. Cut peppers in half and remove stems and seeds.
6. Stuff each pepper half with one fourth of the meat mixture.
7. Place the peppers in air fryer basket and cook for 10 minutes, until peppers are crisp tender.
8. Heat remaining tomato sauce. Serve peppers with warm sauce spooned over top.

Natchitoches Meat Pies

Servings: 8

Cooking Time: 12 Minutes

Ingredients:

- Filling
- ½ pound lean ground beef
- ¼ cup finely chopped onion
- ¼ cup finely chopped green bell pepper
- ⅛ teaspoon salt
- ½ teaspoon garlic powder
- ½ teaspoon red pepper flakes
- 1 tablespoon low sodium Worcestershire sauce
- Crust
- 2 cups self-rising flour
- ¼ cup butter, finely diced
- 1 cup milk
- Egg Wash
- 1 egg
- 1 tablespoon water or milk
- oil for misting or cooking spray

Directions:

1. Mix all filling ingredients well and shape into 4 small patties.
2. Cook patties in air fryer basket at 390°F for 10 to 12minutes or until well done.
3. Place patties in large bowl and use fork and knife to crumble meat into very small pieces. Set aside.
4. To make the crust, use a pastry blender or fork to cut the butter into the flour until well mixed. Add milk and stir until dough stiffens.
5. Divide dough into 8 equal portions.
6. On a lightly floured surface, roll each portion of dough into a circle. The circle should be thin and about 5 inches in diameter, but don't worry about getting a perfect shape. Uneven circles result in a rustic look that many people prefer.
7. Spoon 2 tablespoons of meat filling onto each dough circle.
8. Brush egg wash all the way around the edge of dough circle, about ½-inch deep.
9. Fold each circle in half and press dough with tines of a dinner fork to seal the edges all the way around.
10. Brush tops of sealed meat pies with egg wash.
11. Cook filled pies in a single layer in air fryer basket at 360°F for 4minutes. Spray tops with oil or cooking spray, turn pies over, and spray bottoms with oil or cooking spray. Cook for an additional 2minutes.
12. Repeat previous step to cook remaining pies.

Barbecue-style Beef Cube Steak

Servings: 2

Cooking Time: 14 Minutes

Ingredients:

- 2 4-ounce beef cube steak(s)
- 2 cups (about 8 ounces) Fritos (original flavor) or a generic corn chip equivalent, crushed to crumbs (see here)
- 6 tablespoons Purchased smooth barbecue sauce, any flavor (gluten-free, if a concern)

Directions:

1. Preheat the air fryer to 375°F .

2. Spread the Fritos crumbs in a shallow soup plate or a small pie plate. Rub the barbecue sauce onto both sides of the steak(s). Dredge the steak(s) in the Fritos crumbs to coat well and thoroughly, turning several times and pressing down to get the little bits to adhere to the meat.
3. When the machine is at temperature, set the steak(s) in the basket. Leave as much air space between them as possible if you're working with more than one piece of beef. Air-fry undisturbed for 12 minutes, or until lightly brown and crunchy. If the machine is at 360°F, you may need to add 2 minutes to the cooking time.
4. Use kitchen tongs to transfer the steak(s) to a wire rack. Cool for 5 minutes before serving.

Easy Tex-mex Chimichangas

Servings: 2

Cooking Time: 8 Minutes

Ingredients:

- ¼ pound Thinly sliced deli roast beef, chopped
- ½ cup (about 2 ounces) Shredded Cheddar cheese or shredded Tex-Mex cheese blend
- ¼ cup Jarred salsa verde or salsa rojo
- ½ teaspoon Ground cumin
- ½ teaspoon Dried oregano
- 2 Burrito-size (12-inch) flour tortilla(s), not corn tortillas (gluten-free, if a concern)
- ⅔ cup Canned refried beans
- Vegetable oil spray

Directions:

1. Preheat the air fryer to 375°F .
2. Stir the roast beef, cheese, salsa, cumin, and oregano in a bowl until well mixed.
3. Lay a tortilla on a clean, dry work surface. Spread ⅓ cup of the refried beans in the center lower third of the tortilla(s), leaving an inch on either side of the spread beans.
4. For one chimichanga, spread all of the roast beef mixture on top of the beans. For two, spread half of the roast beef mixture on each tortilla.
5. At either "end" of the filling mixture, fold the sides of the tortilla up and over the filling, partially covering it. Starting with the unfolded side of the tortilla just below the filling, roll the tortilla closed. Fold and roll the second filled tortilla, as necessary.
6. Coat the exterior of the tortilla(s) with vegetable oil spray. Set the chimichanga(s) seam side down in the basket, with at least ½ inch air space between them if you're working with two. Air-fry undisturbed for 8 minutes, or until the tortilla is lightly browned and crisp.
7. Use kitchen tongs to gently transfer the chimichanga(s) to a wire rack. Cool for at last 5 minutes or up to 20 minutes before serving.

Zesty London Broil

Servings: 4

Cooking Time: 28 Minutes

Ingredients:

- ⅔ cup ketchup
- ¼ cup honey
- ¼ cup olive oil
- 2 tablespoons apple cider vinegar
- 2 tablespoons Worcestershire sauce
- 2 tablespoons minced onion
- ½ teaspoon paprika
- 1 teaspoon salt
- 1 teaspoon freshly ground black pepper
- 2 pounds London broil, top round or flank steak (about 1-inch thick)

Directions:

1. Combine the ketchup, honey, olive oil, apple cider vinegar, Worcestershire sauce, minced onion, paprika, salt and pepper in a small bowl and whisk together.
2. Generously pierce both sides of the meat with a fork or meat tenderizer and place it in a shallow dish. Pour the marinade mixture over the steak, making sure all sides of the meat get coated with the marinade. Cover and refrigerate overnight.
3. Preheat the air fryer to 400°F.
4. Transfer the London broil to the air fryer basket and air-fry for 28 minutes, depending on how rare or well done you like your steak. Flip the steak over halfway through the cooking time.
5. Remove the London broil from the air fryer and let it rest for five minutes on a cutting board. To serve, thinly slice the meat against the grain and transfer to a serving platter.

Meat Loaves

Servings: 4
Cooking Time: 19 Minutes

Ingredients:

- Sauce
- ¼ cup white vinegar
- ¼ cup brown sugar
- 2 tablespoons Worcestershire sauce
- ½ cup ketchup
- Meat Loaves
- 1 pound very lean ground beef
- ⅔ cup dry bread (approx. 1 slice torn into small pieces)
- 1 egg
- ⅓ cup minced onion
- 1 teaspoon salt
- 2 tablespoons ketchup

Directions:

1. In a small saucepan, combine all sauce ingredients and bring to a boil. Remove from heat and stir to ensure that brown sugar dissolves completely.
2. In a large bowl, combine the beef, bread, egg, onion, salt, and ketchup. Mix well.
3. Divide meat mixture into 4 portions and shape each into a thick, round patty. Patties will be about 3 to 3½ inches in diameter, and all four should fit easily into the air fryer basket at once.
4. Cook at 360°F for 18 minutes, until meat is well done. Baste tops of mini loaves with a small amount of sauce, and cook 1 minute.
5. Serve hot with additional sauce on the side.

Lemon-butter Veal Cutlets

Servings: 2
Cooking Time: 4 Minutes

Ingredients:

- 3 strips Butter (see step 2)
- 3 Thinly pounded 2-ounce veal leg cutlets (less than ¼ inch thick)
- ¼ teaspoon Lemon-pepper seasoning

Directions:

1. Preheat the air fryer to 400°F.
2. Run a vegetable peeler lengthwise along a hard, cold stick of butter, making 2, 3, or 4 long strips as the recipe requires for the number of cutlets you're making.
3. Lay the veal cutlets on a clean, dry cutting board or work surface. Sprinkle about ⅛ teaspoon lemon-pepper seasoning over each. Set a strip of butter on top of each cutlet.
4. When the machine is at temperature, set the topped cutlets in the basket so that they don't overlap or even touch. Air-fry undisturbed for 4 minutes without turning.
5. Use a nonstick-safe spatula to transfer the cutlets to a serving plate or plates, taking care to keep as much of the butter on top as possible. Remove the basket from the drawer or from over the baking tray. Carefully pour the browned butter over the cutlets.

Perfect Pork Chops

Servings: 3
Cooking Time: 10 Minutes

Ingredients:

- ¾ teaspoon Mild paprika
- ¾ teaspoon Dried thyme
- ¾ teaspoon Onion powder
- ¼ teaspoon Garlic powder
- ¼ teaspoon Table salt
- ¼ teaspoon Ground black pepper
- 3 6-ounce boneless center-cut pork loin chops
- Vegetable oil spray

Directions:

1. Preheat the air fryer to 400°F.
2. Mix the paprika, thyme, onion powder, garlic powder, salt, and pepper in a small bowl until well combined. Massage this mixture into both sides of the chops. Generously coat both sides of the chops with vegetable oil spray.
3. When the machine is at temperature, set the chops in the basket with as much air space between them as possible. Air-fry undisturbed for 10 minutes, or until an instant-read meat thermometer inserted into the thickest part of a chop registers 145°F.
4. Use kitchen tongs to transfer the chops to a cutting board or serving plates. Cool for 5 minutes before serving.

Vietnamese Shaking Beef

Servings: 3

Cooking Time: 7 Minutes

Ingredients:

- 1 pound Beef tenderloin, cut into 1-inch cubes
- 1 tablespoon Regular or low-sodium soy sauce or gluten-free tamari sauce
- 1 tablespoon Fish sauce (gluten-free, if a concern)
- 1 tablespoon Dark brown sugar
- 1½ teaspoons Ground black pepper
- 3 Medium scallions, trimmed and thinly sliced
- 2 tablespoons Butter
- 1½ teaspoons Minced garlic

Directions:

1. Mix the beef, soy or tamari sauce, fish sauce, and brown sugar in a bowl until well combined. Cover and refrigerate for at least 2 hours or up to 8 hours, tossing the beef at least twice in the marinade.
2. Put a 6-inch round or square cake pan in an air-fryer basket for a small batch, a 7-inch round or square cake pan for a medium batch, or an 8-inch round or square cake pan for a large one. Or put one of these on the rack of a toaster oven–style air fryer. Heat the machine with the pan in it to 400°F. When the machine it at temperature, let the pan sit in the heat for 2 to 3 minutes so that it gets very hot.
3. Use a slotted spoon to transfer the beef to the pan, leaving any marinade behind in the bowl. Spread the meat into as close to an even layer as you can. Air-fry undisturbed for 5 minutes. Meanwhile, discard the marinade, if any.
4. Add the scallions, butter, and garlic to the beef. Air-fry for 2 minutes, tossing and rearranging the beef and scallions repeatedly, perhaps every 20 seconds.
5. Remove the basket from the machine and let the meat cool in the pan for a couple of minutes before serving.

Pork Cutlets With Aloha Salsa

Servings: 4

Cooking Time: 9 Minutes

Ingredients:

- Aloha Salsa
- 1 cup fresh pineapple, chopped in small pieces
- ¼ cup red onion, finely chopped
- ¼ cup green or red bell pepper, chopped
- ½ teaspoon ground cinnamon
- 1 teaspoon low-sodium soy sauce
- ⅛ teaspoon crushed red pepper
- ⅛ teaspoon ground black pepper
- 2 eggs
- 2 tablespoons milk
- ¼ cup flour
- ¼ cup panko breadcrumbs
- 4 teaspoons sesame seeds
- 1 pound boneless, thin pork cutlets (⅜- to ½-inch thick)
- lemon pepper and salt
- ¼ cup cornstarch
- oil for misting or cooking spray

Directions:

1. In a medium bowl, stir together all ingredients for salsa. Cover and refrigerate while cooking pork.
2. Preheat air fryer to 390°F.
3. Beat together eggs and milk in shallow dish.
4. In another shallow dish, mix together the flour, panko, and sesame seeds.
5. Sprinkle pork cutlets with lemon pepper and salt to taste. Most lemon pepper seasoning contains salt, so go easy adding extra.
6. Dip pork cutlets in cornstarch, egg mixture, and then panko coating. Spray both sides with oil or cooking spray.
7. Cook cutlets for 3minutes. Turn cutlets over, spraying both sides, and continue cooking for 6 minutes or until well done.
8. Serve fried cutlets with salsa on the side.

Venison Backstrap

Servings: 4
Cooking Time: 10 Minutes

Ingredients:

- 2 eggs
- ¼ cup milk
- 1 cup whole wheat flour
- ½ teaspoon salt
- ¼ teaspoon pepper
- 1 pound venison backstrap, sliced
- salt and pepper
- oil for misting or cooking spray

Directions:

1. Beat together eggs and milk in a shallow dish.
2. In another shallow dish, combine the flour, salt, and pepper. Stir to mix well.
3. Sprinkle venison steaks with additional salt and pepper to taste. Dip in flour, egg wash, then in flour again, pressing in coating.
4. Spray steaks with oil or cooking spray on both sides.
5. Cooking in 2 batches, place steaks in the air fryer basket in a single layer. Cook at 360°F for 8minutes. Spray with oil, turn over, and spray other side. Cook for 2 minutes longer, until coating is crispy brown and meat is done to your liking.
6. Repeat to cook remaining venison.

Bacon, Blue Cheese And Pear Stuffed Pork Chops

Servings: 3
Cooking Time: 24 Minutes

Ingredients:

- 4 slices bacon, chopped
- 1 tablespoon butter
- ½ cup finely diced onion
- ⅓ cup chicken stock
- 1½ cups seasoned stuffing cubes
- 1 egg, beaten
- ½ teaspoon dried thyme
- ½ teaspoon salt
- ⅛ teaspoon black pepper
- 1 pear, finely diced
- ⅓ cup crumbled blue cheese
- 3 boneless center-cut pork chops (2-inch thick)
- olive oil
- salt and freshly ground black pepper

Directions:

1. Preheat the air fryer to 400°F.
2. Place the bacon into the air fryer basket and air-fry for 6 minutes, stirring halfway through the cooking time. Remove the bacon and set it aside on a paper towel. Pour out the grease from the bottom of the air fryer.
3. To make the stuffing, melt the butter in a medium saucepan over medium heat on the stovetop. Add the onion and sauté for a few minutes, until it starts to soften. Add the chicken stock and simmer for 1 minute. Remove the pan from the heat and add the stuffing cubes. Stir until the stock has been absorbed. Add the egg, dried thyme, salt and freshly ground black pepper, and stir until combined. Fold in the diced pear and crumbled blue cheese.
4. Place the pork chops on a cutting board. Using the palm of your hand to hold the chop flat and steady, slice into the side of the pork chop to make a pocket in the center of the chop. Leave about an inch of chop uncut and make sure you don't cut all the way through the pork chop. Brush both sides of the pork chops with olive oil and season with salt and freshly ground black pepper. Stuff each pork chop with a third of the stuffing, packing the stuffing tightly inside the pocket.
5. Preheat the air fryer to 360°F.
6. Spray or brush the sides of the air fryer basket with oil. Place the pork chops in the air fryer basket with the open stuffed edge of the pork chop facing the outside edges of the basket.
7. Air-fry the pork chops for 18 minutes, turning the pork chops over halfway through the cooking time. When the chops are done, let them rest for 5 minutes and then transfer to a serving platter.

Bacon Wrapped Filets Mignons

Servings: 4

Cooking Time: 18 Minutes

Ingredients:

- 4 slices bacon (not thick cut)
- 4 (8-ounce) filets mignons
- 1 tablespoon fresh thyme leaves
- salt and freshly ground black pepper

Directions:

1. Preheat the air fryer to 400°F.
2. Lay the bacon slices down on a cutting board and sprinkle the thyme leaves on the bacon slices. Remove any string tying the filets and place the steaks down on their sides on top of the bacon slices. Roll the bacon around the side of the filets and secure the bacon to the fillets with a toothpick or two.
3. Season the steaks generously with salt and freshly ground black pepper and transfer the steaks to the air fryer.
4. Air-fry for 18 minutes, turning the steaks over halfway through the cooking process. This should cook your steaks to about medium, depending on how thick they are. If you'd prefer your steaks medium-rare or medium-well, simply add or subtract two minutes from the cooking time. Remove the steaks from the air fryer and let them rest for 5 minutes before removing the toothpicks and serving. (Just enough time to quickly air-fry some vegetables to go with them!)

Crispy Pierogi With Kielbasa And Onions

Servings: 3

Cooking Time: 20 Minutes

Ingredients:

- 6 Frozen potato and cheese pierogi, thawed (about 12 pierogi to 1 pound)
- ½ pound Smoked kielbasa, sliced into ½-inch-thick rounds
- ¾ cup Very roughly chopped sweet onion, preferably Vidalia
- Vegetable oil spray

Directions:

1. Preheat the air fryer to 375°F .
2. Put the pierogi, kielbasa rounds, and onion in a large bowl. Coat them with vegetable oil spray, toss well, spray again, and toss until everything is glistening.
3. When the machine is at temperature, dump the contents of the bowl it into the basket. (Items may be leaning against each other and even on top of each other.) Air-fry, tossing and rearranging everything twice so that all covered surfaces get exposed, for 20 minutes, or until the sausages have begun to brown and the pierogi are crisp.
4. Pour the contents of the basket onto a serving platter. Wait a minute or two just to take make sure nothing's searing hot before serving.

Pork & Beef Egg Rolls

Servings: 8

Cooking Time: 8 Minutes

Ingredients:

- ¼ pound very lean ground beef
- ¼ pound lean ground pork
- 1 tablespoon soy sauce
- 1 teaspoon olive oil
- ½ cup grated carrots
- 2 green onions, chopped
- 2 cups grated Napa cabbage
- ¼ cup chopped water chestnuts
- ¼ teaspoon salt
- ¼ teaspoon garlic powder
- ¼ teaspoon black pepper
- 1 egg
- 1 tablespoon water
- 8 egg roll wraps
- oil for misting or cooking spray

Directions:

1. In a large skillet, brown beef and pork with soy sauce. Remove cooked meat from skillet, drain, and set aside.
2. Pour off any excess grease from skillet. Add olive oil, carrots, and onions. Sauté until barely tender, about 1 minute.
3. Stir in cabbage, cover, and cook for 1 minute or just until cabbage slightly wilts. Remove from heat.

4. In a large bowl, combine the cooked meats and vegetables, water chestnuts, salt, garlic powder, and pepper. Stir well. If needed, add more salt to taste.
5. Beat together egg and water in a small bowl.
6. Fill egg roll wrappers, using about ¼ cup of filling for each wrap. Roll up and brush all over with egg wash to seal. Spray very lightly with olive oil or cooking spray.
7. Place 4 egg rolls in air fryer basket and cook at 390°F for 4minutes. Turn over and cook 4 more minutes, until golden brown and crispy.
8. Repeat to cook remaining egg rolls.

Beef And Spinach Braciole

Servings: 4
Cooking Time: 92 Minutes

Ingredients:

- 7-inch oven-safe baking pan or casserole
- ½ onion, finely chopped
- 1 teaspoon olive oil
- ⅓ cup red wine
- 2 cups crushed tomatoes
- 1 teaspoon Italian seasoning
- ½ teaspoon garlic powder
- ¼ teaspoon crushed red pepper flakes
- 2 tablespoons chopped fresh parsley
- 2 top round steaks (about 1½ pounds)
- salt and freshly ground black pepper
- 2 cups fresh spinach, chopped
- 1 clove minced garlic
- ½ cup roasted red peppers, julienned
- ½ cup grated pecorino cheese
- ¼ cup pine nuts, toasted and rough chopped
- 2 tablespoons olive oil

Directions:

1. Preheat the air fryer to 400°F.
2. Toss the onions and olive oil together in a 7-inch metal baking pan or casserole dish. Air-fry at 400°F for 5 minutes, stirring a couple times during the cooking process. Add the red wine, crushed tomatoes, Italian seasoning, garlic powder, red pepper flakes and parsley and stir. Cover the pan tightly with aluminum foil, lower the air fryer temperature to 350°F and continue to air-fry for 15 minutes.
3. While the sauce is simmering, prepare the beef. Using a meat mallet, pound the beef until it is ¼-inch thick. Season both sides of the beef with salt and pepper. Combine the spinach, garlic, red peppers, pecorino cheese, pine nuts and olive oil in a medium bowl. Season with salt and freshly ground black pepper. Spread the mixture evenly over the steaks. Starting at one of the short ends, roll the beef around the filling, tucking in the sides as you roll to ensure the filling is completely enclosed. Secure the beef rolls with toothpicks.
4. Remove the baking pan with the sauce from the air fryer and set it aside. Preheat the air fryer to 400°F.
5. Brush or spray the beef rolls with a little olive oil and air-fry at 400°F for 12 minutes, rotating the beef during the cooking process for even browning. When the beef is browned, submerge the rolls into the sauce in the baking pan, cover the pan with foil and return it to the air fryer. Air-fry at 250°F for 60 minutes.
6. Remove the beef rolls from the sauce. Cut each roll into slices and serve with pasta, ladling some of the sauce overtop.

Peppered Steak Bites

Servings: 4
Cooking Time: 14 Minutes

Ingredients:

- 1 pound sirloin steak, cut into 1-inch cubes
- ½ teaspoon coarse sea salt
- 1 teaspoon coarse black pepper
- 2 teaspoons Worcestershire sauce
- ½ teaspoon garlic powder
- ¼ teaspoon red pepper flakes
- ¼ cup chopped parsley

Directions:

1. Preheat the air fryer to 390°F.
2. In a large bowl, place the steak cubes and toss with the salt, pepper, Worcestershire sauce, garlic powder, and red pepper flakes.
3. Pour the steak into the air fryer basket and cook for 10 to 14 minutes, depending on how well done you prefer your bites. Starting at the 8-minute mark, toss the steak bites every 2 minutes to check for doneness.

4. When the steak is cooked, remove it from the basket to a serving bowl and top with the chopped parsley. Allow the steak to rest for 5 minutes before serving.

Pork Chops

Servings: 2

Cooking Time: 16 Minutes

Ingredients:

- 2 bone-in, centercut pork chops, 1-inch thick (10 ounces each)
- 2 teaspoons Worcestershire sauce
- salt and pepper
- cooking spray

Directions:

1. Rub the Worcestershire sauce into both sides of pork chops.
2. Season with salt and pepper to taste.
3. Spray air fryer basket with cooking spray and place the chops in basket side by side.
4. Cook at 360°F for 16 minutes or until well done. Let rest for 5minutes before serving.

Crispy Five-spice Pork Belly

Servings: 6

Cooking Time: 60-75 Minutes

Ingredients:

- 1½ pounds Pork belly with skin
- 3 tablespoons Shaoxing (Chinese cooking rice wine), dry sherry, or white grape juice
- 1½ teaspoons Granulated white sugar
- ¾ teaspoon Five-spice powder (see the headnote)
- 1¼ cups Coarse sea salt or kosher salt

Directions:

1. Preheat the air fryer to 350°F .
2. Set the pork belly skin side up on a cutting board. Use a meat fork to make dozens and dozens of tiny holes all across the surface of the skin. You can hardly make too many holes. These will allow the skin to bubble up and keep it from becoming hard as it roasts.
3. Turn the pork belly over so that one of its longer sides faces you. Make four evenly spaced vertical slits in the meat. The slits should go about halfway into the meat toward the fat.
4. Mix the Shaoxing or its substitute, sugar, and five-spice powder in a small bowl until the sugar dissolves. Massage this mixture across the meat and into the cuts.
5. Turn the pork belly over again. Blot dry any moisture on the skin. Make a double-thickness aluminum foil tray by setting two 10-inch-long pieces of foil on top of another. Set the pork belly skin side up in the center of this tray. Fold the sides of the tray up toward the pork, crimping the foil as you work to make a high-sided case all around the pork belly. Seal the foil to the meat on all sides so that only the skin is exposed.
6. Pour the salt onto the skin and pat it down and in place to create a crust. Pick up the foil tray with the pork in it and set it in the basket.
7. Air-fry undisturbed for 35 minutes for a small batch, 45 minutes for a medium batch, or 50 minutes for a large batch.
8. Remove the foil tray with the pork belly still in it. Warning: The foil tray is full of scalding-hot fat. Discard the fat in the tray (not down the drain!), as well as the tray itself. Transfer the pork belly to a cutting board.
9. Raise the air fryer temperature to 375°F (or 380°F or 390°F, if one of these is the closest setting). Brush the salt crust off the pork, removing any visible salt from the sides of the meat, too.
10. When the machine is at temperature, return the pork belly skin side up to the basket. Air-fry undisturbed for 25 minutes, or until crisp and very well browned. If the machine is at 390°F, you may be able to shave 5 minutes off the cooking time so that the skin doesn't blacken.
11. Use a nonstick-safe spatula, and perhaps a silicone baking mitt, to transfer the pork belly to a wire rack. Cool for 10 minutes before serving.

Pizza Tortilla Rolls

Servings: 4
Cooking Time: 8 Minutes

Ingredients:

- 1 teaspoon butter
- ½ medium onion, slivered
- ½ red or green bell pepper, julienned
- 4 ounces fresh white mushrooms, chopped
- 8 flour tortillas (6- or 7-inch size)
- ½ cup pizza sauce
- 8 thin slices deli ham
- 24 pepperoni slices (about 1½ ounces)
- 1 cup shredded mozzarella cheese (about 4 ounces)
- oil for misting or cooking spray

Directions:

1. Place butter, onions, bell pepper, and mushrooms in air fryer baking pan. Cook at 390°F for 3minutes. Stir and cook 4 minutes longer until just crisp and tender. Remove pan and set aside.
2. To assemble rolls, spread about 2 teaspoons of pizza sauce on one half of each tortilla. Top with a slice of ham and 3 slices of pepperoni. Divide sautéed vegetables among tortillas and top with cheese.
3. Roll up tortillas, secure with toothpicks if needed, and spray with oil.
4. Place 4 rolls in air fryer basket and cook for 4minutes. Turn and cook 4 minutes, until heated through and lightly browned.
5. Repeat step 4 to cook remaining pizza rolls.

Teriyaki Country-style Pork Ribs

Servings: 3
Cooking Time: 30 Minutes

Ingredients:

- 3 tablespoons Regular or low-sodium soy sauce or gluten-free tamari sauce
- 3 tablespoons Honey
- ¾ teaspoon Ground dried ginger
- ¾ teaspoon Garlic powder
- 3 8-ounce boneless country-style pork ribs
- Vegetable oil spray

Directions:

1. Preheat the air fryer to 350°F .
2. Mix the soy or tamari sauce, honey, ground ginger, and garlic powder in another bowl until uniform.
3. Smear about half of this teriyaki sauce over all sides of the country-style ribs. Reserve the remainder of the teriyaki sauce. Generously coat the meat with vegetable oil spray.
4. When the machine is at temperature, place the country-style ribs in the basket with as much air space between them as possible. Air-fry undisturbed for 15 minutes. Turn the country-style ribs (but keep the space between them) and brush them all over with the remaining teriyaki sauce. Continue air-frying undisturbed for 15 minutes, or until an instant-read meat thermometer inserted into the center of one rib registers at least 145°F.
5. Use kitchen tongs to transfer the country-style ribs to a wire rack. Cool for 5 minutes before serving.

Brie And Cranberry Burgers

Servings: 3
Cooking Time: 9 Minutes

Ingredients:

- 1 pound ground beef (80% lean)
- 1 tablespoon chopped fresh thyme
- 1 tablespoon Worcestershire sauce
- ½ teaspoon salt
- freshly ground black pepper
- 1 (4-ounce) wheel of Brie cheese, sliced
- handful of arugula
- 3 or 4 brioche hamburger buns (or potato hamburger buns), toasted
- ¼ to ½ cup whole berry cranberry sauce

Directions:

1. Combine the beef, thyme, Worcestershire sauce, salt and pepper together in a large bowl and mix well. Divide the meat into 4 (¼-pound) portions or 3 larger portions and then form them into burger patties, being careful not to over-handle the meat.
2. Preheat the air fryer to 390°F and pour a little water into the bottom of the air fryer drawer. (This will help prevent the grease that drips into the bottom drawer from burning and smoking.)

3. Transfer the burgers to the air fryer basket. Air-fry the burgers at 390°F for 5 minutes. Flip the burgers over and air-fry for another 2 minutes. Top each burger with a couple slices of brie and air-fry for another minute or two, just to soften the cheese.
4. Build the burgers by placing a few leaves of arugula on the bottom bun, adding the burger and a spoonful of cranberry sauce on top. Top with the other half of the hamburger bun and enjoy.

Corned Beef Hash

Servings: 6
Cooking Time: 15 Minutes

Ingredients:

- 3 cups (about 14 ounces) Frozen unseasoned hash brown cubes (no need to thaw)
- 9 ounces Deli corned beef, cut into ¾-inch-thick slices, then cubed
- ¾ cup Roughly chopped yellow or white onion
- ¾ cup Stemmed, cored, and roughly chopped red bell pepper
- 2½ tablespoons Olive oil
- ¼ teaspoon Dried thyme
- ¼ teaspoon Dried sage leaves
- Up to a ⅛ teaspoon Cayenne

Directions:

1. Preheat the air fryer to 400°F.
2. Mix all the ingredients in a large or very large bowl until the potato cubes and corned beef are coated in the spices.
3. Spread the mixture in the basket in as close to an even layer as you can. Air-fry for 15 minutes, tossing and rearranging the pieces at the 5- and 10-minute marks to expose covered bits, until the potatoes are browned, even crisp, and the mixture is very fragrant.
4. Pour the contents of the basket onto a serving platter or divide between serving plates. Cool for a couple of minutes before serving.

Meatball Subs

Servings: 4
Cooking Time: 11 Minutes

Ingredients:

- Marinara Sauce
- 1 15-ounce can diced tomatoes
- 1 teaspoon garlic powder
- 1 teaspoon dried basil
- ½ teaspoon oregano
- ⅛ teaspoon salt
- 1 tablespoon robust olive oil
- Meatballs
- ¼ pound ground turkey
- ¾ pound very lean ground beef
- 1 tablespoon milk
- ½ cup torn bread pieces
- 1 egg
- ¼ teaspoon salt
- ½ teaspoon dried onion
- 1 teaspoon garlic powder
- ¼ teaspoon smoked paprika
- ¼ teaspoon crushed red pepper
- 1½ teaspoons dried parsley
- ¼ teaspoon oregano
- 2 teaspoons Worcestershire sauce
- Sandwiches
- 4 large whole-grain sub or hoagie rolls, split
- toppings, sliced or chopped:
- mushrooms
- jalapeño or banana peppers
- red or green bell pepper
- red onions
- grated cheese

Directions:

1. Place all marinara ingredients in saucepan and bring to a boil. Lower heat and simmer 10minutes, uncovered.
2. Combine all meatball ingredients in large bowl and stir. Mixture should be well blended but don't overwork it. Excessive mixing will toughen the meatballs.
3. Divide meat into 16 equal portions and shape into balls.
4. Cook the balls at 360°F until meat is done and juices run clear, about 11 minutes.
5. While meatballs are cooking, taste marinara. If you prefer stronger flavors, add more seasoning and simmer another 5minutes.

6. When meatballs finish cooking, drain them on paper towels.

7. To assemble subs, place 4 meatballs on each sub roll, spoon sauce over meat, and add preferred toppings. Serve with additional marinara for dipping.

California Burritos

Servings: 4
Cooking Time: 17 Minutes

Ingredients:

- 1 pound sirloin steak, sliced thin
- 1 teaspoon dried oregano
- 1 teaspoon ground cumin
- ½ teaspoon garlic powder
- 16 tater tots
- ⅓ cup sour cream
- ½ lime, juiced
- 2 tablespoons hot sauce
- 1 large avocado, pitted
- 1 teaspoon salt, divided
- 4 large (8- to 10-inch) flour tortillas
- ½ cup shredded cheddar cheese or Monterey jack
- 2 tablespoons avocado oil

Directions:

1. Preheat the air fryer to 380°F.
2. Season the steak with oregano, cumin, and garlic powder. Place the steak on one side of the air fryer and the tater tots on the other side. (It's okay for them to touch, because the flavors will all come together in the burrito.) Cook for 8 minutes, toss, and cook an additional 4 to 6 minutes.
3. Meanwhile, in a small bowl, stir together the sour cream, lime juice, and hot sauce.
4. In another small bowl, mash together the avocado and season with ½ teaspoon of the salt, to taste.
5. To assemble the burrito, lay out the tortillas, equally divide the meat amongst the tortillas. Season the steak equally with the remaining ½ teaspoon salt. Then layer the mashed avocado and sour cream mixture on top. Top each tortilla with 4 tater tots and finish each with 2 tablespoons cheese. Roll up the sides and, while holding in the sides, roll up the burrito. Place the burritos in the air fryer basket and brush with avocado oil (working in batches as needed); cook for 3 minutes or until lightly golden on the outside.

Steak Fingers

Servings: 4
Cooking Time: 8 Minutes

Ingredients:

- 4 small beef cube steaks
- salt and pepper
- ½ cup flour
- oil for misting or cooking spray

Directions:

1. Cut cube steaks into 1-inch-wide strips.
2. Sprinkle lightly with salt and pepper to taste.
3. Roll in flour to coat all sides.
4. Spray air fryer basket with cooking spray or oil.
5. Place steak strips in air fryer basket in single layer, very close together but not touching. Spray top of steak strips with oil or cooking spray.
6. Cook at 390°F for 4minutes, turn strips over, and spray with oil or cooking spray.
7. Cook 4 more minutes and test with fork for doneness. Steak fingers should be crispy outside with no red juices inside. If needed, cook an additional 4 minutes or until well done. (Don't eat beef cube steak rare.)
8. Repeat steps 5 through 7 to cook remaining strips.

Air-fried Roast Beef With Rosemary Roasted Potatoes

Servings: 8
Cooking Time: 60 Minutes

Ingredients:

- 1 (5-pound) top sirloin roast
- salt and freshly ground black pepper
- 1 teaspoon dried thyme
- 2 pounds red potatoes, halved or quartered
- 2 teaspoons olive oil
- 1 teaspoon very finely chopped fresh rosemary, plus more for garnish

Directions:

1. Start by making sure your roast will fit into the air fryer basket without touching the top element. Trim it if

you have to in order to get it to fit nicely in your air fryer. (You can always save the trimmings for another use, like a beef sandwich.)
2. Preheat the air fryer to 360°F.
3. Season the beef all over with salt, pepper and thyme. Transfer the seasoned roast to the air fryer basket.
4. Air-fry at 360°F for 20 minutes. Turn the roast over and continue to air-fry at 360°F for another 20 minutes.
5. Toss the potatoes with the olive oil, salt, pepper and fresh rosemary. Turn the roast over again in the air fryer basket and toss the potatoes in around the sides of the roast. Air-fry the roast and potatoes at 360°F for another 20 minutes. Check the internal temperature of the roast with an instant-read thermometer, and continue to roast until the beef is 5° lower than your desired degree of doneness. (Rare – 130°F, Medium – 150°F, Well done – 170°F.) Let the roast rest for 5 to 10 minutes before slicing and serving. While the roast is resting, continue to air-fry the potatoes if desired for extra browning and crispiness.
6. Slice the roast and serve with the potatoes, adding a little more fresh rosemary if desired.

Easy Carnitas

Servings: 3
Cooking Time: 25 Minutes

Ingredients:

- 1½ pounds Boneless country-style pork ribs, cut into 2-inch pieces
- ¼ cup Orange juice
- 2 tablespoons Brine from a jar of pickles, any type, even pickled jalapeño rings (gluten-free, if a concern)
- 2 teaspoons Minced garlic
- 2 teaspoons Minced fresh oregano leaves
- ¾ teaspoon Ground cumin
- ¾ teaspoon Table salt
- ¾ teaspoon Ground black pepper

Directions:

1. Mix the country-style pork rib pieces, orange juice, pickle brine, garlic, oregano, cumin, salt, and pepper in a large bowl. Cover and refrigerate for at least 2 hours or up to 10 hours, stirring the mixture occasionally.
2. Preheat the air fryer to 400°F. Set the rib pieces in their bowl on the counter as the machine heats.
3. Use kitchen tongs to transfer the rib pieces to the basket, arranging them in one layer. Some may touch. Air-fry for 25 minutes, turning and rearranging the pieces at the 10- and 20-minute marks to make sure all surfaces have been exposed to the air currents, until browned and sizzling.
4. Use clean kitchen tongs to transfer the rib pieces to a wire rack. Cool for a couple of minutes before serving.

Bread And Breakfast

Blueberry Muffins

Servings: 8
Cooking Time: 14 Minutes

Ingredients:

- 1⅓ cups flour
- ½ cup sugar
- 2 teaspoons baking powder
- ¼ teaspoon salt
- ⅓ cup canola oil
- 1 egg
- ½ cup milk
- ⅔ cup blueberries, fresh or frozen and thawed
- 8 foil muffin cups including paper liners

Directions:

1. Preheat air fryer to 330°F.
2. In a medium bowl, stir together flour, sugar, baking powder, and salt.
3. In a separate bowl, combine oil, egg, and milk and mix well.
4. Add egg mixture to dry ingredients and stir just until moistened.
5. Gently stir in blueberries.
6. Spoon batter evenly into muffin cups.
7. Place 4 muffin cups in air fryer basket and bake at 330°F for 14 minutes or until tops spring back when touched lightly.
8. Repeat previous step to cook remaining muffins.

Pumpkin Loaf

Servings: 6
Cooking Time: 22 Minutes

Ingredients:

- cooking spray
- 1 large egg
- ½ cup granulated sugar
- ⅓ cup oil
- ½ cup canned pumpkin (not pie filling)
- ½ teaspoon vanilla
- ⅔ cup flour plus 1 tablespoon
- ½ teaspoon baking powder
- ½ teaspoon baking soda
- ½ teaspoon salt
- 1 teaspoon pumpkin pie spice
- ¼ teaspoon cinnamon

Directions:

1. Spray 6 x 6-inch baking dish lightly with cooking spray.
2. Place baking dish in air fryer basket and preheat air fryer to 330°F.
3. In a large bowl, beat eggs and sugar together with a hand mixer.
4. Add oil, pumpkin, and vanilla and mix well.
5. Sift together all dry ingredients. Add to pumpkin mixture and beat well, about 1 minute.
6. Pour batter in baking dish and cook at 330°F for 22 minutes or until toothpick inserted in center of loaf comes out clean.

French Toast Sticks

Servings: 4
Cooking Time: 7 Minutes

Ingredients:

- 2 eggs
- ½ cup milk
- ⅛ teaspoon salt
- ½ teaspoon pure vanilla extract
- ¾ cup crushed cornflakes
- 6 slices sandwich bread, each slice cut into 4 strips
- oil for misting or cooking spray
- maple syrup or honey

Directions:

1. In a small bowl, beat together eggs, milk, salt, and vanilla.
2. Place crushed cornflakes on a plate or in a shallow dish.
3. Dip bread strips in egg mixture, shake off excess, and roll in cornflake crumbs.
4. Spray both sides of bread strips with oil.
5. Place bread strips in air fryer basket in single layer.
6. Cook at 390°F for 7minutes or until they're dark golden brown.

7. Repeat steps 5 and 6 to cook remaining French toast sticks.
8. Serve with maple syrup or honey for dipping.

Orange Rolls

Servings: 8
Cooking Time: 10 Minutes

Ingredients:

- parchment paper
- 3 ounces low-fat cream cheese
- 1 tablespoon low-fat sour cream or plain yogurt (not Greek yogurt)
- 2 teaspoons sugar
- ¼ teaspoon pure vanilla extract
- ¼ teaspoon orange extract
- 1 can (8 count) organic crescent roll dough
- ¼ cup chopped walnuts
- ¼ cup dried cranberries
- ¼ cup shredded, sweetened coconut
- butter-flavored cooking spray
- Orange Glaze
- ½ cup powdered sugar
- 1 tablespoon orange juice
- ¼ teaspoon orange extract
- dash of salt

Directions:

1. Cut a circular piece of parchment paper slightly smaller than the bottom of your air fryer basket. Set aside.
2. In a small bowl, combine the cream cheese, sour cream or yogurt, sugar, and vanilla and orange extracts. Stir until smooth.
3. Preheat air fryer to 300°F.
4. Separate crescent roll dough into 8 triangles and divide cream cheese mixture among them. Starting at wide end, spread cheese mixture to within 1 inch of point.
5. Sprinkle nuts and cranberries evenly over cheese mixture.
6. Starting at wide end, roll up triangles, then sprinkle with coconut, pressing in lightly to make it stick. Spray tops of rolls with butter-flavored cooking spray.
7. Place parchment paper in air fryer basket, and place 4 rolls on top, spaced evenly.
8. Cook for 10minutes, until rolls are golden brown and cooked through.
9. Repeat steps 7 and 8 to cook remaining 4 rolls. You should be able to use the same piece of parchment paper twice.
10. In a small bowl, stir together ingredients for glaze and drizzle over warm rolls.

Pancake Muffins

Servings: 4
Cooking Time: 8 Minutes

Ingredients:

- 1 cup flour
- 2 tablespoons sugar (optional)
- ½ teaspoon baking soda
- 1 teaspoon baking powder
- ¼ teaspoon salt
- 1 egg, beaten
- 1 cup buttermilk
- 2 tablespoons melted butter
- 1 teaspoon pure vanilla extract
- 24 foil muffin cups
- cooking spray
- Suggested Fillings
- 1 teaspoon of jelly or fruit preserves
- 1 tablespoon or less fresh blueberries; chopped fresh strawberries; chopped frozen cherries; dark chocolate chips; chopped walnuts, pecans, or other nuts; cooked, crumbled bacon or sausage

Directions:

1. In a large bowl, stir together flour, optional sugar, baking soda, baking powder, and salt.
2. In a small bowl, combine egg, buttermilk, butter, and vanilla. Mix well.
3. Pour egg mixture into dry ingredients and stir to mix well but don't overbeat.
4. Double up the muffin cups and remove the paper liners from the top cups. Spray the foil cups lightly with cooking spray.
5. Place 6 sets of muffin cups in air fryer basket. Pour just enough batter into each cup to cover the bottom.

Sprinkle with desired filling. Pour in more batter to cover the filling and fill the cups about ¾ full.

6. Cook at 330°F for 8minutes.
7. Repeat steps 5 and 6 for the remaining 6 pancake muffins.

Mediterranean Egg Sandwich

Servings: 1
Cooking Time: 8 Minutes

Ingredients:

- 1 large egg
- 5 baby spinach leaves, chopped
- 1 tablespoon roasted bell pepper, chopped
- 1 English muffin
- 1 thin slice prosciutto or Canadian bacon

Directions:

1. Spray a ramekin with cooking spray or brush the inside with extra-virgin olive oil.
2. In a small bowl, whisk together the egg, baby spinach, and bell pepper.
3. Split the English muffin in half and spray the inside lightly with cooking spray or brush with extra-virgin olive oil.
4. Preheat the air fryer to 350°F for 2 minutes. Place the egg ramekin and open English muffin into the air fryer basket, and cook at 350°F for 5 minutes. Open the air fryer drawer and add the prosciutto or bacon; cook for an additional 1 minute.
5. To assemble the sandwich, place the egg on one half of the English muffin, top with prosciutto or bacon, and place the remaining piece of English muffin on top.

Parmesan Garlic Naan

Servings: 6
Cooking Time: 4 Minutes

Ingredients:

- 1 cup bread flour
- 1 teaspoon baking powder
- ⅛ teaspoon salt
- 1 teaspoon garlic powder
- 2 tablespoon shredded parmesan cheese
- 1 cup plain 2% fat Greek yogurt
- 1 tablespoon extra-virgin olive oil

Directions:

1. Preheat the air fryer to 400°F.
2. In a medium bowl, mix the flour, baking powder, salt, garlic powder, and cheese. Mix the yogurt into the flour, using your hands to combine if necessary.
3. On a flat surface covered with flour, divide the dough into 6 equal balls and roll each out into a 4-inch-diameter circle.
4. Lightly brush both sides of each naan with olive oil and place one naan at a time into the basket. Cook for 3 to 4 minutes (or until the bread begins to rise and brown on the outside). Remove and repeat for the remaining breads.
5. Serve warm.

Tuscan Toast

Servings: 4
Cooking Time: 5 Minutes

Ingredients:

- ¼ cup butter
- ½ teaspoon lemon juice
- ½ clove garlic
- ½ teaspoon dried parsley flakes
- 4 slices Italian bread, 1-inch thick

Directions:

1. Place butter, lemon juice, garlic, and parsley in a food processor. Process about 1 minute, or until garlic is pulverized and ingredients are well blended.
2. Spread garlic butter on both sides of bread slices.
3. Place bread slices upright in air fryer basket. (They can lie flat but cook better standing on end.)
4. Cook at 390°F for 5minutes or until toasty brown.

Whole-grain Cornbread

Servings: 6
Cooking Time: 25 Minutes

Ingredients:

- 1 cup stoneground cornmeal
- ½ cup brown rice flour
- 1 teaspoon sugar
- 2 teaspoons baking powder

- ¼ teaspoon salt
- 1 cup milk
- 2 tablespoons oil
- 2 eggs
- cooking spray

Directions:

1. Preheat the air fryer to 360°F.
2. In a medium mixing bowl, mix cornmeal, brown rice flour, sugar, baking powder, and salt together.
3. Add the remaining ingredients and beat with a spoon until batter is smooth.
4. Spray air fryer baking pan with nonstick cooking spray and add the cornbread batter.
5. Bake at 360°F for 25 minutes, until center is done.

Brown Sugar Grapefruit

Servings: 2

Cooking Time: 4 Minutes

Ingredients:

- 1 grapefruit
- 2 to 4 teaspoons brown sugar

Directions:

1. Preheat the air fryer to 400°F.
2. While the air fryer is Preheating, cut the grapefruit in half horizontally (in other words not through the stem or blossom end of the grapefruit). Slice the bottom of the grapefruit to help it sit flat on the counter if necessary. Using a sharp paring knife (serrated is great), cut around the grapefruit between the flesh of the fruit and the peel. Then, cut each segment away from the membrane so that it is sitting freely in the fruit.
3. Sprinkle 1 to 2 teaspoons of brown sugar on each half of the prepared grapefruit. Set up a rack in the air fryer basket (use an air fryer rack or make your own rack with some crumpled up aluminum foil). You don't have to use a rack, but doing so will get the grapefruit closer to the element so that the brown sugar can caramelize a little better. Transfer the grapefruit half to the rack in the air fryer basket. Depending on how big your grapefruit are and what size air fryer you have, you may need to do each half separately to make sure they sit flat.
4. Air-fry at 400°F for 4 minutes.
5. Remove and let it cool for just a minute before enjoying.

Strawberry Toast

Servings: 4

Cooking Time: 8 Minutes

Ingredients:

- 4 slices bread, ½-inch thick
- butter-flavored cooking spray
- 1 cup sliced strawberries
- 1 teaspoon sugar

Directions:

1. Spray one side of each bread slice with butter-flavored cooking spray. Lay slices sprayed side down.
2. Divide the strawberries among the bread slices.
3. Sprinkle evenly with the sugar and place in the air fryer basket in a single layer.
4. Cook at 390°F for 8minutes. The bottom should look brown and crisp and the top should look glazed.

Bread Boat Eggs

Servings: 4

Cooking Time: 10 Minutes

Ingredients:

- 4 pistolette rolls
- 1 teaspoon butter
- ¼ cup diced fresh mushrooms
- ½ teaspoon dried onion flakes
- 4 eggs
- ½ teaspoon salt
- ¼ teaspoon dried dill weed
- ¼ teaspoon dried parsley
- 1 tablespoon milk

Directions:

1. Cut a rectangle in the top of each roll and scoop out center, leaving ½-inch shell on the sides and bottom.
2. Place butter, mushrooms, and dried onion in air fryer baking pan and cook for 1 minute. Stir and cook 3 moreminutes.
3. In a medium bowl, beat together the eggs, salt, dill, parsley, and milk. Pour mixture into pan with mushrooms.

4. Cook at 390°F for 2minutes. Stir. Continue cooking for 3 or 4minutes, stirring every minute, until eggs are scrambled to your liking.
5. Remove baking pan from air fryer and fill rolls with scrambled egg mixture.
6. Place filled rolls in air fryer basket and cook at 390°F for 2 to 3minutes or until rolls are lightly browned.

Cheddar Cheese Biscuits

Servings: 8
Cooking Time: 22 Minutes

Ingredients:

- 2⅓ cups self-rising flour
- 2 tablespoons sugar
- ½ cup butter (1 stick), frozen for 15 minutes
- ½ cup grated Cheddar cheese, plus more to melt on top
- 1⅓ cups buttermilk
- 1 cup all-purpose flour, for shaping
- 1 tablespoon butter, melted

Directions:

1. Line a buttered 7-inch metal cake pan with parchment paper or a silicone liner.
2. Combine the flour and sugar in a large mixing bowl. Grate the butter into the flour. Add the grated cheese and stir to coat the cheese and butter with flour. Then add the buttermilk and stir just until you can no longer see streaks of flour. The dough should be quite wet.
3. Spread the all-purpose (not self-rising) flour out on a small cookie sheet. With a spoon, scoop 8 evenly sized balls of dough into the flour, making sure they don't touch each other. With floured hands, coat each dough ball with flour and toss them gently from hand to hand to shake off any excess flour. Place each floured dough ball into the prepared pan, right up next to the other. This will help the biscuits rise up, rather than spreading out.
4. Preheat the air fryer to 380°F.
5. Transfer the cake pan to the basket of the air fryer, lowering it into the basket using a sling made of aluminum foil (fold a piece of aluminum foil into a strip about 2-inches wide by 24-inches long). Let the ends of the aluminum foil sling hang across the cake pan before returning the basket to the air fryer.
6. Air-fry for 20 minutes. Check the biscuits a couple of times to make sure they are not getting too brown on top. If they are, re-arrange the aluminum foil strips to cover any brown parts. After 20 minutes, check the biscuits by inserting a toothpick into the center of the biscuits. It should come out clean. If it needs a little more time, continue to air-fry for a couple of extra minutes. Brush the tops of the biscuits with some melted butter and sprinkle a little more grated cheese on top if desired. Pop the basket back into the air fryer for another 2 minutes. Remove the cake pan from the air fryer using the aluminum sling. Let the biscuits cool for just a minute or two and then turn them out onto a plate and pull apart. Serve immediately.

English Scones

Servings: 8
Cooking Time: 8 Minutes

Ingredients:

- 2 cups all-purpose flour
- 1 tablespoon baking powder
- ½ teaspoon salt
- 2 tablespoons sugar
- ¼ cup unsalted butter
- ⅔ cup plus 1 tablespoon whole milk, divided

Directions:

1. Preheat the air fryer to 380°F.
2. In a large bowl, whisk together the flour, baking powder, salt, and sugar. Using a pastry blender or your fingers, cut in the butter until pea-size crumbles appear. Make a well in the center and pour in ⅔ cup of the milk. Quickly mix the batter until a ball forms. Knead the dough 3 times.
3. Place the dough onto a floured surface and, using your hands or a rolling pin, flatten the dough until it's ¾ inch thick. Using a biscuit cutter or drinking glass, cut out 10 circles, reforming the dough and flattening as needed to use up the batter.
4. Brush the tops lightly with the remaining 1 tablespoon of milk.
5. Place the scones into the air fryer basket. Cook for 8 minutes or until golden brown and cooked in the center.

Cheesy Olive And Roasted Pepper Bread

Servings: 8

Cooking Time: 7 Minutes

Ingredients:

- 7-inch round bread boule
- olive oil
- ½ cup mayonnaise
- 2 tablespoons butter, melted
- 1 cup grated mozzarella or Fontina cheese
- ¼ cup grated Parmesan cheese
- ½ teaspoon dried oregano
- ½ cup black olives, sliced
- ½ cup green olives, sliced
- ½ cup coarsely chopped roasted red peppers
- 2 tablespoons minced red onion
- freshly ground black pepper

Directions:

1. Preheat the air fryer to 370°F.
2. Cut the bread boule in half horizontally. If your bread boule has a rounded top, trim the top of the boule so that the top half will lie flat with the cut side facing up. Lightly brush both sides of the boule halves with olive oil.
3. Place one half of the boule into the air fryer basket with the center cut side facing down. Air-fry at 370°F for 2 minutes to lightly toast the bread. Repeat with the other half of the bread boule.
4. Combine the mayonnaise, butter, mozzarella cheese, Parmesan cheese and dried oregano in a small bowl. Fold in the black and green olives, roasted red peppers and red onion and season with freshly ground black pepper. Spread the cheese mixture over the untoasted side of the bread, covering the entire surface.
5. Air-fry at 350°F for 5 minutes until the cheese is melted and browned. Repeat with the other half. Cut into slices and serve warm.

Spinach-bacon Rollups

Servings: 4

Cooking Time: 9 Minutes

Ingredients:

- 4 flour tortillas (6- or 7-inch size)
- 4 slices Swiss cheese
- 1 cup baby spinach leaves
- 4 slices turkey bacon

Directions:

1. Preheat air fryer to 390°F.
2. On each tortilla, place one slice of cheese and ¼ cup of spinach.
3. Roll up tortillas and wrap each with a strip of bacon. Secure each end with a toothpick.
4. Place rollups in air fryer basket, leaving a little space in between them.
5. Cook for 4minutes. Turn and rearrange rollups (for more even cooking) and cook for 5minutes longer, until bacon is crisp.

Walnut Pancake

Servings: 4

Cooking Time: 20 Minutes

Ingredients:

- 3 tablespoons butter, divided into thirds
- 1 cup flour
- 1½ teaspoons baking powder
- ¼ teaspoon salt
- 2 tablespoons sugar
- ¾ cup milk
- 1 egg, beaten
- 1 teaspoon pure vanilla extract
- ½ cup walnuts, roughly chopped
- maple syrup or fresh sliced fruit, for serving

Directions:

1. Place 1 tablespoon of the butter in air fryer baking pan. Cook at 330°F for 3minutes to melt.
2. In a small dish or pan, melt the remaining 2 tablespoons of butter either in the microwave or on the stove.
3. In a medium bowl, stir together the flour, baking powder, salt, and sugar. Add milk, beaten egg, the 2 tablespoons of melted butter, and vanilla. Stir until combined but do not beat. Batter may be slightly lumpy.
4. Pour batter over the melted butter in air fryer baking pan. Sprinkle nuts evenly over top.
5. Cook for 20minutes or until toothpick inserted in center comes out clean. Turn air fryer off, close the machine, and let pancake rest for 2minutes.

6. Remove pancake from pan, slice, and serve with syrup or fresh fruit.

Country Gravy

Servings: 2

Cooking Time: 7 Minutes

Ingredients:

- ¼ pound pork sausage, casings removed
- 1 tablespoon butter
- 2 tablespoons flour
- 2 cups whole milk
- ½ teaspoon salt
- freshly ground black pepper
- 1 teaspoon fresh thyme leaves

Directions:

1. Preheat a saucepan over medium heat. Add and brown the sausage, crumbling it into small pieces as it cooks. Add the butter and flour, stirring well to combine. Continue to cook for 2 minutes, stirring constantly.
2. Slowly pour in the milk, whisking as you do, and bring the mixture to a boil to thicken. Season with salt and freshly ground black pepper, lower the heat and simmer until the sauce has thickened to your desired consistency – about 5 minutes. Stir in the fresh thyme, season to taste and serve hot.

Cinnamon Sugar Donut Holes

Servings: 12

Cooking Time: 6 Minutes

Ingredients:

- 1 cup all-purpose flour
- 6 tablespoons cane sugar, divided
- 1 teaspoon baking powder
- 3 teaspoons ground cinnamon, divided
- ¼ teaspoon salt
- 1 large egg
- 1 teaspoon vanilla extract
- 2 tablespoons melted butter

Directions:

1. Preheat the air fryer to 370°F.
2. In a small bowl, combine the flour, 2 tablespoons of the sugar, the baking powder, 1 teaspoon of the cinnamon, and the salt. Mix well.
3. In a larger bowl, whisk together the egg, vanilla extract, and butter.
4. Slowly add the dry ingredients into the wet until all the ingredients are uniformly combined. Set the bowl inside the refrigerator for at least 30 minutes.
5. Before you're ready to cook, in a small bowl, mix together the remaining 4 tablespoons of sugar and 2 teaspoons of cinnamon.
6. Liberally spray the air fryer basket with olive oil mist so the donut holes don't stick to the bottom. Note: You do not want to use parchment paper in this recipe; it may burn if your air fryer is hotter than others.
7. Remove the dough from the refrigerator and divide it into 12 equal donut holes. You can use a 1-ounce serving scoop if you have one.
8. Roll each donut hole in the sugar and cinnamon mixture; then place in the air fryer basket. Repeat until all the donut holes are covered in the sugar and cinnamon mixture.
9. When the basket is full, cook for 6 minutes. Remove the donut holes from the basket using oven-safe tongs and let cool 5 minutes. Repeat until all 12 are cooked.

Peach Fritters

Servings: 8

Cooking Time: 6 Minutes

Ingredients:

- 1½ cups bread flour
- 1 teaspoon active dry yeast
- ¼ cup sugar
- ¼ teaspoon salt
- ½ cup warm milk
- ½ teaspoon vanilla extract
- 2 egg yolks
- 2 tablespoons melted butter
- 2 cups small diced peaches (fresh or frozen)
- 1 tablespoon butter
- 1 teaspoon ground cinnamon
- 1 to 2 tablespoons sugar
- Glaze

- ¾ cup powdered sugar
- 4 teaspoons milk

Directions:

1. Combine the flour, yeast, sugar and salt in a bowl. Add the milk, vanilla, egg yolks and melted butter and combine until the dough starts to come together. Transfer the dough to a floured surface and knead it by hand for 2 minutes. Shape the dough into a ball, place it in a large oiled bowl, cover with a clean kitchen towel and let the dough rise in a warm place for 1 to 1½ hours, or until the dough has doubled in size.
2. While the dough is rising, melt one tablespoon of butter in a medium saucepan on the stovetop. Add the diced peaches, cinnamon and sugar to taste. Cook the peaches for about 5 minutes, or until they soften. Set the peaches aside to cool.
3. When the dough has risen, transfer it to a floured surface and shape it into a 12-inch circle. Spread the peaches over half of the circle and fold the other half of the dough over the top. With a knife or a board scraper, score the dough by making slits in the dough in a diamond shape. Push the knife straight down into the dough and peaches, rather than slicing through. You should cut through the top layer of dough, but not the bottom. Roll the dough up into a log from one short end to the other. It should be roughly 8 inches long. Some of the peaches will be sticking out of the dough – don't worry, these are supposed to be a little random. Cut the log into 8 equal slices. Place the dough disks on a floured cookie sheet, cover with a clean kitchen towel and let rise in a warm place for 30 minutes.
4. Preheat the air fryer to 370°F.
5. Air-fry 2 or 3 fritters at a time at 370°F, for 3 minutes. Flip them over and continue to air-fry for another 2 to 3 minutes, until they are golden brown.
6. Combine the powdered sugar and milk together in a small bowl. Whisk vigorously until smooth. Allow the fritters to cool for at least 10 minutes and then brush the glaze over both the bottom and top of each one. Serve warm or at room temperature.

Christmas Eggnog Bread

Servings: 6

Cooking Time: 18 Minutes

Ingredients:

- 1 cup flour, plus more for dusting
- ¼ cup sugar
- 1 teaspoon baking powder
- ¼ teaspoon salt
- ¼ teaspoon nutmeg
- ½ cup eggnog
- 1 egg yolk
- 1 tablespoon butter, plus 1 teaspoon, melted
- ¼ cup pecans
- ¼ cup chopped candied fruit (cherries, pineapple, or mixed fruits)
- cooking spray

Directions:

1. Preheat air fryer to 360°F.
2. In a medium bowl, stir together the flour, sugar, baking powder, salt, and nutmeg.
3. Add eggnog, egg yolk, and butter. Mix well but do not beat.
4. Stir in nuts and fruit.
5. Spray a 6 x 6-inch baking pan with cooking spray and dust with flour.
6. Spread batter into prepared pan and cook at 360°F for 18 minutes or until top is dark golden brown and bread starts to pull away from sides of pan.

Western Omelet

Servings: 2

Cooking Time: 22 Minutes

Ingredients:

- ¼ cup chopped onion
- ¼ cup chopped bell pepper, green or red
- ¼ cup diced ham
- 1 teaspoon butter
- 4 large eggs
- 2 tablespoons milk
- ⅛ teaspoon salt
- ¾ cup grated sharp Cheddar cheese

Directions:

1. Place onion, bell pepper, ham, and butter in air fryer baking pan. Cook at 390°F for 1 minute and stir. Continue cooking 5minutes, until vegetables are tender.
2. Beat together eggs, milk, and salt. Pour over vegetables and ham in baking pan. Cook at 360°F for 15minutes or until eggs set and top has browned slightly.
3. Sprinkle grated cheese on top of omelet. Cook 1 minute or just long enough to melt the cheese.

Green Onion Pancakes

Servings: 4
Cooking Time: 8 Minutes

Ingredients:

- 2 cup all-purpose flour
- ½ teaspoon salt
- ¾ cup hot water
- 1 tablespoon vegetable oil
- 1 tablespoon butter, melted
- 2 cups finely chopped green onions
- 1 tablespoon black sesame seeds, for garnish

Directions:

1. In a large bowl, whisk together the flour and salt. Make a well in the center and pour in the hot water. Quickly stir the flour mixture together until a dough forms. Knead the dough for 5 minutes; then cover with a warm, wet towel and set aside for 30 minutes to rest.
2. In a small bowl, mix together the vegetable oil and melted butter.
3. On a floured surface, place the dough and cut it into 8 pieces. Working with 1 piece of dough at a time, use a rolling pin to roll out the dough until it's ¼ inch thick; then brush the surface with the oil and butter mixture and sprinkle with green onions. Next, fold the dough in half and then in half again. Roll out the dough again until it's ¼ inch thick and brush with the oil and butter mixture and green onions. Fold the dough in half and then in half again and roll out one last time until it's ¼ inch thick. Repeat this technique with all 8 pieces.
4. Meanwhile, preheat the air fryer to 400°F.
5. Place 1 or 2 pancakes into the air fryer basket (or as many as will fit in your fryer), and cook for 2 minutes or until crispy and golden brown. Repeat until all the pancakes are cooked. Top with black sesame seeds for garnish, if desired.

Soft Pretzels

Servings: 12
Cooking Time: 6 Minutes

Ingredients:

- 2 teaspoons yeast
- 1 cup water, warm
- 1 teaspoon sugar
- 1 teaspoon salt
- 2½ cups all-purpose flour
- 2 tablespoons butter, melted
- 1 cup boiling water
- 1 tablespoon baking soda
- coarse sea salt
- melted butter

Directions:

1. Combine the yeast and water in a small bowl. Combine the sugar, salt and flour in the bowl of a stand mixer. With the mixer running and using the dough hook, drizzle in the yeast mixture and melted butter and knead dough until smooth and elastic – about 10 minutes. Shape into a ball and let the dough rise for 1 hour.
2. Punch the dough down to release any air and decide what size pretzels you want to make.
3. a. To make large pretzels, divide the dough into 12 portions.
4. b. To make medium sized pretzels, divide the dough into 24 portions.
5. c. To make mini pretzel knots, divide the dough into 48 portions.
6. Roll each portion into a skinny rope using both hands on the counter and rolling from the center to the ends of the rope. Spin the rope into a pretzel shape (or tie the rope into a knot) and place the tied pretzels on a parchment lined baking sheet.
7. Preheat the air fryer to 350°F.
8. Combine the boiling water and baking soda in a shallow bowl and whisk to dissolve (this mixture will bubble, but it will settle down). Let the water cool so that you can put your hands in it. Working in batches,

dip the pretzels (top side down) into the baking soda-water mixture and let them soak for 30 seconds to a minute. (This step is what gives pretzels their texture and helps them to brown faster.) Then, remove the pretzels carefully and return them (top side up) to the baking sheet. Sprinkle the coarse salt on the top.

9. Air-fry in batches for 3 minutes per side. When the pretzels are finished, brush them generously with the melted butter and enjoy them warm with some spicy mustard.

Banana Bread

Servings: 6

Cooking Time: 20 Minutes

Ingredients:

- cooking spray
- 1 cup white wheat flour
- ½ teaspoon baking powder
- ¼ teaspoon salt
- ¼ teaspoon baking soda
- 1 egg
- ½ cup mashed ripe banana
- ¼ cup plain yogurt
- ¼ cup pure maple syrup
- 2 tablespoons coconut oil
- ½ teaspoon pure vanilla extract

Directions:

1. Preheat air fryer to 330°F.
2. Lightly spray 6 x 6-inch baking dish with cooking spray.
3. In a medium bowl, mix together the flour, baking powder, salt, and soda.
4. In a separate bowl, beat the egg and add the mashed banana, yogurt, syrup, oil, and vanilla. Mix until well combined.
5. Pour liquid mixture into dry ingredients and stir gently to blend. Do not beat. Batter may be slightly lumpy.
6. Pour batter into baking dish and cook at 330°F for 20 minutes or until toothpick inserted in center of loaf comes out clean.

Cheddar-ham-corn Muffins

Servings: 8

Cooking Time: 8 Minutes

Ingredients:

- ¾ cup yellow cornmeal
- ¼ cup flour
- 1½ teaspoons baking powder
- ¼ teaspoon salt
- 1 egg, beaten
- 2 tablespoons canola oil
- ½ cup milk
- ½ cup shredded sharp Cheddar cheese
- ½ cup diced ham
- 8 foil muffin cups, liners removed and sprayed with cooking spray

Directions:

1. Preheat air fryer to 390°F.
2. In a medium bowl, stir together the cornmeal, flour, baking powder, and salt.
3. Add egg, oil, and milk to dry ingredients and mix well.
4. Stir in shredded cheese and diced ham.
5. Divide batter among the muffin cups.
6. Place 4 filled muffin cups in air fryer basket and bake for 5minutes.
7. Reduce temperature to 330°F and bake for 1 to 2minutes or until toothpick inserted in center of muffin comes out clean.
8. Repeat steps 6 and 7 to cook remaining muffins.

Sweet-hot Pepperoni Pizza

Servings: 2

Cooking Time: 18 Minutes

Ingredients:

- 1 (6- to 8-ounce) pizza dough ball*
- olive oil
- ½ cup pizza sauce
- ¾ cup grated mozzarella cheese
- ½ cup thick sliced pepperoni
- ⅓ cup sliced pickled hot banana peppers
- ¼ teaspoon dried oregano
- 2 teaspoons honey

Directions:

1. Preheat the air fryer to 390°F.
2. Cut out a piece of aluminum foil the same size as the bottom of the air fryer basket. Brush the foil circle with olive oil. Shape the dough into a circle and place it on top of the foil. Dock the dough by piercing it several times with a fork. Brush the dough lightly with olive oil and transfer it into the air fryer basket with the foil on the bottom.
3. Air-fry the plain pizza dough for 6 minutes. Turn the dough over, remove the aluminum foil and brush again with olive oil. Air-fry for an additional 4 minutes.
4. Spread the pizza sauce on top of the dough and sprinkle the mozzarella cheese over the sauce. Top with the pepperoni, pepper slices and dried oregano. Lower the temperature of the air fryer to 350°F and cook for 8 minutes, until the cheese has melted and lightly browned. Transfer the pizza to a cutting board and drizzle with the honey. Slice and serve.

Egg Muffins

Servings: 4
Cooking Time: 11 Minutes

Ingredients:

- 4 eggs
- salt and pepper
- olive oil
- 4 English muffins, split
- 1 cup shredded Colby Jack cheese
- 4 slices ham or Canadian bacon

Directions:

1. Preheat air fryer to 390°F.
2. Beat together eggs and add salt and pepper to taste. Spray air fryer baking pan lightly with oil and add eggs. Cook for 2minutes, stir, and continue cooking for 4minutes, stirring every minute, until eggs are scrambled to your preference. Remove pan from air fryer.
3. Place bottom halves of English muffins in air fryer basket. Take half of the shredded cheese and divide it among the muffins. Top each with a slice of ham and one-quarter of the eggs. Sprinkle remaining cheese on top of the eggs. Use a fork to press the cheese into the egg a little so it doesn't slip off before it melts.
4. Cook at 360°F for 1 minute. Add English muffin tops and cook for 4minutes to heat through and toast the muffins.

Pizza Dough

Servings: 3
Cooking Time: 10 Minutes

Ingredients:

- 4 cups bread flour, pizza ("00") flour or all-purpose flour
- 1 teaspoon active dry yeast
- 2 teaspoons sugar
- 2 teaspoons salt
- 1½ cups water
- 1 tablespoon olive oil

Directions:

1. Combine the flour, yeast, sugar and salt in the bowl of a stand mixer. Add the olive oil to the flour mixture and start to mix using the dough hook attachment. As you're mixing, add 1¼ cups of the water, mixing until the dough comes together. Continue to knead the dough with the dough hook for another 10 minutes, adding enough water to the dough to get it to the right consistency.
2. Transfer the dough to a floured counter and divide it into 3 equal portions. Roll each portion into a ball. Lightly coat each dough ball with oil and transfer to the refrigerator, covered with plastic wrap. You can place them all on a baking sheet, or place each dough ball into its own oiled zipper sealable plastic bag or container. (You can freeze the dough balls at this stage, removing as much air as possible from the oiled bag.) Keep in the refrigerator for at least one day, or as long as five days.
3. When you're ready to use the dough, remove your dough from the refrigerator at least 1 hour prior to baking and let it sit on the counter, covered gently with plastic wrap.

Chocolate Almond Crescent Rolls

Servings: 4

Cooking Time: 8 Minutes

Ingredients:

- 1 (8-ounce) tube of crescent roll dough
- ⅔ cup semi-sweet or bittersweet chocolate chunks
- 1 egg white, lightly beaten
- ¼ cup sliced almonds
- powdered sugar, for dusting
- butter or oil

Directions:

1. Preheat the air fryer to 350°F.
2. Unwrap the crescent roll dough and separate it into triangles with the points facing away from you. Place a row of chocolate chunks along the bottom edge of the dough. (If you are using chips, make it a double row.) Roll the dough up around the chocolate and then place another row of chunks on the dough. Roll again and finish with one or two chocolate chunks. Be sure to leave the end free of chocolate so that it can adhere to the rest of the roll.
3. Brush the tops of the crescent rolls with the lightly beaten egg white and sprinkle the almonds on top, pressing them into the crescent dough so they adhere.
4. Brush the bottom of the air fryer basket with butter or oil and transfer the crescent rolls to the basket. Air-fry at 350°F for 8 minutes. Remove and let the crescent rolls cool before dusting with powdered sugar and serving.

Peppered Maple Bacon Knots

Servings: 6

Cooking Time: 8 Minutes

Ingredients:

- 1 pound maple smoked center-cut bacon
- ¼ cup maple syrup
- ¼ cup brown sugar
- coarsely cracked black peppercorns

Directions:

1. Tie each bacon strip in a loose knot and place them on a baking sheet.
2. Combine the maple syrup and brown sugar in a bowl. Brush each knot generously with this mixture and sprinkle with coarsely cracked black pepper.
3. Preheat the air fryer to 390°F.
4. Air-fry the bacon knots in batches. Place one layer of knots in the air fryer basket and air-fry for 5 minutes. Turn the bacon knots over and air-fry for an additional 3 minutes.
5. Serve warm.

Fried Pb&j

Servings: 4

Cooking Time: 8 Minutes

Ingredients:

- ½ cup cornflakes, crushed
- ¼ cup shredded coconut
- 8 slices oat nut bread or any whole-grain, oversize bread
- 6 tablespoons peanut butter
- 2 medium bananas, cut into ½-inch-thick slices
- 6 tablespoons pineapple preserves
- 1 egg, beaten
- oil for misting or cooking spray

Directions:

1. Preheat air fryer to 360°F.
2. In a shallow dish, mix together the cornflake crumbs and coconut.
3. For each sandwich, spread one bread slice with 1½ tablespoons of peanut butter. Top with banana slices. Spread another bread slice with 1½ tablespoons of preserves. Combine to make a sandwich.
4. Using a pastry brush, brush top of sandwich lightly with beaten egg. Sprinkle with about 1½ tablespoons of crumb coating, pressing it in to make it stick. Spray with oil.
5. Turn sandwich over and repeat to coat and spray the other side.
6. Cooking 2 at a time, place sandwiches in air fryer basket and cook for 6 to 7minutes or until coating is golden brown and crispy. If sandwich doesn't brown enough, spray with a little more oil and cook at 390°F for another minute.
7. Cut cooked sandwiches in half and serve warm.

Chocolate Chip Banana Muffins

Servings: 12

Cooking Time: 14 Minutes

Ingredients:

- 2 medium bananas, mashed
- ¼ cup brown sugar
- 1½ teaspoons vanilla extract
- ⅔ cup milk
- 2 tablespoons butter
- 1 large egg
- 1 cup white whole-wheat flour
- ½ cup old-fashioned oats
- 1 teaspoon baking soda
- ½ teaspoon baking powder
- ⅛ teaspoon sea salt
- ¼ cup mini chocolate chips

Directions:

1. Preheat the air fryer to 330°F.
2. In a large bowl, combine the bananas, brown sugar, vanilla extract, milk, butter, and egg; set aside.
3. In a separate bowl, combine the flour, oats, baking soda, baking powder, and salt.
4. Slowly add the dry ingredients into the wet ingredients, folding in the flour mixture ⅓ cup at a time.
5. Mix in the chocolate chips and set aside.
6. Using silicone muffin liners, fill 6 muffin liners two-thirds full. Carefully place the muffin liners in the air fryer basket and bake for 20 minutes (or until the tops are browned and a toothpick inserted in the center comes out clean). Carefully remove the muffins from the basket and repeat with the remaining batter.
7. Serve warm.

Garlic-cheese Biscuits

Servings: 8

Cooking Time: 8 Minutes

Ingredients:

- 1 cup self-rising flour
- 1 teaspoon garlic powder
- 2 tablespoons butter, diced
- 2 ounces sharp Cheddar cheese, grated
- ½ cup milk
- cooking spray

Directions:

1. Preheat air fryer to 330°F.
2. Combine flour and garlic in a medium bowl and stir together.
3. Using a pastry blender or knives, cut butter into dry ingredients.
4. Stir in cheese.
5. Add milk and stir until stiff dough forms.
6. If dough is too sticky to handle, stir in 1 or 2 more tablespoons of self-rising flour before shaping. Biscuits should be firm enough to hold their shape. Otherwise, they'll stick to the air fryer basket.
7. Divide dough into 8 portions and shape into 2-inch biscuits about ¾-inch thick.
8. Spray air fryer basket with nonstick cooking spray.
9. Place all 8 biscuits in basket and cook at 330°F for 8 minutes.

Zucchini Walnut Bread

Servings: 6

Cooking Time: 30 Minutes

Ingredients:

- ¾ cup all-purpose flour
- ½ teaspoon baking soda
- 1 teaspoon ground cinnamon
- ⅛ teaspoon salt
- 1 large egg
- ⅓ cup packed brown sugar
- ¼ cup canola oil
- 1 teaspoon vanilla extract
- ⅓ cup milk
- 1 medium zucchini, shredded (about 1⅓ cups)
- ⅓ cup chopped walnuts

Directions:

1. Preheat the air fryer to 320°F.
2. In a medium bowl, mix together the flour, baking soda, cinnamon, and salt.
3. In a large bowl, whisk together the egg, brown sugar, oil, vanilla, and milk. Stir in the zucchini.
4. Slowly fold the dry ingredients into the wet ingredients. Stir in the chopped walnuts. Then pour the batter into two 4-inch oven-safe loaf pans.

5. Bake for 30 minutes or until a toothpick inserted into the center comes out clean. Let cool before slicing.
6. NOTE: Store tightly wrapped on the counter for up to 5 days, in the refrigerator for up to 10 days, or in the freezer for 3 months.

Almond Cranberry Granola

Servings: 12
Cooking Time: 9 Minutes

Ingredients:

- 2 tablespoons sesame seeds
- ¼ cup chopped almonds
- ¼ cup sunflower seeds
- ½ cup unsweetened shredded coconut
- 2 tablespoons unsalted butter, melted or at least softened
- 2 tablespoons coconut oil
- ⅓ cup honey
- 2½ cups oats
- ¼ teaspoon sea salt
- ½ cup dried cranberries

Directions:

1. In a large mixing bowl, stir together the sesame seeds, almonds, sunflower seeds, coconut, butter, coconut oil, honey, oats, and salt.
2. Line the air fryer basket with parchment paper. Punch 8 to 10 holes into the parchment paper with a fork so air can circulate. Pour the granola mixture onto the parchment paper.
3. Air fry the granola at 350°F for 9 minutes, stirring every 3 minutes.
4. When cooking is complete, stir in the dried cranberries and allow the mixture to cool. Store in an airtight container up to 2 weeks or freeze for 6 months.

Classic Cinnamon Rolls

Servings: 4
Cooking Time: 6 Minutes

Ingredients:

- 1½ cups all-purpose flour
- 1 tablespoon granulated sugar
- 2 teaspoons baking powder
- ½ teaspoon salt
- 4 tablespoons butter, divided
- ½ cup buttermilk
- 2 tablespoons brown sugar
- 1 teaspoon cinnamon
- 1 cup powdered sugar
- 2 tablespoons milk

Directions:

1. Preheat the air fryer to 360°F.
2. In a large bowl, stir together the flour, sugar, baking powder, and salt. Cut in 3 tablespoons of the butter with a pastry blender or two knives until coarse crumbs remain. Stir in the buttermilk until a dough forms.
3. Place the dough onto a floured surface and roll out into a square shape about ½ inch thick.
4. Melt the remaining 1 tablespoon of butter in the microwave for 20 seconds. Using a pastry brush or your fingers, spread the melted butter onto the dough.
5. In a small bowl, mix together the brown sugar and cinnamon. Sprinkle the mixture across the surface of the dough. Roll the dough up, forming a long log. Using a pastry cutter or sharp knife, cut 10 cinnamon rolls.
6. Carefully place the cinnamon rolls into the air fryer basket. Then bake at 360°F for 6 minutes or until golden brown.
7. Meanwhile, in a small bowl, whisk together the powdered sugar and milk.
8. Plate the cinnamon rolls and drizzle the glaze over the surface before serving.

Pigs In A Blanket

Servings: 10
Cooking Time: 8 Minutes

Ingredients:

- 1 cup all-purpose flour, plus more for rolling
- 1 teaspoon baking powder
- ¼ cup salted butter, cut into small pieces
- ½ cup buttermilk
- 10 fully cooked breakfast sausage links

Directions:

1. In a large mixing bowl, whisk together the flour and baking powder. Using your fingers or a pastry blender, cut in the butter until you have small pea-size crumbles.

2. Using a rubber spatula, make a well in the center of the flour mixture. Pour the buttermilk into the well, and fold the mixture together until you form a dough ball.
3. Place the sticky dough onto a floured surface and, using a floured rolling pin, roll out until ½-inch thick. Using a round biscuit cutter, cut out 10 rounds, reshaping the dough and rolling out, as needed.
4. Place 1 fully cooked breakfast sausage link on the left edge of each biscuit and roll up, leaving the ends slightly exposed.
5. Using a pastry brush, brush the biscuits with the whisked eggs, and spray them with cooking spray.
6. Place the pigs in a blanket into the air fryer basket with at least 1 inch between each biscuit. Set the air fryer to 340°F and cook for 8 minutes.

Cajun Breakfast Potatoes

Servings: 4
Cooking Time: 20 Minutes

Ingredients:

- 1 pound roasting potatoes (like russet), scrubbed clean
- 1 tablespoon vegetable oil
- 2 teaspoons paprika
- ½ teaspoon garlic powder
- ¼ teaspoon onion powder
- ¼ teaspoon ground cumin
- 1 teaspoon thyme
- 1 teaspoon sea salt
- ½ teaspoon black pepper

Directions:

1. Cut the potatoes into 1-inch cubes.
2. In a large bowl, toss the cut potatoes with vegetable oil.
3. Sprinkle paprika, garlic powder, onion powder, cumin, thyme, salt, and pepper onto the potatoes, and toss to coat well.
4. Preheat the air fryer to 400°F for 4 minutes.
5. Add the potatoes to the air fryer basket and bake for 10 minutes. Stir or toss the potatoes and continue baking for an additional 5 minutes. Stir or toss again and continue baking for an additional 5 minutes or until the desired crispness is achieved.

Sweet And Spicy Pumpkin Scones

Servings: 8
Cooking Time: 8 Minutes

Ingredients:

- 2 cups all-purpose flour
- 3 tablespoons packed brown sugar
- ½ teaspoon baking powder
- ¼ teaspoon baking soda
- ½ teaspoon kosher salt
- ½ teaspoon ground cinnamon
- ¼ teaspoon ground ginger
- ¼ teaspoon ground cardamom
- 4 tablespoons cold unsalted butter
- ½ cup plus 2 tablespoons pumpkin puree, divided
- 4 tablespoons milk, divided
- 1 large egg
- 1 cup powdered sugar

Directions:

1. In a large bowl, mix together the flour, brown sugar, baking powder, baking soda, salt, cinnamon, ginger, and cardamom. Using a pastry blender or two knives, cut in the butter until coarse crumbles appear.
2. In a small bowl, whisk together ½ cup of the pumpkin puree, 2 tablespoons of the milk, and the egg until combined. Pour the wet ingredients into the dry ingredients; stir to combine.
3. Form the dough into a ball and place onto a floured service. Press the dough out or use a rolling pin to roll out the dough until ½ inch thick and in a circle. Cut the dough into 8 wedges.
4. Bake at 360°F for 8 to 10 minutes or until completely cooked through. Cook in batches as needed.
5. In a medium bowl, whisk together the powdered sugar, the remaining 2 tablespoons of pumpkin puree, and the remaining 2 tablespoons of milk. When the pumpkin scones have cooled, drizzle the pumpkin glaze over the top before serving.

Sweet Potato-cinnamon Toast

Servings: 6
Cooking Time: 8 Minutes

Ingredients:

- 1 small sweet potato, cut into ⅜-inch slices
- oil for misting
- ground cinnamon

Directions:

1. Preheat air fryer to 390°F.
2. Spray both sides of sweet potato slices with oil. Sprinkle both sides with cinnamon to taste.
3. Place potato slices in air fryer basket in a single layer.
4. Cook for 4minutes, turn, and cook for 4 more minutes or until potato slices are barely fork tender.

Goat Cheese, Beet, And Kale Frittata

Servings: 6
Cooking Time: 20 Minutes

Ingredients:

- 6 large eggs
- ½ teaspoon garlic powder
- ¼ teaspoon black pepper
- ¼ teaspoon salt
- 1 cup chopped kale
- 1 cup cooked and chopped red beets
- ⅓ cup crumbled goat cheese

Directions:

1. Preheat the air fryer to 320°F.
2. In a medium bowl, whisk the eggs with the garlic powder, pepper, and salt. Mix in the kale, beets, and goat cheese.
3. Spray an oven-safe 7-inch springform pan with cooking spray. Pour the egg mixture into the pan and place it in the air fryer basket.
4. Cook for 20 minutes, or until the internal temperature reaches 145°F.
5. When the frittata is cooked, let it set for 5 minutes before removing from the pan.
6. Slice and serve immediately.

Hole In One

Servings: 1
Cooking Time: 7 Minutes

Ingredients:

- 1 slice bread
- 1 teaspoon soft butter
- 1 egg
- salt and pepper
- 1 tablespoon shredded Cheddar cheese
- 2 teaspoons diced ham

Directions:

1. Place a 6 x 6-inch baking dish inside air fryer basket and preheat fryer to 330°F.
2. Using a 2½-inch-diameter biscuit cutter, cut a hole in center of bread slice.
3. Spread softened butter on both sides of bread.
4. Lay bread slice in baking dish and crack egg into the hole. Sprinkle egg with salt and pepper to taste.
5. Cook for 5minutes.
6. Turn toast over and top it with shredded cheese and diced ham.
7. Cook for 2 more minutes or until yolk is done to your liking.

Oat Bran Muffins

Servings: 8
Cooking Time: 12 Minutes

Ingredients:

- ⅔ cup oat bran
- ½ cup flour
- ¼ cup brown sugar
- 1 teaspoon baking powder
- ½ teaspoon baking soda
- ⅛ teaspoon salt
- ½ cup buttermilk
- 1 egg
- 2 tablespoons canola oil
- ½ cup chopped dates, raisins, or dried cranberries
- 24 paper muffin cups
- cooking spray

Directions:

1. Preheat air fryer to 330°F.
2. In a large bowl, combine the oat bran, flour, brown sugar, baking powder, baking soda, and salt.

3. In a small bowl, beat together the buttermilk, egg, and oil.
4. Pour buttermilk mixture into bowl with dry ingredients and stir just until moistened. Do not beat.
5. Gently stir in dried fruit.
6. Use triple baking cups to help muffins hold shape during baking. Spray them with cooking spray, place 4 sets of cups in air fryer basket at a time, and fill each one ¾ full of batter.
7. Cook for 12minutes, until top springs back when lightly touched and toothpick inserted in center comes out clean.
8. Repeat for remaining muffins.

Cinnamon Biscuit Rolls

Servings: 12
Cooking Time: 5 Minutes

Ingredients:

- Dough
- ¼ cup warm water (105–115°F)
- 1 teaspoon active dry yeast
- 1 tablespoon sugar
- ½ cup buttermilk, lukewarm
- 2 cups flour, plus more for dusting
- 1 teaspoon baking powder
- ½ teaspoon salt
- 3 tablespoons cold butter
- Filling
- 1 tablespoon butter, melted
- 1 teaspoon cinnamon
- 2 tablespoons sugar
- Icing
- ⅔ cup powdered sugar
- ¼ teaspoon vanilla
- 2–3 teaspoons milk

Directions:

1. Dissolve yeast and sugar in warm water. Add buttermilk, stir, and set aside.
2. In a large bowl, sift together flour, baking powder, and salt. Using knives or a pastry blender, cut in butter until mixture is well combined and crumbly.
3. Pour in buttermilk mixture and stir with fork until a ball of dough forms.
4. Knead dough on a lightly floured surface for 5minutes. Roll into an 8 x 11-inch rectangle.
5. For the filling, spread the melted butter over the dough.
6. In a small bowl, stir together the cinnamon and sugar, then sprinkle over dough.
7. Starting on a long side, roll up dough so that you have a roll about 11 inches long. Cut into 12 slices with a serrated knife and sawing motion so slices remain round.
8. Place rolls on a plate or cookie sheet about an inch apart and let rise for 30minutes.
9. For icing, mix the powdered sugar, vanilla, and milk. Stir and add additional milk until icing reaches a good spreading consistency.
10. Preheat air fryer to 360°F.
11. Place 6 cinnamon rolls in basket and cook 5 minutes or until top springs back when lightly touched. Repeat to cook remaining 6 rolls.
12. Spread icing over warm rolls and serve.

Apple Fritters

Servings: 6
Cooking Time: 12 Minutes

Ingredients:

- 1 cup all-purpose flour
- 1½ teaspoons baking powder
- ¼ teaspoon salt
- 2 tablespoon brown sugar
- 1 teaspoon vanilla extract
- ¾ cup plain Greek yogurt
- 1 tablespoon cinnamon
- 1 large Granny Smith apple, cored, peeled, and finely chopped
- ¼ cup chopped walnuts
- ½ cup powdered sugar
- 1 tablespoon milk

Directions:

1. Preheat the air fryer to 320°F.
2. In a medium bowl, combine the flour, baking powder, and salt.
3. In a large bowl, add the brown sugar, vanilla, yogurt, cinnamon, apples, and walnuts. Mix the dry ingredients into the wet, using your hands to combine, until all the

ingredients are mixed together. Knead the mixture in the bowl about 4 times.

4. Lightly spray the air fryer basket with olive oil spray.
5. Divide the batter into 6 equally sized balls; then lightly flatten them and place inside the basket. Repeat until all the fritters are formed.
6. Place the basket in the air fryer and cook for 6 minutes, flip, and then cook another 6 minutes.
7. While the fritters are cooking, in a small bowl, mix the powdered sugar with the milk. Set aside.
8. When the cooking completes, remove the air fryer basket and allow the fritters to cool on a wire rack. Drizzle with the homemade glaze and serve.

Broccoli Cornbread

Servings: 6

Cooking Time: 18 Minutes

Ingredients:

- 1 cup frozen chopped broccoli, thawed and drained
- ¼ cup cottage cheese
- 1 egg, beaten
- 2 tablespoons minced onion
- 2 tablespoons melted butter
- ½ cup flour
- ½ cup yellow cornmeal
- 1 teaspoon baking powder
- ½ teaspoon salt
- ¼ cup milk, plus 2 tablespoons
- cooking spray

Directions:

1. Place thawed broccoli in colander and press with a spoon to squeeze out excess moisture.
2. Stir together all ingredients in a large bowl.
3. Spray 6 x 6-inch baking pan with cooking spray.
4. Spread batter in pan and cook at 330°F for 18 minutes or until cornbread is lightly browned and loaf starts to pull away from sides of pan.

Roasted Vegetable Frittata

Servings: 1

Cooking Time: 19 Minutes

Ingredients:

- ½ red or green bell pepper, cut into ½-inch chunks
- 4 button mushrooms, sliced
- ½ cup diced zucchini
- ½ teaspoon chopped fresh oregano or thyme
- 1 teaspoon olive oil
- 3 eggs, beaten
- ½ cup grated Cheddar cheese
- salt and freshly ground black pepper, to taste
- 1 teaspoon butter
- 1 teaspoon chopped fresh parsley

Directions:

1. Preheat the air fryer to 400°F.
2. Toss the peppers, mushrooms, zucchini and oregano with the olive oil and air-fry for 6 minutes, shaking the basket once or twice during the cooking process to redistribute the ingredients.
3. While the vegetables are cooking, beat the eggs well in a bowl, stir in the Cheddar cheese and season with salt and freshly ground black pepper. Add the air-fried vegetables to this bowl when they have finished cooking.
4. Place a 6- or 7-inch non-stick metal cake pan into the air fryer basket with the butter using an aluminum sling to lower the pan into the basket. (Fold a piece of aluminum foil into a strip about 2-inches wide by 24-inches long.) Air-fry for 1 minute at 380°F to melt the butter. Remove the cake pan and rotate the pan to distribute the butter and grease the pan. Pour the egg mixture into the cake pan and return the pan to the air fryer, using the aluminum sling.
5. Air-fry at 380°F for 12 minutes, or until the frittata has puffed up and is lightly browned. Let the frittata sit in the air fryer for 5 minutes to cool to an edible temperature and set up. Remove the cake pan from the air fryer, sprinkle with parsley and serve immediately.

French Toast And Turkey Sausage Roll-ups

Servings: 3
Cooking Time: 24 Minutes

Ingredients:

- 6 links turkey sausage
- 6 slices of white bread, crusts removed*
- 2 eggs
- ½ cup milk
- ½ teaspoon ground cinnamon
- ½ teaspoon vanilla extract
- 1 tablespoon butter, melted
- powdered sugar (optional)
- maple syrup

Directions:

1. Preheat the air fryer to 380°F and pour a little water into the bottom of the air fryer drawer. (This will help prevent the grease that drips into the bottom drawer from burning and smoking.)
2. Air-fry the sausage links at 380°F for 8 to 10 minutes, turning them a couple of times during the cooking process. (If you have pre-cooked sausage links, omit this step.)
3. Roll each sausage link in a piece of bread, pressing the finished seam tightly to seal shut.
4. Preheat the air fryer to 370°F.
5. Combine the eggs, milk, cinnamon, and vanilla in a shallow dish. Dip the sausage rolls in the egg mixture and let them soak in the egg for 30 seconds. Spray or brush the bottom of the air fryer basket with oil and transfer the sausage rolls to the basket, seam side down.
6. Air-fry the rolls at 370°F for 9 minutes. Brush melted butter over the bread, flip the rolls over and air-fry for an additional 5 minutes. Remove the French toast roll-ups from the basket and dust with powdered sugar, if using. Serve with maple syrup and enjoy.

Fry Bread

Servings: 4
Cooking Time: 5 Minutes

Ingredients:

- 1 cup flour
- 2 teaspoons baking powder
- ¼ teaspoon salt
- ¼ cup lukewarm milk
- 1 teaspoon oil
- 2–3 tablespoons water
- oil for misting or cooking spray

Directions:

1. Stir together flour, baking powder, and salt. Gently mix in the milk and oil. Stir in 1 tablespoon water. If needed, add more water 1 tablespoon at a time until stiff dough forms. Dough shouldn't be sticky, so use only as much as you need.
2. Divide dough into 4 portions and shape into balls. Cover with a towel and let rest for 10minutes.
3. Preheat air fryer to 390°F.
4. Shape dough as desired:
5. a. Pat into 3-inch circles. This will make a thicker bread to eat plain or with a sprinkle of cinnamon or honey butter. You can cook all 4 at once.
6. b. Pat thinner into rectangles about 3 x 6 inches. This will create a thinner bread to serve as a base for dishes such as Indian tacos. The circular shape is more traditional, but rectangles allow you to cook 2 at a time in your air fryer basket.
7. Spray both sides of dough pieces with oil or cooking spray.
8. Place the 4 circles or 2 of the dough rectangles in the air fryer basket and cook at 390°F for 3minutes. Spray tops, turn, spray other side, and cook for 2 more minutes. If necessary, repeat to cook remaining bread.
9. Serve piping hot as is or allow to cool slightly and add toppings to create your own Native American tacos.

Carrot Orange Muffins

Servings: 12
Cooking Time: 12 Minutes

Ingredients:

- 1½ cups all-purpose flour
- ½ cup granulated sugar
- ½ teaspoon ground cinnamon
- 2 teaspoons baking powder
- ¼ teaspoon baking soda
- ½ teaspoon salt

- 2 large eggs
- ¼ cup vegetable oil
- ⅓ cup orange marmalade
- 2 cups grated carrots

Directions:

1. Preheat the air fryer to 320°F.
2. In a large bowl, whisk together the flour, sugar, cinnamon, baking powder, baking soda, and salt; set aside.
3. In a separate bowl, whisk together the eggs, vegetable oil, orange marmalade, and grated carrots.
4. Make a well in the dry ingredients; then pour the wet ingredients into the well of the dry ingredients. Using a rubber spatula, mix the ingredients for 1 minute or until slightly lumpy.
5. Using silicone muffin liners, fill 6 muffin liners two-thirds full.
6. Carefully place the muffin liners in the air fryer basket and bake for 12 minutes (or until the tops are browned and a toothpick inserted in the center comes out clean). Carefully remove the muffins from the basket and repeat with remaining batter.
7. Serve warm.

Mini Pita Breads

Servings: 8

Cooking Time: 6 Minutes

Ingredients:

- 2 teaspoons active dry yeast
- 1 tablespoon sugar
- 1¼ to 1½ cups warm water (90° - 110°F)
- 3¼ cups all-purpose flour
- 2 teaspoons salt
- 1 tablespoon olive oil, plus more for brushing
- kosher salt (optional)

Directions:

1. Dissolve the yeast, sugar and water in the bowl of a stand mixer. Let the mixture sit for 5 minutes to make sure the yeast is active – it should foam a little. (If there's no foaming, discard and start again with new yeast.) Combine the flour and salt in a bowl, and add it to the water, along with the olive oil. Mix with the dough hook until combined. Add a little more flour if needed to get the dough to pull away from the sides of the mixing bowl, or add a little more water if the dough seems too dry.
2. Knead the dough until it is smooth and elastic (about 8 minutes in the mixer or 15 minutes by hand). Transfer the dough to a lightly oiled bowl, cover and let it rise in a warm place until doubled in bulk. Divide the dough into 8 portions and roll each portion into a circle about 4-inches in diameter. Don't roll the balls too thin, or you won't get the pocket inside the pita.
3. Preheat the air fryer to 400°F.
4. Brush both sides of the dough with olive oil, and sprinkle with kosher salt if desired. Air-fry one at a time at 400°F for 6 minutes, flipping it over when there are two minutes left in the cooking time.

Ham And Cheddar Gritters

Servings: 6

Cooking Time: 12 Minutes

Ingredients:

- 4 cups water
- 1 cup quick-cooking grits
- ¼ teaspoon salt
- 2 tablespoons butter
- 2 cups grated Cheddar cheese, divided
- 1 cup finely diced ham
- 1 tablespoon chopped chives
- salt and freshly ground black pepper
- 1 egg, beaten
- 2 cups panko breadcrumbs
- vegetable oil

Directions:

1. Bring the water to a boil in a saucepan. Whisk in the grits and ¼ teaspoon of salt, and cook for 7 minutes until the grits are soft. Remove the pan from the heat and stir in the butter and 1 cup of the grated Cheddar cheese. Transfer the grits to a bowl and let them cool for just 10 to 15 minutes.
2. Stir the ham, chives and the rest of the cheese into the grits and season with salt and pepper to taste. Add the beaten egg and refrigerate the mixture for 30 minutes. (Try not to chill the grits much longer than 30 minutes, or the mixture will be too firm to shape into patties.)

3. While the grit mixture is chilling, make the country gravy and set it aside.
4. Place the panko breadcrumbs in a shallow dish. Measure out ¼-cup portions of the grits mixture and shape them into patties. Coat all sides of the patties with the panko breadcrumbs, patting them with your hands so the crumbs adhere to the patties. You should have about 16 patties. Spray both sides of the patties with oil.
5. Preheat the air fryer to 400°F.
6. In batches of 5 or 6, air-fry the fritters for 8 minutes. Using a flat spatula, flip the fritters over and air-fry for another 4 minutes.
7. Serve hot with country gravy.

Hush Puffins

Servings: 20
Cooking Time: 8 Minutes

Ingredients:

- 1 cup buttermilk
- ¼ cup butter, melted
- 2 eggs
- 1½ cups all-purpose flour
- 1½ cups cornmeal
- ⅓ cup sugar
- 1 teaspoon baking soda
- 1 teaspoon salt
- 4 scallions, minced
- vegetable oil

Directions:

1. Combine the buttermilk, butter and eggs in a large mixing bowl. In a second bowl combine the flour, cornmeal, sugar, baking soda and salt. Add the dry ingredients to the wet ingredients, stirring just to combine. Stir in the minced scallions and refrigerate the batter for 30 minutes.
2. Shape the batter into 2-inch balls. Brush or spray the balls with oil.
3. Preheat the air fryer to 360°F.
4. Air-fry the hush puffins in two batches at 360°F for 8 minutes, turning them over after 6 minutes of the cooking process.
5. Serve warm with butter.

Southern Sweet Cornbread

Servings: 6
Cooking Time: 17 Minutes

Ingredients:

- cooking spray
- ½ cup white cornmeal
- ½ cup flour
- 2 teaspoons baking powder
- ½ teaspoon salt
- 4 teaspoons sugar
- 1 egg
- 2 tablespoons oil
- ½ cup milk

Directions:

1. Preheat air fryer to 360°F.
2. Spray air fryer baking pan with nonstick cooking spray.
3. In a medium bowl, stir together the cornmeal, flour, baking powder, salt, and sugar.
4. In a small bowl, beat together the egg, oil, and milk. Stir into dry ingredients until well combined.
5. Pour batter into prepared baking pan.
6. Cook at 360°F for 17 minutes or until toothpick inserted in center comes out clean or with crumbs clinging.

Western Frittata

Servings: 1
Cooking Time: 19 Minutes

Ingredients:

- ½ red or green bell pepper, cut into ½-inch chunks
- 1 teaspoon olive oil
- 3 eggs, beaten
- ¼ cup grated Cheddar cheese
- ¼ cup diced cooked ham
- salt and freshly ground black pepper, to taste
- 1 teaspoon butter
- 1 teaspoon chopped fresh parsley

Directions:

1. Preheat the air fryer to 400°F.

2. Toss the peppers with the olive oil and air-fry for 6 minutes, shaking the basket once or twice during the cooking process to redistribute the ingredients.
3. While the vegetables are cooking, beat the eggs well in a bowl, stir in the Cheddar cheese and ham, and season with salt and freshly ground black pepper. Add the air-fried peppers to this bowl when they have finished cooking.
4. Place a 6- or 7-inch non-stick metal cake pan into the air fryer basket with the butter using an aluminum sling to lower the pan into the basket. (Fold a piece of aluminum foil into a strip about 2-inches wide by 24-inches long.) Air-fry for 1 minute at 380°F to melt the butter. Remove the cake pan and rotate the pan to distribute the butter and grease the pan. Pour the egg mixture into the cake pan and return the pan to the air fryer, using the aluminum sling.
5. Air-fry at 380°F for 12 minutes, or until the frittata has puffed up and is lightly browned. Let the frittata sit in the air fryer for 5 minutes to cool to an edible temperature and set up. Remove the cake pan from the air fryer, sprinkle with parsley and serve immediately.

Not-so-english Muffins

Servings: 4
Cooking Time: 10 Minutes

Ingredients:

- 2 strips turkey bacon, cut in half crosswise
- 2 whole-grain English muffins, split
- 1 cup fresh baby spinach, long stems removed
- ¼ ripe pear, peeled and thinly sliced
- 4 slices Provolone cheese

Directions:

1. Place bacon strips in air fryer basket and cook for 2minutes. Check and separate strips if necessary so they cook evenly. Cook for 4 more minutes, until crispy. Remove and drain on paper towels.
2. Place split muffin halves in air fryer basket and cook at 390°F for 2minutes, just until lightly browned.
3. Open air fryer and top each muffin with a quarter of the baby spinach, several pear slices, a strip of bacon, and a slice of cheese.
4. Cook at 360°F for 2minutes, until cheese completely melts.

Scones

Servings: 9
Cooking Time: 8 Minutes Per Batch

Ingredients:

- 2 cups self-rising flour, plus ¼ cup for kneading
- ⅓ cup granulated sugar
- ¼ cup butter, cold
- 1 cup milk

Directions:

1. Preheat air fryer at 360°F.
2. In large bowl, stir together flour and sugar.
3. Cut cold butter into tiny cubes, and stir into flour mixture with fork.
4. Stir in milk until soft dough forms.
5. Sprinkle ¼ cup of flour onto wax paper and place dough on top. Knead lightly by folding and turning the dough about 6 to 8 times.
6. Pat dough into a 6 x 6-inch square.
7. Cut into 9 equal squares.
8. Place all squares in air fryer basket or as many as will fit in a single layer, close together but not touching.
9. Cook at 360°F for 8minutes. When done, scones will be lightly browned on top and will spring back when pressed gently with a dull knife.
10. Repeat steps 8 and 9 to cook remaining scones.

Cinnamon Rolls With Cream Cheese Glaze

Servings: 8
Cooking Time: 9 Minutes

Ingredients:

- 1 pound frozen bread dough, thawed
- ¼ cup butter, melted and cooled
- ¾ cup brown sugar
- 1½ tablespoons ground cinnamon
- Cream Cheese Glaze:
- 4 ounces cream cheese, softened
- 2 tablespoons butter, softened
- 1¼ cups powdered sugar

- ½ teaspoon vanilla

Directions:

1. Let the bread dough come to room temperature on the counter. On a lightly floured surface roll the dough into a 13-inch by 11-inch rectangle. Position the rectangle so the 13-inch side is facing you. Brush the melted butter all over the dough, leaving a 1-inch border uncovered along the edge farthest away from you.
2. Combine the brown sugar and cinnamon in a small bowl. Sprinkle the mixture evenly over the buttered dough, keeping the 1-inch border uncovered. Roll the dough into a log starting with the edge closest to you. Roll the dough tightly, making sure to roll evenly and push out any air pockets. When you get to the uncovered edge of the dough, press the dough onto the roll to seal it together.
3. Cut the log into 8 pieces slicing slowly with a sawing motion so you don't flatten the dough. Turn the slices on their sides and cover with a clean kitchen towel. Let the rolls sit in the warmest part of your kitchen for 1½ to 2 hours to rise.
4. To make the glaze, place the cream cheese and butter in a microwave-safe bowl. Soften the mixture in the microwave for 30 seconds at a time until it is easy to stir. Gradually add the powdered sugar and stir to combine. Add the vanilla extract and whisk until smooth. Set aside.
5. When the rolls have risen, Preheat the air fryer to 350°F.
6. Transfer 4 of the rolls to the air fryer basket. Air-fry for 5 minutes. Turn the rolls over and air-fry for another 4 minutes. Repeat with the remaining 4 rolls.
7. Let the rolls cool for a couple of minutes before glazing. Spread large dollops of cream cheese glaze on top of the warm cinnamon rolls, allowing some of the glaze to drip down the side of the rolls. Serve warm and enjoy!

Crunchy French Toast Sticks

Servings: 2

Cooking Time: 9 Minutes

Ingredients:

- 2 eggs, beaten
- ¾ cup milk
- ½ teaspoon vanilla extract
- ½ teaspoon ground cinnamon
- 1½ cups crushed crunchy cinnamon cereal, or any cereal flakes
- 4 slices Texas Toast (or other bread that you can slice into 1-inch thick slices)
- maple syrup, for serving
- vegetable oil or melted butter

Directions:

1. Combine the eggs, milk, vanilla and cinnamon in a shallow bowl. Place the crushed cereal in a second shallow bowl.
2. Trim the crusts off the slices of bread and cut each slice into 3 sticks. Dip the sticks of bread into the egg mixture, turning them over to coat all sides. Let the bread sticks absorb the egg mixture for ten seconds or so, but don't let them get too wet. Roll the bread sticks in the cereal crumbs, pressing the cereal gently onto all sides so that it adheres to the bread.
3. Preheat the air fryer to 400°F.
4. Spray or brush the air fryer basket with oil or melted butter. Place the coated sticks in the basket. It's ok to stack a few on top of the others in the opposite direction.
5. Air-fry for 9 minutes. Turn the sticks over a couple of times during the cooking process so that the sticks crisp evenly. Serve warm with the maple syrup or some berries.

Spinach And Artichoke White Pizza

Servings: 2

Cooking Time: 18 Minutes

Ingredients:

- olive oil
- 3 cups fresh spinach
- 2 cloves garlic, minced, divided
- 1 (6- to 8-ounce) pizza dough ball*
- ½ cup grated mozzarella cheese
- ¼ cup grated Fontina cheese
- ¼ cup artichoke hearts, coarsely chopped
- 2 tablespoons grated Parmesan cheese
- ¼ teaspoon dried oregano
- salt and freshly ground black pepper

Directions:

1. Heat the oil in a medium sauté pan on the stovetop. Add the spinach and half the minced garlic to the pan and sauté for a few minutes, until the spinach has wilted. Remove the sautéed spinach from the pan and set it aside.
2. Preheat the air fryer to 390°F.
3. Cut out a piece of aluminum foil the same size as the bottom of the air fryer basket. Brush the foil circle with olive oil. Shape the dough into a circle and place it on top of the foil. Dock the dough by piercing it several times with a fork. Brush the dough lightly with olive oil and transfer it into the air fryer basket with the foil on the bottom.
4. Air-fry the plain pizza dough for 6 minutes. Turn the dough over, remove the aluminum foil and brush again with olive oil. Air-fry for an additional 4 minutes.
5. Sprinkle the mozzarella and Fontina cheeses over the dough. Top with the spinach and artichoke hearts. Sprinkle the Parmesan cheese and dried oregano on top and drizzle with olive oil. Lower the temperature of the air fryer to 350°F and cook for 8 minutes, until the cheese has melted and is lightly browned. Season to taste with salt and freshly ground black pepper.

Strawberry Bread

Servings: 6

Cooking Time: 28 Minutes

Ingredients:

- ½ cup frozen strawberries in juice, completely thawed (do not drain)
- 1 cup flour
- ½ cup sugar
- 1 teaspoon cinnamon
- ½ teaspoon baking soda
- ⅛ teaspoon salt
- 1 egg, beaten
- ⅓ cup oil
- cooking spray

Directions:

1. Cut any large berries into smaller pieces no larger than ½ inch.
2. Preheat air fryer to 330°F.
3. In a large bowl, stir together the flour, sugar, cinnamon, soda, and salt.
4. In a small bowl, mix together the egg, oil, and strawberries. Add to dry ingredients and stir together gently.
5. Spray 6 x 6-inch baking pan with cooking spray.
6. Pour batter into prepared pan and cook at 330°F for 28 minutes.
7. When bread is done, let cool for 10minutes before removing from pan.

Breakfast Pot Pies

Servings: 4

Cooking Time: 20 Minutes

Ingredients:

- 1 refrigerated pie crust
- ½ pound pork breakfast sausage
- ¼ cup diced onion
- 1 garlic clove, minced
- ½ teaspoon ground black pepper
- ¼ teaspoon salt
- 1 cup chopped bell peppers
- 1 cup roasted potatoes
- 2 cups milk
- 2 to 3 tablespoons all-purpose flour

Directions:

1. Flatten the store-bought pie crust out on an even surface. Cut 4 equal circles that are slightly larger than the circumference of ramekins (by about ¼ inch). Set aside.
2. In a medium pot, sauté the breakfast sausage with the onion, garlic, black pepper, and salt. When browned, add in the bell peppers and potatoes and cook an additional 3 to 4 minutes to soften the bell peppers. Remove from the heat and portion equally into the ramekins.
3. To the same pot (without washing it), add the milk. Heat over medium-high heat until boiling. Slowly reduce to a simmer and stir in the flour, 1 tablespoon at a time, until the gravy thickens and coats the back of a wooden spoon (about 5 minutes).

4. Remove from the heat and equally portion ½ cup of gravy into each ramekin on top of the sausage and potato mixture.
5. Place the circle pie crusts on top of the ramekins, lightly pressing them down on the perimeter of each ramekin with the prongs of a fork. Gently poke the prongs into the center top of the pie crust a few times to create holes for the steam to escape as the pie cooks.
6. Bake in the air fryer for 6 minutes (or until the tops are golden brown).
7. Remove and let cool 5 minutes before serving.

White Wheat Walnut Bread

Servings: 8
Cooking Time: 25 Minutes

Ingredients:

- 1 cup lukewarm water (105–115°F)
- 1 packet RapidRise yeast
- 1 tablespoon light brown sugar
- 2 cups whole-grain white wheat flour
- 1 egg, room temperature, beaten with a fork
- 2 teaspoons olive oil
- ½ teaspoon salt
- ½ cup chopped walnuts
- cooking spray

Directions:

1. In a small bowl, mix the water, yeast, and brown sugar.
2. Pour yeast mixture over flour and mix until smooth.
3. Add the egg, olive oil, and salt and beat with a wooden spoon for 2minutes.
4. Stir in chopped walnuts. You will have very thick batter rather than stiff bread dough.
5. Spray air fryer baking pan with cooking spray and pour in batter, smoothing the top.
6. Let batter rise for 15minutes.
7. Preheat air fryer to 360°F.
8. Cook bread for 25 minutes, until toothpick pushed into center comes out with crumbs clinging. Let bread rest for 10minutes before removing from pan.

Bacon, Broccoli And Swiss Cheese Bread Pudding

Servings: 2
Cooking Time: 48 Minutes

Ingredients:

- ½ pound thick cut bacon, cut into ¼-inch pieces
- 3 cups brioche bread or rolls, cut into ½-inch cubes
- 3 eggs
- 1 cup milk
- ½ teaspoon salt
- freshly ground black pepper
- 1 cup frozen broccoli florets, thawed and chopped
- 1½ cups grated Swiss cheese

Directions:

1. Preheat the air fryer to 400°F.
2. Air-fry the bacon for 6 minutes until crispy, shaking the basket a few times while it cooks to help it cook evenly. Remove the bacon and set it aside on a paper towel.
3. Air-fry the brioche bread cubes for 2 minutes to dry and toast lightly. (If your brioche is a few days old and slightly stale, you can omit this step.)
4. Butter a 6- or 7-inch cake pan. Combine all the ingredients in a large bowl and toss well. Transfer the mixture to the buttered cake pan, cover with aluminum foil and refrigerate the bread pudding overnight, or for at least 8 hours.
5. Remove the casserole from the refrigerator an hour before you plan to cook, and let it sit on the countertop to come to room temperature.
6. Preheat the air fryer to 330°F. Transfer the covered cake pan, to the basket of the air fryer, lowering the dish into the basket using a sling made of aluminum foil (fold a piece of aluminum foil into a strip about 2-inches wide by 24-inches long). Fold the ends of the aluminum foil over the top of the dish before returning the basket to the air fryer. Air-fry for 20 minutes. Remove the foil and air-fry for an additional 20 minutes. If the top starts to brown a little too much before the custard has set, simply return the foil to the pan. The bread pudding has cooked through when a skewer inserted into the center comes out clean.

Vegetable Side Dishes Recipes

Tandoori Cauliflower

Servings: 4

Cooking Time: 10 Minutes

Ingredients:

- ½ cup Plain full-fat yogurt (not Greek yogurt)
- 1½ teaspoons Yellow curry powder, purchased or homemade (see the headnote)
- 1½ teaspoons Lemon juice
- ¾ teaspoon Table salt (optional)
- 4½ cups (about 1 pound 2 ounces) 2-inch cauliflower florets

Directions:

1. Preheat the air fryer to 400°F.
2. Whisk the yogurt, curry powder, lemon juice, and salt (if using) in a large bowl until uniform. Add the florets and stir gently to coat the florets well and evenly. Even better, use your clean, dry hands to get the yogurt mixture down into all the nooks of the florets.
3. When the machine is at temperature, transfer the florets to the basket, spreading them gently into as close to one layer as you can. Air-fry for 10 minutes, tossing and rearranging the florets twice so that any covered or touching parts are exposed to the air currents, until lightly browned and tender if still a bit crunchy.
4. Pour the contents of the basket onto a wire rack. Cool for at least 5 minutes before serving, or serve at room temperature.

Fingerling Potatoes

Servings: 4

Cooking Time: 15 Minutes

Ingredients:

- 1 pound fingerling potatoes
- 1 tablespoon light olive oil
- ½ teaspoon dried parsley
- ½ teaspoon lemon juice
- coarsely ground sea salt

Directions:

1. Cut potatoes in half lengthwise.
2. In a large bowl, combine potatoes, oil, parsley, and lemon juice. Stir well to coat potatoes.
3. Place potatoes in air fryer basket and cook at 360°F for 15 minutes or until lightly browned and tender inside.
4. Sprinkle with sea salt before serving.

Simple Roasted Sweet Potatoes

Servings: 2

Cooking Time: 45 Minutes

Ingredients:

- 2 10- to 12-ounce sweet potato(es)

Directions:

1. Preheat the air fryer to 350°F .
2. Prick the sweet potato(es) in four or five different places with the tines of a flatware fork (not in a line but all around).
3. When the machine is at temperature, set the sweet potato(es) in the basket with as much air space between them as possible. Air-fry undisturbed for 45 minutes, or until soft when pricked with a fork.
4. Use kitchen tongs to transfer the sweet potato(es) to a wire rack. Cool for 5 minutes before serving.

Hasselbacks

Servings: 4

Cooking Time: 41 Minutes

Ingredients:

- 2 large potatoes (approx. 1 pound each)
- oil for misting or cooking spray
- salt, pepper, and garlic powder
- 1½ ounces sharp Cheddar cheese, sliced very thin
- ¼ cup chopped green onions
- 2 strips turkey bacon, cooked and crumbled
- light sour cream for serving (optional)

Directions:

1. Preheat air fryer to 390°F.
2. Scrub potatoes. Cut thin vertical slices ¼-inch thick crosswise about three-quarters of the way down so that bottom of potato remains intact.
3. Fan potatoes slightly to separate slices. Mist with oil and sprinkle with salt, pepper, and garlic powder to taste.

Potatoes will be very stiff, but try to get some of the oil and seasoning between the slices.

4. Place potatoes in air fryer basket and cook for 40 minutes or until centers test done when pierced with a fork.

5. Top potatoes with cheese slices and cook for 30 seconds to 1 minute to melt cheese.

6. Cut each potato in half crosswise, and sprinkle with green onions and crumbled bacon. If you like, add a dollop of sour cream before serving.

Corn On The Cob

Servings: 4

Cooking Time: 12 Minutes

Ingredients:

- 2 large ears fresh corn
- olive oil for misting
- salt (optional)

Directions:

1. Shuck corn, remove silks, and wash.
2. Cut or break each ear in half crosswise.
3. Spray corn with olive oil.
4. Cook at 390°F for 12 minutes or until browned as much as you like.
5. Serve plain or with coarsely ground salt.

Perfect Broccoli

Servings: 4

Cooking Time: 12 Minutes

Ingredients:

- 5 cups (about 1 pound 10 ounces) 1- to 1½-inch fresh broccoli florets (not frozen)
- Olive oil spray
- ¾ teaspoon Table salt

Directions:

1. Preheat the air fryer to 375°F .
2. Put the broccoli florets in a big bowl, coat them generously with olive oil spray, then toss to coat all surfaces, even down into the crannies, spraying them in a couple of times more. Sprinkle the salt on top and toss again.
3. When the machine is at temperature, pour the florets into the basket. Air-fry for 10 minutes, tossing and rearranging the pieces twice so that all the covered or touching bits are eventually exposed to the air currents, until lightly browned but still crunchy. (If the machine is at 360°F, you may have to add 2 minutes to the cooking time.)
4. Pour the florets into a serving bowl. Cool for a minute or two, then serve hot.

Glazed Carrots

Servings: 4

Cooking Time: 10 Minutes

Ingredients:

- 2 teaspoons honey
- 1 teaspoon orange juice
- ½ teaspoon grated orange rind
- ⅛ teaspoon ginger
- 1 pound baby carrots
- 2 teaspoons olive oil
- ¼ teaspoon salt

Directions:

1. Combine honey, orange juice, grated rind, and ginger in a small bowl and set aside.
2. Toss the carrots, oil, and salt together to coat well and pour them into the air fryer basket.
3. Cook at 390°F for 5minutes. Shake basket to stir a little and cook for 4 minutes more, until carrots are barely tender.
4. Pour carrots into air fryer baking pan.
5. Stir the honey mixture to combine well, pour glaze over carrots, and stir to coat.
6. Cook at 360°F for 1 minute or just until heated through.

Fried Okra

Servings: 4

Cooking Time: 8 Minutes

Ingredients:

- 1 pound okra
- 1 large egg
- 1 tablespoon milk
- 1 teaspoon salt, divided
- ½ teaspoon black pepper, divided
- ¼ teaspoon paprika
- ¼ teaspoon thyme
- ½ cup cornmeal
- ½ cup all-purpose flour

Directions:

1. Preheat the air fryer to 400°F.
2. Cut the okra into ½-inch rounds.
3. In a medium bowl, whisk together the egg, milk, ½ teaspoon of the salt, and ¼ teaspoon of black pepper. Place the okra into the egg mixture and toss until well coated.
4. In a separate bowl, mix together the remaining ½ teaspoon of salt, the remaining ¼ teaspoon of black pepper, the paprika, the thyme, the cornmeal, and the flour. Working in small batches, dredge the egg-coated okra in the cornmeal mixture until all the okra has been breaded.
5. Place a single layer of okra in the air fryer basket and spray with cooking spray. Cook for 4 minutes, toss to check for crispness, and cook another 4 minutes. Repeat in batches, as needed.

Sweet Potato Curly Fries

Servings: 4

Cooking Time: 10 Minutes

Ingredients:

- 2 medium sweet potatoes, washed
- 2 tablespoons avocado oil
- ¾ teaspoon salt, divided
- 1 medium avocado
- ½ teaspoon garlic powder
- ½ teaspoon paprika
- ¼ teaspoon black pepper
- ½ juice lime
- 3 tablespoons fresh cilantro

Directions:

1. Preheat the air fryer to 400°F.
2. Using a spiralizer, create curly spirals with the sweet potatoes. Keep the pieces about 1½ inches long. Continue until all the potatoes are used.
3. In a large bowl, toss the curly sweet potatoes with the avocado oil and ½ teaspoon of the salt.
4. Place the potatoes in the air fryer basket and cook for 5 minutes; shake and cook another 5 minutes.
5. While cooking, add the avocado, garlic, paprika, pepper, the remaining ¼ teaspoon of salt, lime juice, and cilantro to a blender and process until smooth. Set aside.
6. When cooking completes, remove the fries and serve warm with the lime avocado sauce.

Roasted Brussels Sprouts With Bacon

Servings: 4

Cooking Time: 20 Minutes

Ingredients:

- 4 slices thick-cut bacon, chopped (about ¼ pound)
- 1 pound Brussels sprouts, halved (or quartered if large)
- freshly ground black pepper

Directions:

1. Preheat the air fryer to 380°F.
2. Air-fry the bacon for 5 minutes, shaking the basket once or twice during the cooking time.
3. Add the Brussels sprouts to the basket and drizzle a little bacon fat from the bottom of the air fryer drawer into the basket. Toss the sprouts to coat with the bacon fat. Air-fry for an additional 15 minutes, or until the Brussels sprouts are tender to a knifepoint.
4. Season with freshly ground black pepper.

Curried Fruit

Servings: 6
Cooking Time: 20 Minutes

Ingredients:

- 1 cup cubed fresh pineapple
- 1 cup cubed fresh pear (firm, not overly ripe)
- 8 ounces frozen peaches, thawed
- 1 15-ounce can dark, sweet, pitted cherries with juice
- 2 tablespoons brown sugar
- 1 teaspoon curry powder

Directions:

1. Combine all ingredients in large bowl. Stir gently to mix in the sugar and curry.
2. Pour into air fryer baking pan and cook at 360°F for 10minutes.
3. Stir fruit and cook 10 more minutes.
4. Serve hot.

Roasted Peppers With Balsamic Vinegar And Basil

Servings: 6
Cooking Time: 12 Minutes

Ingredients:

- 4 Small or medium red or yellow bell peppers
- 3 tablespoons Olive oil
- 1 tablespoon Balsamic vinegar
- Up to 6 Fresh basil leaves, torn up

Directions:

1. Preheat the air fryer to 400°F.
2. When the machine is at temperature, put the peppers in the basket with at least ¼ inch between them. Air-fry undisturbed for 12 minutes, until blistered, even blackened in places.
3. Use kitchen tongs to transfer the peppers to a medium bowl. Cover the bowl with plastic wrap. Set aside at room temperature for 30 minutes.
4. Uncover the bowl and use kitchen tongs to transfer the peppers to a cutting board or work surface. Peel off the filmy exterior skin. If there are blackened bits under it, these can stay on the peppers. Cut off and remove the stem ends. Split open the peppers and discard any seeds and their spongy membranes. Slice the peppers into ½-inch- to 1-inch-wide strips.
5. Put these in a clean bowl and gently toss them with the oil, vinegar, and basil. Serve at once. Or cover and store at room temperature for up to 4 hours or in the refrigerator for up to 5 days.

Buttery Stuffed Tomatoes

Servings: 6
Cooking Time: 15 Minutes

Ingredients:

- 3 8-ounce round tomatoes
- ½ cup plus 1 tablespoon Plain panko bread crumbs (gluten-free, if a concern)
- 3 tablespoons (about ½ ounce) Finely grated Parmesan cheese
- 3 tablespoons Butter, melted and cooled
- 4 teaspoons Stemmed and chopped fresh parsley leaves
- 1 teaspoon Minced garlic
- ¼ teaspoon Table salt
- Up to ¼ teaspoon Red pepper flakes
- Olive oil spray

Directions:

1. Preheat the air fryer to 375°F .
2. Cut the tomatoes in half through their "equators" (that is, not through the stem ends). One at a time, gently squeeze the tomato halves over a trash can, using a clean finger to gently force out the seeds and most of the juice inside, working carefully so that the tomato doesn't lose its round shape or get crushed.
3. Stir the bread crumbs, cheese, butter, parsley, garlic, salt, and red pepper flakes in a bowl until the bread crumbs are moistened and the parsley is uniform throughout the mixture. Pile this mixture into the spaces left in the tomato halves. Press gently to compact the filling. Coat the tops of the tomatoes with olive oil spray.
4. Place the tomatoes cut side up in the basket. They may touch each other. Air-fry for 15 minutes, or until the filling is lightly browned and crunchy.
5. Use nonstick-safe spatula and kitchen tongs for balance to gently transfer the stuffed tomatoes to a platter or a cutting board. Cool for a couple of minutes before serving.

Tuna Platter

Servings: 4

Cooking Time: 9 Minutes

Ingredients:

- 4 new potatoes, boiled in their jackets
- ½ cup vinaigrette dressing, plus 2 tablespoons
- ½ pound fresh green beans, cut in half-inch pieces and steamed
- 1 tablespoon Herbes de Provence
- 1 tablespoon minced shallots
- 1½ tablespoons tarragon vinegar
- 4 tuna steaks, each ¾-inch thick, about 1 pound
- salt and pepper
- Salad
- 8 cups chopped romaine lettuce
- 12 grape tomatoes, halved lengthwise
- ½ cup pitted olives (black, green, nicoise, or combination)
- 2 boiled eggs, peeled and halved lengthwise

Directions:

1. Quarter potatoes and toss with 1 tablespoon salad dressing.
2. Toss the warm beans with the other tablespoon of salad dressing. Set both aside while you prepare the tuna.
3. Mix together the herbs, shallots, and vinegar and rub into all sides of tuna. Season fish to taste with salt and pepper.
4. Cook tuna at 390°F for 7minutes and check. If needed, cook 2 minutes longer, until tuna is barely pink in the center.
5. Spread the lettuce over a large platter.
6. Slice the tuna steaks in ½-inch pieces and arrange them in the center of the lettuce.
7. Place the remaining ingredients around the tuna. Diners create their own plates by selecting what they want from the platter. Pass remainder of salad dressing at the table.

Curried Cauliflower With Cashews And Yogurt

Servings: 2

Cooking Time: 12 Minutes

Ingredients:

- 4 cups cauliflower florets (about half a large head)
- 1 tablespoon olive oil
- salt
- 1 teaspoon curry powder
- ½ cup toasted, chopped cashews
- Cool Yogurt Drizzle
- ¼ cup plain yogurt
- 2 tablespoons sour cream
- 1 teaspoon lemon juice
- pinch cayenne pepper
- salt
- 1 teaspoon honey
- 1 tablespoon chopped fresh cilantro, plus leaves for garnish

Directions:

1. Preheat the air fryer to 400°F.
2. Toss the cauliflower florets with the olive oil, salt and curry powder, coating evenly.
3. Transfer the cauliflower to the air fryer basket and air-fry at 400°F for 12 minutes, shaking the basket a couple of times during the cooking process.
4. While the cauliflower is cooking, make the cool yogurt drizzle by combining all ingredients in a bowl.
5. When the cauliflower is cooked to your liking, serve it warm with the cool yogurt either underneath or drizzled over the top. Scatter the cashews and cilantro leaves around.

Roasted Garlic

Servings: 20

Cooking Time: 40 Minutes

Ingredients:

- 20 Peeled medium garlic cloves
- 2 tablespoons, plus more Olive oil

Directions:

1. Preheat the air fryer to 400°F.
2. Set a 10-inch sheet of aluminum foil on your work surface for a small batch, a 14-inch sheet for a medium batch, or a 16-inch sheet for a large batch. Put the garlic cloves in its center in one layer without bunching the cloves together. (Spread them out a little for even cooking.) Drizzle the small batch with 1 tablespoon oil,

the medium batch with 2 tablespoons, or the large one with 3 tablespoons. Fold up the sides and seal the foil into a packet.

3. When the machine is at temperature, put the packet in the basket. Air-fry for 40 minutes, or until very fragrant. The cloves inside should be golden and soft.

4. Transfer the packet to a cutting board. Cool for 5 minutes, then open and use the cloves hot. Or cool them to room temperature, set them in a small container or jar, pour in enough olive oil to cover them, seal or cover the container, and refrigerate for up to 2 weeks.

Okra

Servings: 4

Cooking Time: 12 Minutes

Ingredients:

- 7–8 ounces fresh okra
- 1 egg
- 1 cup milk
- 1 cup breadcrumbs
- ½ teaspoon salt
- oil for misting or cooking spray

Directions:

1. Remove stem ends from okra and cut in ½-inch slices.
2. In a medium bowl, beat together egg and milk. Add okra slices and stir to coat.
3. In a sealable plastic bag or container with lid, mix together the breadcrumbs and salt.
4. Remove okra from egg mixture, letting excess drip off, and transfer into bag with breadcrumbs.
5. Shake okra in crumbs to coat well.
6. Place all of the coated okra into the air fryer basket and mist with oil or cooking spray. Okra doesn't need to cook in a single layer, nor is it necessary to spray all sides at this point. A good spritz on top will do.
7. Cook at 390°F for 5minutes. Shake basket to redistribute and give it another spritz as you shake.
8. Cook 5 more minutes. Shake and spray again. Cook for 2 minutes longer or until golden brown and crispy.

Moroccan Cauliflower

Servings: 6

Cooking Time: 15 Minutes

Ingredients:

- 1 tablespoon curry powder
- 2 teaspoons smoky paprika
- ½ teaspoon ground cumin
- ½ teaspoon salt
- 1 head cauliflower, cut into bite-size pieces
- ¼ cup red wine vinegar
- 2 tablespoons extra-virgin olive oil
- 2 tablespoons chopped parsley

Directions:

1. Preheat the air fryer to 370°F.
2. In a large bowl, mix the curry powder, paprika, cumin, and salt. Add the cauliflower and stir to coat. Pour the red wine vinegar over the top and continue stirring.
3. Place the cauliflower into the air fryer basket; drizzle olive oil over the top.
4. Cook the cauliflower for 5 minutes, toss, and cook another 5 minutes. Raise the temperature to 400°F and continue cooking for 4 to 6 minutes, or until crispy.

Roasted Herbed Shiitake Mushrooms

Servings: 4

Cooking Time: 5 Minutes

Ingredients:

- 8 ounces shiitake mushrooms, stems removed and caps roughly chopped
- 1 tablespoon olive oil
- ½ teaspoon salt
- freshly ground black pepper
- 1 teaspoon chopped fresh thyme leaves
- 1 teaspoon chopped fresh oregano
- 1 tablespoon chopped fresh parsley

Directions:

1. Preheat the air fryer to 400°F.
2. Toss the mushrooms with the olive oil, salt, pepper, thyme and oregano. Air-fry for 5 minutes, shaking the basket once or twice during the cooking process. The mushrooms will still be somewhat chewy with a meaty

texture. If you'd like them a little more tender, add a couple of minutes to this cooking time.

3. Once cooked, add the parsley to the mushrooms and toss. Season again to taste and serve.

Yellow Squash

Servings: 4

Cooking Time: 10 Minutes

Ingredients:

- 1 large yellow squash (about 1½ cups)
- 2 eggs
- ¼ cup buttermilk
- 1 cup panko breadcrumbs
- ¼ cup white cornmeal
- ½ teaspoon salt
- oil for misting or cooking spray

Directions:

1. Preheat air fryer to 390°F.
2. Cut the squash into ¼-inch slices.
3. In a shallow dish, beat together eggs and buttermilk.
4. In sealable plastic bag or container with lid, combine ¼ cup panko crumbs, white cornmeal, and salt. Shake to mix well.
5. Place the remaining ¾ cup panko crumbs in a separate shallow dish.
6. Dump all the squash slices into the egg/buttermilk mixture. Stir to coat.
7. Remove squash from buttermilk mixture with a slotted spoon, letting excess drip off, and transfer to the panko/cornmeal mixture. Close bag or container and shake well to coat.
8. Remove squash from crumb mixture, letting excess fall off. Return squash to egg/buttermilk mixture, stirring gently to coat. If you need more liquid to coat all the squash, add a little more buttermilk.
9. Remove each squash slice from egg wash and dip in a dish of ¾ cup panko crumbs.
10. Mist squash slices with oil or cooking spray and place in air fryer basket. Squash should be in a single layer, but it's okay if the slices crowd together and overlap a little.
11. Cook at 390°F for 5minutes. Shake basket to break up any that have stuck together. Mist again with oil or spray.
12. Cook 5minutes longer and check. If necessary, mist again with oil and cook an additional two minutes, until squash slices are golden brown and crisp.

Roasted Broccoli And Red Bean Salad

Servings: 3

Cooking Time: 14 Minutes

Ingredients:

- 3 cups (about 1 pound) 1- to 1½-inch fresh broccoli florets (not frozen)
- 1½ tablespoons Olive oil spray
- 1¼ cups Canned red kidney beans, drained and rinsed
- 3 tablespoons Minced yellow or white onion
- 2 tablespoons plus 1 teaspoon Red wine vinegar
- ¾ teaspoon Dried oregano
- ¼ teaspoon Table salt
- ¼ teaspoon Ground black pepper

Directions:

1. Preheat the air fryer to 375°F .
2. Put the broccoli florets in a big bowl, coat them generously with olive oil spray, then toss to coat all surfaces, even down into the crannies, spraying them a couple of times more.
3. Pour the florets into the basket, spreading them into as close to one layer as you can. Air-fry for 12 minutes, tossing and rearranging the florets twice so that any touching or covered parts are eventually exposed to the air currents, until light browned but still a bit firm. (If the machine is at 360°F, you may need to add 2 minutes to the cooking time.)
4. Dump the contents of the basket onto a large cutting board. Cool for a minute or two, then chop the florets into small bits. Scrape these into a bowl and add the kidney beans, onion, vinegar, oregano, salt, and pepper. Toss well and serve warm or at room temperature.

Sweet Potato Puffs

Servings: 18
Cooking Time: 35 Minutes

Ingredients:

- 3 8- to 10-ounce sweet potatoes
- 1 cup Seasoned Italian-style dried bread crumbs
- 3 tablespoons All-purpose flour
- 3 tablespoons Instant mashed potato flakes
- ¾ teaspoon Onion powder
- ¾ teaspoon Table salt
- Olive oil spray

Directions:

1. Preheat the air fryer to 350°F .
2. Prick the sweet potatoes in four or five different places with the tines of a flatware fork (not in a line but all around the sweet potatoes).
3. When the machine is at temperature, set the sweet potatoes in the basket with as much air space between them as possible. Air-fry undisturbed for 20 minutes.
4. Use kitchen tongs to transfer the sweet potatoes to a wire rack. (They will still be firm; they are only partially cooked.) Cool for 10 to 15 minutes. Meanwhile, increase the machine's temperature to 400°F. Spread the bread crumbs on a dinner plate.
5. Peel the sweet potatoes. Shred them through the large holes of a box grater into a large bowl. Stir in the flour, potato flakes, onion powder, and salt until well combined.
6. Scoop up 2 tablespoons of the sweet potato mixture. Form it into a small puff, a cylinder about like a Tater Tot. Set this cylinder in the bread crumbs. Gently roll it around to coat on all sides, even the ends. Set aside on a cutting board and continue making more puffs: 11 more for a small batch, 17 more for a mediùm batch, or 23 more for a large batch.
7. Generously coat the puffs with olive oil spray on all sides. Set the puffs in the basket with as much air space between them as possible. They should not be touching, but even a fraction of an inch will work well. Air-fry undisturbed for 15 minutes, or until lightly browned and crunchy.
8. Gently turn the contents of the basket out onto a wire rack. Cool the puffs for a couple of minutes before serving.

Asiago Broccoli

Servings: 4
Cooking Time: 14 Minutes

Ingredients:

- 1 head broccoli, cut into florets
- 1 tablespoon extra-virgin olive oil
- 1 teaspoon minced garlic
- ¼ teaspoon ground black pepper
- ¼ teaspoon salt
- ¼ cup asiago cheese

Directions:

1. Preheat the air fryer to 360°F.
2. In a medium bowl, toss the broccoli florets with the olive oil, garlic, pepper, and salt. Lightly spray the air fryer basket with olive oil spray.
3. Place the broccoli florets into the basket and cook for 7 minutes. Shake the basket and sprinkle the broccoli with cheese. Cook another 7 minutes.
4. Remove from the basket and serve warm.

Roasted Heirloom Carrots With Orange And Thyme

Servings: 2
Cooking Time: 12 Minutes

Ingredients:

- 10 to 12 heirloom or rainbow carrots (about 1 pound), scrubbed but not peeled
- 1 teaspoon olive oil
- salt and freshly ground black pepper
- 1 tablespoon butter
- 1 teaspoon fresh orange zest
- 1 teaspoon chopped fresh thyme

Directions:

1. Preheat the air fryer to 400°F.
2. Scrub the carrots and halve them lengthwise. Toss them in the olive oil, season with salt and freshly ground black pepper and transfer to the air fryer.

3. Air-fry at 400°F for 12 minutes, shaking the basket every once in a while to rotate the carrots as they cook.
4. As soon as the carrots have finished cooking, add the butter, orange zest and thyme and toss all the ingredients together in the air fryer basket to melt the butter and coat evenly. Serve warm.

Jerk Rubbed Corn On The Cob

Servings: 4
Cooking Time: 6 Minutes

Ingredients:

- 1 teaspoon ground allspice
- 1 teaspoon dried thyme
- ½ teaspoon ground ginger
- ½ teaspoon ground cinnamon
- ¼ teaspoon ground nutmeg
- ⅛ teaspoon ground cayenne pepper
- 1 teaspoon salt
- 2 tablespoons butter, melted
- 4 ears of corn, husked

Directions:

1. Preheat the air fryer to 380°F.
2. Combine all the spices in a bowl. Brush the corn with the melted butter and then sprinkle the spices generously on all sides of each ear of corn.
3. Transfer the ears of corn to the air fryer basket. It's ok if they are crisscrossed on top of each other. Air-fry at 380°F for 6 minutes, rotating the ears as they cook.
4. Brush more butter on at the end and sprinkle with any remaining spice mixture.

Crispy Brussels Sprouts

Servings: 3
Cooking Time: 12 Minutes

Ingredients:

- 1¼ pounds Medium, 2-inch-in-length Brussels sprouts
- 1½ tablespoons Olive oil
- ¾ teaspoon Table salt

Directions:

1. Preheat the air fryer to 400°F.
2. Halve each Brussels sprout through the stem end, pulling off and discarding any discolored outer leaves. Put the sprout halves in a large bowl, add the oil and salt, and stir well to coat evenly, until the Brussels sprouts are glistening.
3. When the machine is at temperature, scrape the contents of the bowl into the basket, gently spreading the Brussels sprout halves into as close to one layer as possible. Air-fry for 12 minutes, gently tossing and rearranging the vegetables twice to get all covered or touching parts exposed to the air currents, until crisp and browned at the edges.
4. Gently pour the contents of the basket onto a wire rack. Cool for a minute or two before serving.

Crispy Herbed Potatoes

Servings: 6
Cooking Time: 20 Minutes

Ingredients:

- 3 medium baking potatoes, washed and cubed
- ½ teaspoon dried thyme
- 1 teaspoon minced dried rosemary
- ½ teaspoon garlic powder
- 1 teaspoon sea salt
- ½ teaspoon black pepper
- 2 tablespoons extra-virgin olive oil
- ¼ cup chopped parsley

Directions:

1. Preheat the air fryer to 390°F.
2. Pat the potatoes dry. In a large bowl, mix together the cubed potatoes, thyme, rosemary, garlic powder, sea salt, and pepper. Drizzle and toss with olive oil.
3. Pour the herbed potatoes into the air fryer basket. Cook for 20 minutes, stirring every 5 minutes.
4. Toss the cooked potatoes with chopped parsley and serve immediately.
5. VARY IT! Potatoes are versatile — add any spice or seasoning mixture you prefer and create your own favorite side dish.

Asparagus Fries

Servings: 4

Cooking Time: 5 Minutes Per Batch

Ingredients:

- 12 ounces fresh asparagus spears with tough ends trimmed off
- 2 egg whites
- ¼ cup water
- ¾ cup panko breadcrumbs
- ¼ cup grated Parmesan cheese, plus 2 tablespoons
- ¼ teaspoon salt
- oil for misting or cooking spray

Directions:

1. Preheat air fryer to 390°F.
2. In a shallow dish, beat egg whites and water until slightly foamy.
3. In another shallow dish, combine panko, Parmesan, and salt.
4. Dip asparagus spears in egg, then roll in crumbs. Spray with oil or cooking spray.
5. Place a layer of asparagus in air fryer basket, leaving just a little space in between each spear. Stack another layer on top, crosswise. Cook at 390°F for 5 minutes, until crispy and golden brown.
6. Repeat to cook remaining asparagus.

Blistered Tomatoes

Servings: 20

Cooking Time: 15 Minutes

Ingredients:

- 1½ pounds Cherry or grape tomatoes
- Olive oil spray
- 1½ teaspoons Balsamic vinegar
- ¼ teaspoon Table salt
- ¼ teaspoon Ground black pepper

Directions:

1. Put the basket in a drawer-style air fryer, or a baking tray in the lower third of a toaster oven–style air fryer. Place a 6-inch round cake pan in the basket or on the tray for a small batch, a 7-inch round cake pan for a medium batch, or an 8-inch round cake pan for a large one. Heat the air fryer to 400°F with the pan in the basket. When the machine is at temperature, keep heating the pan for 5 minutes more.
2. Place the tomatoes in a large bowl, coat them with the olive oil spray, toss gently, then spritz a couple of times more, tossing after each spritz, until the tomatoes are glistening.
3. Pour the tomatoes into the cake pan and air-fry undisturbed for 10 minutes, or until they split and begin to brown.
4. Use kitchen tongs and a nonstick-safe spatula, or silicone baking mitts, to remove the cake pan from the basket. Toss the hot tomatoes with the vinegar, salt, and pepper. Cool in the pan for a few minutes before serving.

Perfect French Fries

Servings: 3

Cooking Time: 37 Minutes

Ingredients:

- 1 pound Large russet potato(es)
- Vegetable oil or olive oil spray
- ½ teaspoon Table salt

Directions:

1. Cut each potato lengthwise into ¼-inch-thick slices. Cut each of these lengthwise into ¼-inch-thick matchsticks.
2. Set the potato matchsticks in a big bowl of cool water and soak for 5 minutes. Drain in a colander set in the sink, then spread the matchsticks out on paper towels and dry them very well.
3. Preheat the air fryer to 225°F (or 230°F, if that's the closest setting).
4. When the machine is at temperature, arrange the matchsticks in an even layer (if overlapping but not compact) in the basket. Air-fry for 20 minutes, tossing and rearranging the fries twice.
5. Pour the contents of the basket into a big bowl. Increase the air fryer's temperature to 325°F (or 330°F, if that's the closest setting).
6. Generously coat the fries with vegetable or olive oil spray. Toss well, then coat them again to make sure they're covered on all sides, tossing (and maybe spraying) a couple of times to make sure.

7. When the machine is at temperature, pour the fries into the basket and air-fry for 12 minutes, tossing and rearranging the fries at least twice.
8. Increase the machine's temperature to 375°F (or 380°F or 390°F, if one of these is the closest setting). Air-fry for 5 minutes more (from the moment you raise the temperature), tossing and rearranging the fries at least twice to keep them from burning and to make sure they all get an even measure of the heat, until brown and crisp.
9. Pour the contents of the basket into a serving bowl. Toss the fries with the salt and serve hot.

Sweet Potato Fries

Servings: 4
Cooking Time: 30 Minutes

Ingredients:

- 2 pounds sweet potatoes
- 1 teaspoon dried marjoram
- 2 teaspoons olive oil
- sea salt

Directions:

1. Peel and cut the potatoes into ¼-inch sticks, 4 to 5 inches long.
2. In a sealable plastic bag or bowl with lid, toss sweet potatoes with marjoram and olive oil. Rub seasonings in to coat well.
3. Pour sweet potatoes into air fryer basket and cook at 390°F for approximately 30 minutes, until cooked through with some brown spots on edges.
4. Season to taste with sea salt.

Fried Cauliflowerwith Parmesan Lemon Dressing

Servings: 2
Cooking Time: 12 Minutes

Ingredients:

- 4 cups cauliflower florets (about half a large head)
- 1 tablespoon olive oil
- salt and freshly ground black pepper
- 1 teaspoon finely chopped lemon zest
- 1 tablespoon fresh lemon juice (about half a lemon)
- ¼ cup grated Parmigiano-Reggiano cheese
- 4 tablespoons extra virgin olive oil
- ¼ teaspoon salt
- lots of freshly ground black pepper
- 1 tablespoon chopped fresh parsley

Directions:

1. Preheat the air fryer to 400°F.
2. Toss the cauliflower florets with the olive oil, salt and freshly ground black pepper. Air-fry for 12 minutes, shaking the basket a couple of times during the cooking process.
3. While the cauliflower is frying, make the dressing. Combine the lemon zest, lemon juice, Parmigiano-Reggiano cheese and olive oil in a small bowl. Season with salt and lots of freshly ground black pepper. Stir in the parsley.
4. Turn the fried cauliflower out onto a serving platter and drizzle the dressing over the top.

Green Peas With Mint

Servings: 4
Cooking Time: 5 Minutes

Ingredients:

- 1 cup shredded lettuce
- 1 10-ounce package frozen green peas, thawed
- 1 tablespoon fresh mint, shredded
- 1 teaspoon melted butter

Directions:

1. Lay the shredded lettuce in the air fryer basket.
2. Toss together the peas, mint, and melted butter and spoon over the lettuce.
3. Cook at 360°F for 5minutes, until peas are warm and lettuce wilts.

Salt And Pepper Baked Potatoes

Servings: 4
Cooking Time: 40 Minutes

Ingredients:

- 1 to 2 tablespoons olive oil
- 4 medium russet potatoes (about 9 to 10 ounces each)
- salt and coarsely ground black pepper

- butter, sour cream, chopped fresh chives, scallions or bacon bits (optional)

Directions:

1. Preheat the air fryer to 400°F.
2. Rub the olive oil all over the potatoes and season them generously with salt and coarsely ground black pepper. Pierce all sides of the potatoes several times with the tines of a fork.
3. Air-fry for 40 minutes, turning the potatoes over halfway through the cooking time.
4. Serve the potatoes, split open with butter, sour cream, fresh chives, scallions or bacon bits.

Chicken Eggrolls

Servings: 10

Cooking Time: 17 Minutes

Ingredients:

- 1 tablespoon vegetable oil
- ¼ cup chopped onion
- 1 clove garlic, minced
- 1 cup shredded carrot
- ½ cup thinly sliced celery
- 2 cups cooked chicken
- 2 cups shredded white cabbage
- ½ cup teriyaki sauce
- 20 egg roll wrappers
- 1 egg, whisked
- 1 tablespoon water

Directions:

1. Preheat the air fryer to 390°F.
2. In a large skillet, heat the oil over medium-high heat. Add in the onion and sauté for 1 minute. Add in the garlic and sauté for 30 seconds. Add in the carrot and celery and cook for 2 minutes. Add in the chicken, cabbage, and teriyaki sauce. Allow the mixture to cook for 1 minute, stirring to combine. Remove from the heat.
3. In a small bowl, whisk together the egg and water for brushing the edges.
4. Lay the eggroll wrappers out at an angle. Place ¼ cup filling in the center. Fold the bottom corner up first and then fold in the corners; roll up to complete eggroll.
5. Place the eggrolls in the air fryer basket, spray with cooking spray, and cook for 8 minutes, turn over, and cook another 2 to 4 minutes.

Florentine Stuffed Tomatoes

Servings: 2

Cooking Time: 12 Minutes

Ingredients:

- 1 cup frozen spinach, thawed and squeezed dry
- ¼ cup toasted pine nuts
- ¼ cup grated mozzarella cheese
- ½ cup crumbled feta cheese
- ½ cup coarse fresh breadcrumbs
- 1 tablespoon olive oil
- salt and freshly ground black pepper
- 2 to 3 beefsteak tomatoes, halved horizontally and insides scooped out

Directions:

1. Combine the spinach, pine nuts, mozzarella and feta cheeses, breadcrumbs, olive oil, salt and freshly ground black pepper in a bowl. Spoon the mixture into the tomato halves. You should have enough filling for 2 to 3 tomatoes, depending on how big they are.
2. Preheat the air fryer to 350°F.
3. Place three or four tomato halves (depending on whether you're using 2 or 3 tomatoes and how big they are) into the air fryer and air-fry for 12 minutes. The tomatoes should be soft but still manageable and the tops should be lightly browned. Repeat with second batch if necessary.
4. Let the tomatoes cool for just a minute or two before serving.

Pork Tenderloin Salad

Servings: 4

Cooking Time: 25 Minutes

Ingredients:

- Pork Tenderloin
- ½ teaspoon smoked paprika
- ¼ teaspoon salt
- ¼ teaspoon garlic powder
- ½ teaspoon onion powder

- ⅛ teaspoon ginger
- 1 teaspoon extra-light olive oil
- ¾ pound pork tenderloin
- Dressing
- 3 tablespoons extra-light olive oil
- 2 tablespoons red wine vinegar
- 2 tablespoons Dijon mustard
- 1 tablespoon honey
- Salad
- ¼ sweet red bell pepper
- 1 large Granny Smith apple
- 8 cups shredded Napa cabbage

Directions:

1. Mix the tenderloin seasonings together with oil and rub all over surface of meat.
2. Place pork tenderloin in the air fryer basket and cook at 390°F for 25minutes, until meat registers 130°F on a meat thermometer.
3. Allow meat to rest while preparing salad and dressing.
4. In a jar, shake all dressing ingredients together until well mixed.
5. Cut the bell pepper into slivers, then core, quarter, and slice the apple crosswise.
6. In a large bowl, toss together the cabbage, bell pepper, apple, and dressing.
7. Divide salad mixture among 4 plates.
8. Slice pork tenderloin into ½-inch slices and divide among the 4 salads.
9. Serve with sweet potato or other vegetable chips.

Zucchini Fries

Servings: 3

Cooking Time: 12 Minutes

Ingredients:

- 1 large Zucchini
- ½ cup All-purpose flour or tapioca flour
- 2 Large egg(s), well beaten
- 1 cup Seasoned Italian-style dried bread crumbs (gluten-free, if a concern)
- Olive oil spray

Directions:

1. Preheat the air fryer to 400°F.
2. Trim the zucchini into a long rectangular block, taking off the ends and four "sides" to make this shape. Cut the block lengthwise into ½-inch-thick slices. Lay these slices flat and cut in half widthwise. Slice each of these pieces into ½-inch-thick batons.
3. Set up and fill three shallow soup plates or small pie plates on your counter: one for the flour, one for the beaten egg(s), and one for the bread crumbs.
4. Set a zucchini baton in the flour and turn it several times to coat all sides. Gently shake off any excess flour, then dip it in the egg(s), turning it to coat. Let any excess egg slip back into the rest, then set the baton in the bread crumbs and turn it several times, pressing gently to coat all sides, even the ends. Set aside on a cutting board and continue coating the remainder of the batons in the same way.
5. Lightly coat the batons on all sides with olive oil spray. Set them in two flat layers in the basket, the top layer at a 90-degree angle to the bottom one, with a little air space between the batons in each layer. In the end, the whole thing will look like a crosshatch pattern. Air-fry undisturbed for 6 minutes.
6. Use kitchen tongs to gently rearrange the batons so that any covered parts are now uncovered. The batons no longer need to be in a crosshatch pattern. Continue air-frying undisturbed for 6 minutes, or until lightly browned and crisp.
7. Gently pour the contents of the basket onto a wire rack. Spread the batons out and cool for only a minute or two before serving.

Mexican-style Roasted Corn

Servings: 3

Cooking Time: 14 Minutes

Ingredients:

- 3 tablespoons Butter, melted and cooled
- 2 teaspoons Minced garlic
- ¾ teaspoon Ground cumin
- Up to ¾ teaspoon Red pepper flakes
- ¼ teaspoon Table salt
- 3 Cold 4-inch lengths husked and de-silked corn on the cob
- Minced fresh cilantro leaves

- Crumbled queso fresco

Directions:

1. Preheat the air fryer to 400°F.
2. Mix the melted butter, garlic, cumin, red pepper flakes, and salt in a large zip-closed plastic bag. Add the cold corn pieces, seal the bag, and massage the butter mixture into the surface of the corn.
3. When the machine is at temperature, take the pieces of corn out of the plastic bag and put them in the basket with as much air space between the pieces as possible. Air-fry undisturbed for 14 minutes, until golden brown and maybe even charred in a few small spots.
4. Use kitchen tongs to gently transfer the pieces of corn to a serving platter. Sprinkle each piece with the cilantro and queso fresco. Serve warm.

Roasted Fennel Salad

Servings: 3

Cooking Time: 20 Minutes

Ingredients:

- 3 cups (about ¾ pound) Trimmed fennel (see the headnote), roughly chopped
- 1½ tablespoons Olive oil
- ¼ teaspoon Table salt
- ¼ teaspoon Ground black pepper
- 1½ tablespoons White balsamic vinegar (see here)

Directions:

1. Preheat the air fryer to 400°F.
2. Toss the fennel, olive oil, salt, and pepper in a large bowl until the fennel is well coated in the oil.
3. When the machine is at temperature, pour the fennel into the basket, spreading it out into as close to one layer as possible. Air-fry for 20 minutes, tossing and rearranging the fennel pieces twice so that any covered or touching parts get exposed to the air currents, until golden at the edges and softened.
4. Pour the fennel into a serving bowl. Add the vinegar while hot. Toss well, then cool a couple of minutes before serving. Or serve at room temperature.

Roasted Cauliflower With Garlic And Capers

Servings: 3

Cooking Time: 10 Minutes

Ingredients:

- 3 cups (about 15 ounces) 1-inch cauliflower florets
- 2 tablespoons Olive oil
- 1½ tablespoons Drained and rinsed capers, chopped
- 2 teaspoons Minced garlic
- ¼ teaspoon Table salt
- Up to ¼ teaspoon Red pepper flakes

Directions:

1. Preheat the air fryer to 375°F .
2. Stir the cauliflower florets, olive oil, capers, garlic, salt, and red pepper flakes in a large bowl until the florets are evenly coated.
3. When the machine is at temperature, put the florets in the basket, spreading them out to as close to one layer as you can. Air-fry for 10 minutes, tossing once to get any covered pieces exposed to the air currents, until tender and lightly browned.
4. Dump the contents of the basket into a serving bowl or onto a serving platter. Cool for a minute or two before serving.

Sesame Carrots And Sugar Snap Peas

Servings: 4

Cooking Time: 16 Minutes

Ingredients:

- 1 pound carrots, peeled sliced on the bias (½-inch slices)
- 1 teaspoon olive oil
- salt and freshly ground black pepper
- ⅓ cup honey
- 1 tablespoon sesame oil
- 1 tablespoon soy sauce
- ½ teaspoon minced fresh ginger
- 4 ounces sugar snap peas (about 1 cup)
- 1½ teaspoons sesame seeds

Directions:

1. Preheat the air fryer to 360°F.

2. Toss the carrots with the olive oil, season with salt and pepper and air-fry for 10 minutes, shaking the basket once or twice during the cooking process.
3. Combine the honey, sesame oil, soy sauce and minced ginger in a large bowl. Add the sugar snap peas and the air-fried carrots to the honey mixture, toss to coat and return everything to the air fryer basket.
4. Turn up the temperature to 400°F and air-fry for an additional 6 minutes, shaking the basket once during the cooking process.
5. Transfer the carrots and sugar snap peas to a serving bowl. Pour the sauce from the bottom of the cooker over the vegetables and sprinkle sesame seeds over top. Serve immediately.

Mushrooms

Servings: 4
Cooking Time: 12 Minutes

Ingredients:

- 8 ounces whole white button mushrooms
- ½ teaspoon salt
- ⅛ teaspoon pepper
- ¼ teaspoon garlic powder
- ¼ teaspoon onion powder
- 5 tablespoons potato starch
- 1 egg, beaten
- ¾ cup panko breadcrumbs
- oil for misting or cooking spray

Directions:

1. Place mushrooms in a large bowl. Add the salt, pepper, garlic and onion powders, and stir well to distribute seasonings.
2. Add potato starch to mushrooms and toss in bowl until well coated.
3. Dip mushrooms in beaten egg, roll in panko crumbs, and mist with oil or cooking spray.
4. Place mushrooms in air fryer basket. You can cook them all at once, and it's okay if a few are stacked.
5. Cook at 390°F for 5minutes. Shake basket, then continue cooking for 7 more minutes, until golden brown and crispy.

Parsnip Fries With Romesco Sauce

Servings: 2
Cooking Time: 24 Minutes

Ingredients:

- Romesco Sauce:
- 1 red bell pepper, halved and seeded
- 1 (1-inch) thick slice of Italian bread, torn into pieces (about 1 to 1½ cups)
- 1 cup almonds, toasted
- olive oil
- ½ Jalapeño pepper, seeded
- 1 tablespoon fresh parsley leaves
- 1 clove garlic
- 2 Roma tomatoes, peeled and seeded (or ⅓ cup canned crushed tomatoes)
- 1 tablespoon red wine vinegar
- ¼ teaspoon smoked paprika
- ½ teaspoon salt
- ¾ cup olive oil
- 3 parsnips, peeled and cut into long strips
- 2 teaspoons olive oil
- salt and freshly ground black pepper

Directions:

1. Preheat the air fryer to 400°F.
2. Place the red pepper halves, cut side down, in the air fryer basket and air-fry for 10 minutes, or until the skin turns black all over. Remove the pepper from the air fryer and let it cool. When it is cool enough to handle, peel the pepper.
3. Toss the torn bread and almonds with a little olive oil and air-fry for 4 minutes, shaking the basket a couple times throughout the cooking time. When the bread and almonds are nicely toasted, remove them from the air fryer and let them cool for just a minute or two.
4. Combine the toasted bread, almonds, roasted red pepper, Jalapeño pepper, parsley, garlic, tomatoes, vinegar, smoked paprika and salt in a food processor or blender. Process until smooth. With the processor running, add the olive oil through the feed tube until the sauce comes together in a smooth paste that is barely pourable.

5. Toss the parsnip strips with the olive oil, salt and freshly ground black pepper and air-fry at 400°F for 10 minutes, shaking the basket a couple times during the cooking process so they brown and cook evenly. Serve the parsnip fries warm with the Romesco sauce to dip into.

Perfect Asparagus

Servings: 3

Cooking Time: 10 Minutes

Ingredients:

- 1 pound Very thin asparagus spears
- 2 tablespoons Olive oil
- 1 teaspoon Coarse sea salt or kosher salt
- ¾ teaspoon Finely grated lemon zest

Directions:

1. Preheat the air fryer to 400°F.
2. Trim just enough off the bottom of the asparagus spears so they'll fit in the basket. Put the spears on a large plate and drizzle them with some of the olive oil. Turn them over and drizzle more olive oil, working to get all the spears coated.
3. When the machine is at temperature, place the spears in one direction in the basket. They may be touching. Air-fry for 10 minutes, tossing and rearranging the spears twice, until tender.
4. Dump the contents of the basket on a serving platter. Spread out the spears. Sprinkle them with the salt and lemon zest while still warm. Serve at once.

Mini Hasselback Potatoes

Servings: 4

Cooking Time: 25 Minutes

Ingredients:

- 1½ pounds baby Yukon Gold potatoes (about 10)
- 5 tablespoons butter, cut into very thin slices
- salt and freshly ground black pepper
- 1 tablespoon vegetable oil
- ¼ cup grated Parmesan cheese (optional)
- chopped fresh parsley or chives

Directions:

1. Preheat the air fryer to 400°F.
2. Make six to eight deep vertical slits across the top of each potato about three quarters of the way down. Make sure the slits are deep enough to allow the slices to spread apart a little, but don't cut all the way through the potato. Place a thin slice of butter between each of the slices and season generously with salt and pepper.
3. Transfer the potatoes to the air fryer basket. Pack them in next to each other. It's alright if some of the potatoes sit on top or rest on another potato. Air-fry for 20 minutes.
4. Spray or brush the potatoes with a little vegetable oil and sprinkle the Parmesan cheese on top. Air-fry for an additional 5 minutes. Garnish with chopped parsley or chives and serve hot.

Acorn Squash Halves With Maple Butter Glaze

Servings: 2

Cooking Time: 33 Minutes

Ingredients:

- 1 medium (1 to 1¼ pounds) Acorn squash
- Vegetable oil spray
- ¼ teaspoon Table salt
- 1½ tablespoons Butter, melted
- 1½ tablespoons Maple syrup

Directions:

1. Preheat the air fryer to 325°F (or 330°F, if that's the closest setting).
2. Cut a squash in half through the stem end. Use a flatware spoon (preferably, a serrated grapefruit spoon) to scrape out and discard the seeds and membranes in each half. Use a paring knife to make a crisscross pattern of cuts about ½ inch apart and ¼ inch deep across the "meat" of the squash. If working with a second squash, repeat this step for that one.
3. Generously coat the cut side of the squash halves with vegetable oil spray. Sprinkle the halves with the salt. Set them in the basket cut side up with at least ¼ inch between them. Air-fry undisturbed for 30 minutes.
4. Increase the machine's temperature to 400°F. Mix the melted butter and syrup in a small bowl until uniform. Brush this mixture over the cut sides of the

squash(es), letting it pool in the center. Air-fry undisturbed for 3 minutes, or until the glaze is bubbling.

5. Use a nonstick-safe spatula and kitchen tongs to transfer the squash halves cut side up to a wire rack. Cool for 5 to 10 minutes before serving.

Mashed Potato Tots

Servings: 18

Cooking Time: 10 Minutes

Ingredients:

- 1 medium potato or 1 cup cooked mashed potatoes
- 1 tablespoon real bacon bits
- 2 tablespoons chopped green onions, tops only
- ¼ teaspoon onion powder
- 1 teaspoon dried chopped chives
- salt
- 2 tablespoons flour
- 1 egg white, beaten
- ½ cup panko breadcrumbs
- oil for misting or cooking spray

Directions:

1. If using cooked mashed potatoes, jump to step 4.
2. Peel potato and cut into ½-inch cubes. (Small pieces cook more quickly.) Place in saucepan, add water to cover, and heat to boil. Lower heat slightly and continue cooking just until tender, about 10minutes.
3. Drain potatoes and place in ice cold water. Allow to cool for a minute or two, then drain well and mash.
4. Preheat air fryer to 390°F.
5. In a large bowl, mix together the potatoes, bacon bits, onions, onion powder, chives, salt to taste, and flour. Add egg white and stir well.
6. Place panko crumbs on a sheet of wax paper.
7. For each tot, use about 2 teaspoons of potato mixture. To shape, drop the measure of potato mixture onto panko crumbs and push crumbs up and around potatoes to coat edges. Then turn tot over to coat other side with crumbs.
8. Mist tots with oil or cooking spray and place in air fryer basket, crowded but not stacked.
9. Cook at 390°F for 10 minutes, until browned and crispy.
10. Repeat steps 8 and 9 to cook remaining tots.

Cheesy Texas Toast

Servings: 2

Cooking Time: 4 Minutes

Ingredients:

- 2 1-inch-thick slice(s) Italian bread (each about 4 inches across)
- 4 teaspoons Softened butter
- 2 teaspoons Minced garlic
- ¼ cup (about ¾ ounce) Finely grated Parmesan cheese

Directions:

1. Preheat the air fryer to 400°F.
2. Spread one side of a slice of bread with 2 teaspoons butter. Sprinkle with 1 teaspoon minced garlic, followed by 2 tablespoons grated cheese. Repeat this process if you're making one or more additional toasts.
3. When the machine is at temperature, put the bread slice(s) cheese side up in the basket (with as much air space between them as possible if you're making more than one). Air-fry undisturbed for 4 minutes, or until browned and crunchy.
4. Use a nonstick-safe spatula to transfer the toasts cheese side up to a wire rack. Cool for 5 minutes before serving.

Crispy, Cheesy Leeks

Servings: 4

Cooking Time: 15 Minutes

Ingredients:

- 2 Medium leek(s), about 9 ounces each
- Olive oil spray
- ¼ cup Seasoned Italian-style dried bread crumbs (gluten-free, if a concern)
- ¼ cup (about ¾ ounce) Finely grated Parmesan cheese
- 2 tablespoons Olive oil

Directions:

1. Preheat the air fryer to 350°F .
2. Trim off the root end of the leek(s) as well as the dark green top(s), leaving about a 5-inch usable section. Split the leek section(s) in half lengthwise. Set the leek halves cut side up on your work surface. Pull out and

remove in one piece the semicircles that make up the inner structure of the leek, about halfway down. Set the removed "inside" next to the outer leek "shells" on your cutting board. Generously coat them all on all sides (particularly the "bottoms") with olive oil spray.

3. Set the leeks and their insides cut side up in the basket with as much air space between them as possible. Air-fry undisturbed for 12 minutes.
4. Meanwhile, mix the bread crumbs, cheese, and olive oil in a small bowl until well combined.
5. After 12 minutes in the air fryer, sprinkle this mixture inside the leek shells and on top of the leek insides. Increase the machine's temperature to 375°F (or 380°F or 390°F, if one of these is the closest setting). Air-fry undisturbed for 3 minutes, or until the topping is lightly browned.
6. Use a nonstick-safe spatula to transfer the leeks to a serving platter. Cool for a few minutes before serving warm.

Home Fries

Servings: 4
Cooking Time: 20 Minutes

Ingredients:

- 3 pounds potatoes, cut into 1-inch cubes
- ½ teaspoon oil
- salt and pepper

Directions:

1. In a large bowl, mix the potatoes and oil thoroughly.
2. Cook at 390°F for 10minutes and shake the basket to redistribute potatoes.
3. Cook for an additional 10 minutes, until brown and crisp.
4. Season with salt and pepper to taste.

Perfect Broccolini

Servings: 4
Cooking Time: 15 Minutes

Ingredients:

- 1 pound Broccolini
- Olive oil spray
- Coarse sea salt or kosher salt

Directions:

1. Preheat the air fryer to 375°F .
2. Place the broccolini on a cutting board. Generously coat it with olive oil spray, turning the vegetables and rearranging them before spraying a couple of times more, to make sure everything's well coated, even the flowery bits in their heads.
3. When the machine is at temperature, pile the broccolini in the basket, spreading it into as close to one layer as you can. Air-fry for 5 minutes, tossing once to get any covered or touching parts exposed to the air currents, until the leaves begin to get brown and even crisp. Watch carefully and use this visual cue to know the moment to stop the cooking.
4. Transfer the broccolini to a platter. Spread out the pieces and sprinkle them with salt to taste.

Fried Green Tomatoes With Sriracha Mayo

Servings: 4
Cooking Time: 12 Minutes

Ingredients:

- 3 green tomatoes
- salt and freshly ground black pepper
- ⅓ cup all-purpose flour*
- 2 eggs
- ½ cup buttermilk
- 1 cup panko breadcrumbs*
- 1 cup cornmeal
- olive oil, in a spray bottle
- fresh thyme sprigs or chopped fresh chives
- Sriracha Mayo
- ½ cup mayonnaise
- 1 to 2 tablespoons sriracha hot sauce
- 1 tablespoon milk

Directions:

1. Cut the tomatoes in ¼-inch slices. Pat them dry with a clean kitchen towel and season generously with salt and pepper.
2. Set up a dredging station using three shallow dishes. Place the flour in the first shallow dish, whisk the eggs

and buttermilk together in the second dish, and combine the panko breadcrumbs and cornmeal in the third dish.

3. Preheat the air fryer to 400°F.
4. Dredge the tomato slices in flour to coat on all sides. Then dip them into the egg mixture and finally press them into the breadcrumbs to coat all sides of the tomato.
5. Spray or brush the air-fryer basket with olive oil. Transfer 3 to 4 tomato slices into the basket and spray the top with olive oil. Air-fry the tomatoes at 400°F for 8 minutes. Flip them over, spray the other side with oil and air-fry for an additional 4 minutes until golden brown.
6. While the tomatoes are cooking, make the sriracha mayo. Combine the mayonnaise, 1 tablespoon of the sriracha hot sauce and milk in a small bowl. Stir well until the mixture is smooth. Add more sriracha sauce to taste.
7. When the tomatoes are done, transfer them to a cooling rack or a platter lined with paper towels so the bottom does not get soggy. Before serving, carefully stack the all the tomatoes into air fryer and air-fry at 350°F for 1 to 2 minutes to heat them back up.
8. Serve the fried green tomatoes hot with the sriracha mayo on the side. Season one last time with salt and freshly ground black pepper and garnish with sprigs of fresh thyme or chopped fresh chives.

Roasted Brussels Sprouts

Servings: 4
Cooking Time: 25 Minutes

Ingredients:

- ½ cup balsamic vinegar
- 2 tablespoons honey
- 1 pound Brussels sprouts, halved lengthwise
- 2 slices bacon, chopped
- ½ teaspoon garlic powder
- 1 teaspoon salt
- 1 tablespoon extra-virgin olive oil
- ¼ cup grated Parmesan cheese

Directions:

1. Preheat the air fryer to 370°F.
2. In a small saucepan, heat the vinegar and honey for 8 to 10 minutes over medium-low heat, or until the balsamic vinegar reduces by half to create a thick balsamic glazing sauce.
3. While the balsamic glaze is reducing, in a large bowl, toss together the Brussels sprouts, bacon, garlic powder, salt, and olive oil. Pour the mixture into the air fryer basket and cook for 10 minutes; check for doneness. Cook another 2 to 5 minutes or until slightly crispy and tender.
4. Pour the balsamic glaze into a serving bowl and add the cooked Brussels sprouts to the dish, stirring to coat. Top with grated Parmesan cheese and serve.

Cauliflower

Servings: 4
Cooking Time: 6 Minutes

Ingredients:

- ½ cup water
- 1 10-ounce package frozen cauliflower (florets)
- 1 teaspoon lemon pepper seasoning

Directions:

1. Pour the water into air fryer drawer.
2. Pour the frozen cauliflower into the air fryer basket and sprinkle with lemon pepper seasoning.
3. Cook at 390°F for approximately 6 minutes.

Stuffed Avocados

Servings: 4
Cooking Time: 8 Minutes

Ingredients:

- 1 cup frozen shoepeg corn, thawed
- 1 cup cooked black beans
- ¼ cup diced onion
- ½ teaspoon cumin
- 2 teaspoons lime juice, plus extra for serving
- salt and pepper
- 2 large avocados, split in half, pit removed

Directions:

1. Mix together the corn, beans, onion, cumin, and lime juice. Season to taste with salt and pepper.
2. Scoop out some of the flesh from center of each avocado and set aside. Divide corn mixture evenly between the cavities.

3. Set avocado halves in air fryer basket and cook at 360°F for 8 minutes, until corn mixture is hot.
4. Season the avocado flesh that you scooped out with a squirt of lime juice, salt, and pepper. Spoon it over the cooked halves.

Rosemary New Potatoes

Servings: 4
Cooking Time: 6 Minutes

Ingredients:

- 3 large red potatoes (enough to make 3 cups sliced)
- ¼ teaspoon ground rosemary
- ¼ teaspoon ground thyme
- ⅛ teaspoon salt
- ⅛ teaspoon ground black pepper
- 2 teaspoons extra-light olive oil

Directions:

1. Preheat air fryer to 330°F.
2. Place potatoes in large bowl and sprinkle with rosemary, thyme, salt, and pepper.
3. Stir with a spoon to distribute seasonings evenly.
4. Add oil to potatoes and stir again to coat well.
5. Cook at 330°F for 4minutes. Stir and break apart any that have stuck together.
6. Cook an additional 2 minutes or until fork-tender.

Honey-roasted Parsnips

Servings: 3
Cooking Time: 23 Minutes

Ingredients:

- 1½ pounds Medium parsnips, peeled
- Olive oil spray
- 1 tablespoon Honey
- 1½ teaspoons Water
- ¼ teaspoon Table salt

Directions:

1. Preheat the air fryer to 350°F .
2. If the thick end of a parsnip is more than ½ inch in diameter, cut the parsnip just below where it swells to its large end, then slice the large section in half lengthwise. If the parsnips are larger than the basket (or basket attachment), trim off the thin end so the parsnips will fit. Generously coat the parsnips on all sides with olive oil spray.
3. When the machine is at temperature, set the parsnips in the basket with as much air space between them as possible. Air-fry undisturbed for 20 minutes.
4. Whisk the honey, water, and salt in a small bowl until smooth. Brush this mixture over the parsnips. Air-fry undisturbed for 3 minutes more, or until the glaze is lightly browned.
5. Use kitchen tongs to transfer the parsnips to a wire rack or a serving platter. Cool for a couple of minutes before serving.

Latkes

Servings: 12
Cooking Time: 13 Minutes

Ingredients:

- 1 russet potato
- ¼ onion
- 2 eggs, lightly beaten
- ⅓ cup flour*
- ½ teaspoon baking powder
- 1 teaspoon salt
- freshly ground black pepper
- canola or vegetable oil, in a spray bottle
- chopped chives, for garnish
- apple sauce
- sour cream

Directions:

1. Shred the potato and onion with a coarse box grater or a food processor with the shredding blade. Place the shredded vegetables into a colander or mesh strainer and squeeze or press down firmly to remove the excess water.
2. Transfer the onion and potato to a large bowl and add the eggs, flour, baking powder, salt and black pepper. Mix to combine and then shape the mixture into patties, about ¼-cup of mixture each. Brush or spray both sides of the latkes with oil.
3. Preheat the air fryer to 400°F.
4. Air-fry the latkes in batches. Transfer one layer of the latkes to the air fryer basket and air-fry at 400°F for 12 to 13 minutes, flipping them over halfway through the cooking time. Transfer the finished latkes to a platter

and cover with aluminum foil, or place them in a warm oven to keep warm.

5. Garnish the latkes with chopped chives and serve with sour cream and applesauce.

Mashed Sweet Potato Tots

Servings: 18

Cooking Time: 12 Minutes

Ingredients:

- 1 cup cooked mashed sweet potatoes
- 1 egg white, beaten
- ⅛ teaspoon ground cinnamon
- 1 dash nutmeg
- 2 tablespoons chopped pecans
- 1½ teaspoons honey
- salt
- ½ cup panko breadcrumbs
- oil for misting or cooking spray

Directions:

1. Preheat air fryer to 390°F.
2. In a large bowl, mix together the potatoes, egg white, cinnamon, nutmeg, pecans, honey, and salt to taste.
3. Place panko crumbs on a sheet of wax paper.
4. For each tot, use about 2 teaspoons of sweet potato mixture. To shape, drop the measure of potato mixture onto panko crumbs and push crumbs up and around potatoes to coat edges. Then turn tot over to coat other side with crumbs.
5. Mist tots with oil or cooking spray and place in air fryer basket in single layer.
6. Cook at 390°F for 12 minutes, until browned and crispy.
7. Repeat steps 5 and 6 to cook remaining tots.

Shoestring Butternut Squash Fries

Servings: 3

Cooking Time: 16 Minutes

Ingredients:

- 1 pound 2 ounces Spiralized butternut squash strands
- Vegetable oil spray
- To taste Coarse sea salt or kosher salt

Directions:

1. Preheat the air fryer to 375°F .
2. Place the spiralized squash in a big bowl. Coat the strands with vegetable oil spray, toss well, coat again, and toss several times to make sure all the strands have been oiled.
3. When the machine is at temperature, pour the strands into the basket and spread them out into as even a layer as possible. Air-fry for 16 minutes, tossing and rearranging the strands every 4 minutes, or until they're lightly browned and crisp.
4. Pour the contents of the basket into a serving bowl, add salt to taste, and toss well before serving hot.

Cheesy Potato Skins

Servings: 6

Cooking Time: 54 Minutes

Ingredients:

- 3 6- to 8-ounce small russet potatoes
- 3 Thick-cut bacon strips, halved widthwise (gluten-free, if a concern)
- ¾ teaspoon Mild paprika
- ¼ teaspoon Garlic powder
- ¼ teaspoon Table salt
- ¼ teaspoon Ground black pepper
- ½ cup plus 1 tablespoon (a little over 2 ounces) Shredded Cheddar cheese
- 3 tablespoons Thinly sliced trimmed chives
- 6 tablespoons (a little over 1 ounce) Finely grated Parmesan cheese

Directions:

1. Preheat the air fryer to 375°F .
2. Prick each potato in four places with a fork (not four places in a line but four places all around the potato). Set the potatoes in the basket with as much air space between them as possible. Air-fry undisturbed for 45 minutes, or until the potatoes are tender when pricked with a fork.
3. Use kitchen tongs to gently transfer the potatoes to a wire rack. Cool for 15 minutes. Maintain the machine's temperature.
4. Lay the bacon strip halves in the basket in one layer. They may touch but should not overlap. Air-fry

undisturbed for 5 minutes, until crisp. Use those same tongs to transfer the bacon pieces to the wire rack. If there's a great deal of rendered bacon fat in the basket's bottom or on a tray under the basket attachment, pour this into a bowl, cool, and discard. Don't throw it down the drain!

5. Cut the potatoes in half lengthwise (not just slit them open but actually cut in half). Use a flatware spoon to scoop the hot, soft middles into a bowl, leaving ½ inch of potato all around the inside of the spud next to the skin. Sprinkle the inside of the potato "shells" evenly with paprika, garlic powder, salt, and pepper.
6. Chop the bacon pieces into small bits. Sprinkle these along with the Cheddar and chives evenly inside the potato shells. Crumble 2 to 3 tablespoons of the soft potato insides over the filling mixture. Divide the grated Parmesan evenly over the tops of the potatoes.
7. Set the stuffed potatoes in the basket with as much air space between them as possible. Air-fry undisturbed for 4 minutes, until the cheese melts and lightly browns.
8. Use kitchen tongs to gently transfer the stuffed potato halves to a wire rack. Cool for 5 minutes before serving.

Roasted Eggplant Halves With Herbed Ricotta

Servings: 3

Cooking Time: 20 Minutes

Ingredients:

- 3 5- to 6-ounce small eggplants, stemmed
- Olive oil spray
- ¼ teaspoon Table salt
- ¼ teaspoon Ground black pepper
- ½ cup Regular or low-fat ricotta
- 1½ tablespoons Minced fresh basil leaves
- 1¼ teaspoons Minced fresh oregano leaves
- Honey

Directions:

1. Preheat the air fryer to 325°F (or 330°F, if that's the closest setting).
2. Cut the eggplants in half lengthwise. Set them cut side up on your work surface. Using the tip of a paring knife, make a series of slits about three-quarters down into the flesh of each eggplant half; work at a 45-degree angle to the (former) stem across the vegetable and make the slits about ½ inch apart. Make a second set of equidistant slits at a 90-degree angle to the first slits, thus creating a crosshatch pattern in the vegetable.
3. Generously coat the cut sides of the eggplants with olive oil spray. Sprinkle the salt and pepper over the cut surfaces.
4. Set the eggplant halves cut side up in the basket with as much air space between them as possible. Air-fry undisturbed for 20 minutes, or until soft and golden.
5. Use kitchen tongs to gently transfer the eggplant halves to serving plates or a platter. Cool for 5 minutes.
6. Whisk the ricotta, basil, and oregano in a small bowl until well combined. Top the eggplant halves with this mixture. Drizzle the halves with honey to taste before serving warm.

Wilted Brussels Sprout Slaw

Servings: 4

Cooking Time: 18 Minutes

Ingredients:

- 2 Thick-cut bacon strip(s), halved widthwise (gluten-free, if a concern)
- 4½ cups (about 1 pound 2 ounces) Bagged shredded Brussels sprouts
- ¼ teaspoon Table salt
- 2 tablespoons White balsamic vinegar (see here)
- 2 teaspoons Worcestershire sauce (gluten-free, if a concern)
- 1 teaspoon Dijon mustard (gluten-free, if a concern)
- ¼ teaspoon Ground black pepper

Directions:

1. Preheat the air fryer to 375°F .
2. When the machine is at temperature, lay the bacon strip halves in the basket in one layer and air-fry for 10 minutes, or until crisp.
3. Use kitchen tongs to transfer the bacon pieces to a wire rack. Put the shredded Brussels sprouts in a large bowl. Drain any fat from the basket or the tray under the basket onto the Brussels sprouts. Add the salt and toss well to coat.

4. Put the Brussels sprout shreds in the basket, spreading them out into as close to an even layer as you can. Air-fry for 8 minutes, tossing the basket's contents at least three times, until wilted and lightly browned.
5. Pour the contents of the basket into a serving bowl. Chop the bacon and add it to the Brussels sprouts. Add the vinegar, Worcestershire sauce, mustard, and pepper. Toss well to blend the dressing and coat the Brussels sprout shreds. Serve warm.

Buttery Rolls

Servings: 6

Cooking Time: 14 Minutes

Ingredients:

- 6½ tablespoons Room-temperature whole or low-fat milk
- 3 tablespoons plus 1 teaspoon Butter, melted and cooled
- 3 tablespoons plus 1 teaspoon (or 1 medium egg, well beaten) Pasteurized egg substitute, such as Egg Beaters
- 1½ tablespoons Granulated white sugar
- 1¼ teaspoons Instant yeast
- ¼ teaspoon Table salt
- 2 cups, plus more for dusting All-purpose flour
- Vegetable oil
- Additional melted butter, for brushing

Directions:

1. Stir the milk, melted butter, pasteurized egg substitute (or whole egg), sugar, yeast, and salt in a medium bowl to combine. Stir in the flour just until the mixture makes a soft dough.
2. Lightly flour a clean, dry work surface. Turn the dough out onto the work surface. Knead the dough for 5 minutes to develop the gluten.
3. Lightly oil the inside of a clean medium bowl. Gather the dough into a compact ball and set it in the bowl. Turn the dough over so that its surface has oil on it all over. Cover the bowl tightly with plastic wrap and set aside in a warm, draft-free place until the dough has doubled in bulk, about 1½ hours.
4. Punch down the dough, then turn it out onto a clean, dry work surface. Divide it into 5 even balls for a small batch, 6 balls for a medium batch, or 8 balls for a large one.
5. For a small batch, lightly oil the inside of a 6-inch round cake pan and set the balls around its perimeter, separating them as much as possible.
6. For a medium batch, lightly oil the inside of a 7-inch round cake pan and set the balls in it with one ball at its center, separating them as much as possible.
7. For a large batch, lightly oil the inside of an 8-inch round cake pan and set the balls in it with one at the center, separating them as much as possible.
8. Cover with plastic wrap and set aside to rise for 30 minutes.
9. Preheat the air fryer to 350°F .
10. Uncover the pan and brush the rolls with a little melted butter, perhaps ½ teaspoon per roll. When the machine is at temperature, set the cake pan in the basket. Air-fry undisturbed for 14 minutes, or until the rolls have risen and browned.
11. Using kitchen tongs and a nonstick-safe spatula, two hot pads, or silicone baking mitts, transfer the cake pan from the basket to a wire rack. Cool the rolls in the pan for a minute or two. Turn the rolls out onto a wire rack, set them top side up again, and cool for at least another couple of minutes before serving warm.

Sandwiches And Burgers Recipes

Best-ever Roast Beef Sandwiches

Servings: 6

Cooking Time: 30-50 Minutes

Ingredients:

- 2½ teaspoons Olive oil
- 1½ teaspoons Dried oregano
- 1½ teaspoons Dried thyme
- 1½ teaspoons Onion powder
- 1½ teaspoons Table salt
- 1½ teaspoons Ground black pepper
- 3 pounds Beef eye of round
- 6 Round soft rolls, such as Kaiser rolls or hamburger buns (gluten-free, if a concern), split open lengthwise
- ¾ cup Regular, low-fat, or fat-free mayonnaise (gluten-free, if a concern)
- 6 Romaine lettuce leaves, rinsed
- 6 Round tomato slices (¼ inch thick)

Directions:

1. Preheat the air fryer to 350°F .
2. Mix the oil, oregano, thyme, onion powder, salt, and pepper in a small bowl. Spread this mixture all over the eye of round.
3. When the machine is at temperature, set the beef in the basket and air-fry for 30 to 50 minutes (the range depends on the size of the cut), turning the meat twice, until an instant-read meat thermometer inserted into the thickest piece of the meat registers 130°F for rare, 140°F for medium, or 150°F for well-done.
4. Use kitchen tongs to transfer the beef to a cutting board. Cool for 10 minutes. If serving now, carve into ⅛-inch-thick slices. Spread each roll with 2 tablespoons mayonnaise and divide the beef slices between the rolls. Top with a lettuce leaf and a tomato slice and serve. Or set the beef in a container, cover, and refrigerate for up to 3 days to make cold roast beef sandwiches anytime.

Black Bean Veggie Burgers

Servings: 3

Cooking Time: 10 Minutes

Ingredients:

- 1 cup Drained and rinsed canned black beans
- ⅓ cup Pecan pieces
- ⅓ cup Rolled oats (not quick-cooking or steel-cut; gluten-free, if a concern)
- 2 tablespoons (or 1 small egg) Pasteurized egg substitute, such as Egg Beaters (gluten-free, if a concern)
- 2 teaspoons Red ketchup-like chili sauce, such as Heinz
- ¼ teaspoon Ground cumin
- ¼ teaspoon Dried oregano
- ¼ teaspoon Table salt
- ¼ teaspoon Ground black pepper
- Olive oil
- Olive oil spray

Directions:

1. Preheat the air fryer to 400°F.
2. Put the beans, pecans, oats, egg substitute or egg, chili sauce, cumin, oregano, salt, and pepper in a food processor. Cover and process to a coarse paste that will hold its shape like sugar-cookie dough, adding olive oil in 1-teaspoon increments to get the mixture to blend smoothly. The amount of olive oil is actually dependent on the internal moisture content of the beans and the oats. Figure on about 1 tablespoon (three 1-teaspoon additions) for the smaller batch, with proportional increases for the other batches. A little too much olive oil can't hurt, but a dry paste will fall apart as it cooks and a far-too-wet paste will stick to the basket.
3. Scrape down and remove the blade. Using clean, wet hands, form the paste into two 4-inch patties for the small batch, three 4-inch patties for the medium, or four 4-inch patties for the large batch, setting them one by one on a cutting board. Generously coat both sides of the patties with olive oil spray.
4. Set them in the basket in one layer. Air-fry undisturbed for 10 minutes, or until lightly browned and crisp at the edges.
5. Use a nonstick-safe spatula, and perhaps a flatware fork for balance, to transfer the burgers to a wire rack. Cool for 5 minutes before serving.

Asian Glazed Meatballs

Servings: 4

Cooking Time: 10 Minutes

Ingredients:

- 1 large shallot, finely chopped
- 2 cloves garlic, minced
- 1 tablespoon grated fresh ginger
- 2 teaspoons fresh thyme, finely chopped
- 1½ cups brown mushrooms, very finely chopped (a food processor works well here)
- 2 tablespoons soy sauce
- freshly ground black pepper
- 1 pound ground beef
- ½ pound ground pork
- 3 egg yolks
- 1 cup Thai sweet chili sauce (spring roll sauce)
- ¼ cup toasted sesame seeds
- 2 scallions, sliced

Directions:

1. Combine the shallot, garlic, ginger, thyme, mushrooms, soy sauce, freshly ground black pepper, ground beef and pork, and egg yolks in a bowl and mix the ingredients together. Gently shape the mixture into 24 balls, about the size of a golf ball.
2. Preheat the air fryer to 380°F.
3. Working in batches, air-fry the meatballs for 8 minutes, turning the meatballs over halfway through the cooking time. Drizzle some of the Thai sweet chili sauce on top of each meatball and return the basket to the air fryer, air-frying for another 2 minutes. Reserve the remaining Thai sweet chili sauce for serving.
4. As soon as the meatballs are done, sprinkle with toasted sesame seeds and transfer them to a serving platter. Scatter the scallions around and serve warm.

Turkey Burgers

Servings: 3

Cooking Time: 23 Minutes

Ingredients:

- 1 pound 2 ounces Ground turkey
- 6 tablespoons Frozen chopped spinach, thawed and squeezed dry
- 3 tablespoons Plain panko bread crumbs (gluten-free, if a concern)
- 1 tablespoon Dijon mustard (gluten-free, if a concern)
- 1½ teaspoons Minced garlic
- ¾ teaspoon Table salt
- ¾ teaspoon Ground black pepper
- Olive oil spray
- 3 Kaiser rolls (gluten-free, if a concern), split open

Directions:

1. Preheat the air fryer to 375°F .
2. Gently mix the ground turkey, spinach, bread crumbs, mustard, garlic, salt, and pepper in a large bowl until well combined, trying to keep some of the fibers of the ground turkey intact. Form into two 5-inch-wide patties for the small batch, three 5-inch patties for the medium batch, or four 5-inch patties for the large. Coat each side of the patties with olive oil spray.
3. Set the patties in in the basket in one layer and air-fry undisturbed for 20 minutes, or until an instant-read meat thermometer inserted into the center of a burger registers 165°F. You may need to add 2 minutes to the cooking time if the air fryer is at 360°F.
4. Use a nonstick-safe spatula, and perhaps a flatware fork for balance, to transfer the burgers to a cutting board. Set the buns cut side down in the basket in one layer (working in batches as necessary) and air-fry for 1 minute, to toast a bit and warm up. Serve the burgers warm in the buns.

White Bean Veggie Burgers

Servings: 3

Cooking Time: 13 Minutes

Ingredients:

- 1⅓ cups Drained and rinsed canned white beans
- 3 tablespoons Rolled oats (not quick-cooking or steel-cut; gluten-free, if a concern)
- 3 tablespoons Chopped walnuts
- 2 teaspoons Olive oil
- 2 teaspoons Lemon juice
- 1½ teaspoons Dijon mustard (gluten-free, if a concern)
- ¾ teaspoon Dried sage leaves

- ¼ teaspoon Table salt
- Olive oil spray
- 3 Whole-wheat buns or gluten-free whole-grain buns (if a concern), split open

Directions:

1. Preheat the air fryer to 400°F.
2. Place the beans, oats, walnuts, oil, lemon juice, mustard, sage, and salt in a food processor. Cover and process to make a coarse paste that will hold its shape, about like wet sugar-cookie dough, stopping the machine to scrape down the inside of the canister at least once.
3. Scrape down and remove the blade. With clean and wet hands, form the bean paste into two 4-inch patties for the small batch, three 4-inch patties for the medium, or four 4-inch patties for the large batch. Generously coat the patties on both sides with olive oil spray.
4. Set them in the basket with some space between them and air-fry undisturbed for 12 minutes, or until lightly brown and crisp at the edges. The tops of the burgers will feel firm to the touch.
5. Use a nonstick-safe spatula, and perhaps a flatware fork for balance, to transfer the burgers to a cutting board. Set the buns cut side down in the basket in one layer (working in batches as necessary) and air-fry undisturbed for 1 minute, to toast a bit and warm up. Serve the burgers warm in the buns.

Chicken Apple Brie Melt

Servings: 3

Cooking Time: 13 Minutes

Ingredients:

- 3 5- to 6-ounce boneless skinless chicken breasts
- Vegetable oil spray
- 1½ teaspoons Dried herbes de Provence
- 3 ounces Brie, rind removed, thinly sliced
- 6 Thin cored apple slices
- 3 French rolls (gluten-free, if a concern)
- 2 tablespoons Dijon mustard (gluten-free, if a concern)

Directions:

1. Preheat the air fryer to 375°F .
2. Lightly coat all sides of the chicken breasts with vegetable oil spray. Sprinkle the breasts evenly with the herbes de Provence.
3. When the machine is at temperature, set the breasts in the basket and air-fry undisturbed for 10 minutes.
4. Top the chicken breasts with the apple slices, then the cheese. Air-fry undisturbed for 2 minutes, or until the cheese is melty and bubbling.
5. Use a nonstick-safe spatula and kitchen tongs, for balance, to transfer the breasts to a cutting board. Set the rolls in the basket and air-fry for 1 minute to warm through. (Putting them in the machine without splitting them keeps the insides very soft while the outside gets a little crunchy.)
6. Transfer the rolls to the cutting board. Split them open lengthwise, then spread 1 teaspoon mustard on each cut side. Set a prepared chicken breast on the bottom of a roll and close with its top, repeating as necessary to make additional sandwiches. Serve warm.

Chicken Spiedies

Servings: 3

Cooking Time: 12 Minutes

Ingredients:

- 1¼ pounds Boneless skinless chicken thighs, trimmed of any fat blobs and cut into 2-inch pieces
- 3 tablespoons Red wine vinegar
- 2 tablespoons Olive oil
- 2 tablespoons Minced fresh mint leaves
- 2 tablespoons Minced fresh parsley leaves
- 2 teaspoons Minced fresh dill fronds
- ¾ teaspoon Fennel seeds
- ¾ teaspoon Table salt
- Up to a ¼ teaspoon Red pepper flakes
- 3 Long soft rolls, such as hero, hoagie, or Italian sub rolls (gluten-free, if a concern), split open lengthwise
- 4½ tablespoons Regular or low-fat mayonnaise (not fat-free; gluten-free, if a concern)
- 1½ tablespoons Distilled white vinegar
- 1½ teaspoons Ground black pepper

Directions:

1. Mix the chicken, vinegar, oil, mint, parsley, dill, fennel seeds, salt, and red pepper flakes in a zip-closed

plastic bag. Seal, gently massage the marinade ingredients into the meat, and refrigerate for at least 2 hours or up to 6 hours. (Longer than that and the meat can turn rubbery.)

2. Set the plastic bag out on the counter (to make the contents a little less frigid). Preheat the air fryer to 400°F.

3. When the machine is at temperature, use kitchen tongs to set the chicken thighs in the basket (discard any remaining marinade) and air-fry undisturbed for 6 minutes. Turn the thighs over and continue air-frying undisturbed for 6 minutes more, until well browned, cooked through, and even a little crunchy.

4. Dump the contents of the basket onto a wire rack and cool for 2 or 3 minutes. Divide the chicken evenly between the rolls. Whisk the mayonnaise, vinegar, and black pepper in a small bowl until smooth. Drizzle this sauce over the chicken pieces in the rolls.

Thai-style Pork Sliders

Servings: 4

Cooking Time: 15 Minutes

Ingredients:

- 11 ounces Ground pork
- 2½ tablespoons Very thinly sliced scallions, white and green parts
- 4 teaspoons Minced peeled fresh ginger
- 2½ teaspoons Fish sauce (gluten-free, if a concern)
- 2 teaspoons Thai curry paste (see the headnote; gluten-free, if a concern)
- 2 teaspoons Light brown sugar
- ¾ teaspoon Ground black pepper
- 4 Slider buns (gluten-free, if a concern)

Directions:

1. Preheat the air fryer to 375°F .

2. Gently mix the pork, scallions, ginger, fish sauce, curry paste, brown sugar, and black pepper in a bowl until well combined. With clean, wet hands, form about ⅓ cup of the pork mixture into a slider about 2½ inches in diameter. Repeat until you use up all the meat—3 sliders for the small batch, 4 for the medium, and 6 for the large. (Keep wetting your hands to help the patties adhere.)

3. When the machine is at temperature, set the sliders in the basket in one layer. Air-fry undisturbed for 14 minutes, or until the sliders are golden brown and caramelized at their edges and an instant-read meat thermometer inserted into the center of a slider registers 160°F.

4. Use a nonstick-safe spatula, and perhaps a flatware fork for balance, to transfer the sliders to a cutting board. Set the buns cut side down in the basket in one layer (working in batches as necessary) and air-fry undisturbed for 1 minute, to toast a bit and warm up. Serve the sliders warm in the buns.

Perfect Burgers

Servings: 3

Cooking Time: 13 Minutes

Ingredients:

- 1 pound 2 ounces 90% lean ground beef
- 1½ tablespoons Worcestershire sauce (gluten-free, if a concern)
- ½ teaspoon Ground black pepper
- 3 Hamburger buns (gluten-free if a concern), split open

Directions:

1. Preheat the air fryer to 375°F .

2. Gently mix the ground beef, Worcestershire sauce, and pepper in a bowl until well combined but preserving as much of the meat's fibers as possible. Divide this mixture into two 5-inch patties for the small batch, three 5-inch patties for the medium, or four 5-inch patties for the large. Make a thumbprint indentation in the center of each patty, about halfway through the meat.

3. Set the patties in the basket in one layer with some space between them. Air-fry undisturbed for 10 minutes, or until an instant-read meat thermometer inserted into the center of a burger registers 160°F (a medium-well burger). You may need to add 2 minutes cooking time if the air fryer is at 360°F.

4. Use a nonstick-safe spatula, and perhaps a flatware fork for balance, to transfer the burgers to a cutting board. Set the buns cut side down in the basket in one layer (working in batches as necessary) and air-fry undisturbed for 1 minute, to toast a bit and warm up. Serve the burgers in the warm buns.

Sausage And Pepper Heros

Servings: 3

Cooking Time: 11 Minutes

Ingredients:

- 3 links (about 9 ounces total) Sweet Italian sausages (gluten-free, if a concern)
- 1½ Medium red or green bell pepper(s), stemmed, cored, and cut into ½-inch-wide strips
- 1 medium Yellow or white onion(s), peeled, halved, and sliced into thin half-moons
- 3 Long soft rolls, such as hero, hoagie, or Italian sub rolls (gluten-free, if a concern), split open lengthwise
- For garnishing Balsamic vinegar
- For garnishing Fresh basil leaves

Directions:

1. Preheat the air fryer to 400°F.
2. When the machine is at temperature, set the sausage links in the basket in one layer and air-fry undisturbed for 5 minutes.
3. Add the pepper strips and onions. Continue air-frying, tossing and rearranging everything about once every minute, for 5 minutes, or until the sausages are browned and an instant-read meat thermometer inserted into one of the links registers 160°F.
4. Use a nonstick-safe spatula and kitchen tongs to transfer the sausages and vegetables to a cutting board. Set the rolls cut side down in the basket in one layer (working in batches as necessary) and air-fry undisturbed for 1 minute, to toast the rolls a bit and warm them up. Set 1 sausage with some pepper strips and onions in each warm roll, sprinkle balsamic vinegar over the sandwich fillings, and garnish with basil leaves.

Dijon Thyme Burgers

Servings: 3

Cooking Time: 18 Minutes

Ingredients:

- 1 pound lean ground beef
- ⅓ cup panko breadcrumbs
- ¼ cup finely chopped onion
- 3 tablespoons Dijon mustard
- 1 tablespoon chopped fresh thyme
- 4 teaspoons Worcestershire sauce
- 1 teaspoon salt
- freshly ground black pepper
- Topping (optional):
- 2 tablespoons Dijon mustard
- 1 tablespoon dark brown sugar
- 1 teaspoon Worcestershire sauce
- 4 ounces sliced Swiss cheese, optional

Directions:

1. Combine all the burger ingredients together in a large bowl and mix well. Divide the meat into 4 equal portions and then form the burgers, being careful not to over-handle the meat. One good way to do this is to throw the meat back and forth from one hand to another, packing the meat each time you catch it. Flatten the balls into patties, making an indentation in the center of each patty with your thumb (this will help it stay flat as it cooks) and flattening the sides of the burgers so that they will fit nicely into the air fryer basket.
2. Preheat the air fryer to 370°F.
3. If you don't have room for all four burgers, air-fry two or three burgers at a time for 8 minutes. Flip the burgers over and air-fry for another 6 minutes.
4. While the burgers are cooking combine the Dijon mustard, dark brown sugar, and Worcestershire sauce in a small bowl and mix well. This optional topping to the burgers really adds a boost of flavor at the end. Spread the Dijon topping evenly on each burger. If you cooked the burgers in batches, return the first batch to the cooker at this time – it's ok to place the fourth burger on top of the others in the center of the basket. Air-fry the burgers for another 3 minutes.
5. Finally, if desired, top each burger with a slice of Swiss cheese. Lower the air fryer temperature to 330°F and air-fry for another minute to melt the cheese. Serve the burgers on toasted brioche buns, dressed the way you like them.

Thanksgiving Turkey Sandwiches

Servings: 3

Cooking Time: 10 Minutes

Ingredients:

- 1½ cups Herb-seasoned stuffing mix (not cornbread-style; gluten-free, if a concern)
- 1 Large egg white(s)
- 2 tablespoons Water
- 3 5- to 6-ounce turkey breast cutlets
- Vegetable oil spray
- 4½ tablespoons Purchased cranberry sauce, preferably whole berry
- ⅛ teaspoon Ground cinnamon
- ⅛ teaspoon Ground dried ginger
- 4½ tablespoons Regular, low-fat, or fat-free mayonnaise (gluten-free, if a concern)
- 6 tablespoons Shredded Brussels sprouts
- 3 Kaiser rolls (gluten-free, if a concern), split open

Directions:

1. Preheat the air fryer to 375°F .
2. Put the stuffing mix in a heavy zip-closed bag, seal it, lay it flat on your counter, and roll a rolling pin over the bag to crush the stuffing mix to the consistency of rough sand. (Or you can pulse the stuffing mix to the desired consistency in a food processor.)
3. Set up and fill two shallow soup plates or small pie plates on your counter: one for the egg white(s), whisked with the water until foamy; and one for the ground stuffing mix.
4. Dip a cutlet in the egg white mixture, coating both sides and letting any excess egg white slip back into the rest. Set the cutlet in the ground stuffing mix and coat it evenly on both sides, pressing gently to coat well on both sides. Lightly coat the cutlet on both sides with vegetable oil spray, set it aside, and continue dipping and coating the remaining cutlets in the same way.
5. Set the cutlets in the basket and air-fry undisturbed for 10 minutes, or until crisp and brown. Use kitchen tongs to transfer the cutlets to a wire rack to cool for a few minutes.
6. Meanwhile, stir the cranberry sauce with the cinnamon and ginger in a small bowl. Mix the shredded Brussels sprouts and mayonnaise in a second bowl until the vegetable is evenly coated.
7. Build the sandwiches by spreading about 1½ tablespoons of the cranberry mixture on the cut side of the bottom half of each roll. Set a cutlet on top, then spread about 3 tablespoons of the Brussels sprouts mixture evenly over the cutlet. Set the other half of the roll on top and serve warm.

Lamb Burgers

Servings: 3

Cooking Time: 17 Minutes

Ingredients:

- 1 pound 2 ounces Ground lamb
- 3 tablespoons Crumbled feta
- 1 teaspoon Minced garlic
- 1 teaspoon Tomato paste
- ¾ teaspoon Ground coriander
- ¾ teaspoon Ground dried ginger
- Up to ⅛ teaspoon Cayenne
- Up to a ⅛ teaspoon Table salt (optional)
- 3 Kaiser rolls or hamburger buns (gluten-free, if a concern), split open

Directions:

1. Preheat the air fryer to 375°F .
2. Gently mix the ground lamb, feta, garlic, tomato paste, coriander, ginger, cayenne, and salt (if using) in a bowl until well combined, trying to keep the bits of cheese intact. Form this mixture into two 5-inch patties for the small batch, three 5-inch patties for the medium, or four 5-inch patties for the large.
3. Set the patties in the basket in one layer and air-fry undisturbed for 16 minutes, or until an instant-read meat thermometer inserted into one burger registers 160°F. (The cheese is not an issue with the temperature probe in this recipe as it was for the Inside-Out Cheeseburgers, because the feta is so well mixed into the ground meat.)
4. Use a nonstick-safe spatula, and perhaps a flatware fork for balance, to transfer the burgers to a cutting board. Set the buns cut side down in the basket in one layer (working in batches as necessary) and air-fry undisturbed for 1 minute, to toast a bit and warm up. Serve the burgers warm in the buns.

Chicken Club Sandwiches

Servings: 3

Cooking Time: 15 Minutes

Ingredients:

- 3 5- to 6-ounce boneless skinless chicken breasts
- 6 Thick-cut bacon strips (gluten-free, if a concern)
- 3 Long soft rolls, such as hero, hoagie, or Italian sub rolls (gluten-free, if a concern)
- 3 tablespoons Regular, low-fat, or fat-free mayonnaise (gluten-free, if a concern)
- 3 Lettuce leaves, preferably romaine or iceberg
- 6 ¼-inch-thick tomato slices

Directions:

1. Preheat the air fryer to 375°F .
2. Wrap each chicken breast with 2 strips of bacon, spiraling the bacon around the meat, slightly overlapping the strips on each revolution. Start the second strip of bacon farther down the breast but on a line with the start of the first strip so they both end at a lined-up point on the chicken breast.
3. When the machine is at temperature, set the wrapped breasts bacon-seam side down in the basket with space between them. Air-fry undisturbed for 12 minutes, until the bacon is browned, crisp, and cooked through and an instant-read meat thermometer inserted into the center of a breast registers 165°F. You may need to add 2 minutes in the air fryer if the temperature is at 360°F.
4. Use kitchen tongs to transfer the breasts to a wire rack. Split the rolls open lengthwise and set them cut side down in the basket. Air-fry for 1 minute, or until warmed through.
5. Use kitchen tongs to transfer the rolls to a cutting board. Spread 1 tablespoon mayonnaise on the cut side of one half of each roll. Top with a chicken breast, lettuce leaf, and tomato slice. Serve warm.

Inside-out Cheeseburgers

Servings: 3

Cooking Time: 9-11 Minutes

Ingredients:

- 1 pound 2 ounces 90% lean ground beef
- ¾ teaspoon Dried oregano
- ¾ teaspoon Table salt
- ¾ teaspoon Ground black pepper
- ¼ teaspoon Garlic powder
- 6 tablespoons (about 1½ ounces) Shredded Cheddar, Swiss, or other semi-firm cheese, or a purchased blend of shredded cheeses
- 3 Hamburger buns (gluten-free, if a concern), split open

Directions:

1. Preheat the air fryer to 375°F .
2. Gently mix the ground beef, oregano, salt, pepper, and garlic powder in a bowl until well combined without turning the mixture to mush. Form it into two 6-inch patties for the small batch, three for the medium, or four for the large.
3. Place 2 tablespoons of the shredded cheese in the center of each patty. With clean hands, fold the sides of the patty up to cover the cheese, then pick it up and roll it gently into a ball to seal the cheese inside. Gently press it back into a 5-inch burger without letting any cheese squish out. Continue filling and preparing more burgers, as needed.
4. Place the burgers in the basket in one layer and air-fry undisturbed for 8 minutes for medium or 10 minutes for well-done. (An instant-read meat thermometer won't work for these burgers because it will hit the mostly melted cheese inside and offer a hotter temperature than the surrounding meat.)
5. Use a nonstick-safe spatula, and perhaps a flatware fork for balance, to transfer the burgers to a cutting board. Set the buns cut side down in the basket in one layer (working in batches as necessary) and air-fry undisturbed for 1 minute, to toast a bit and warm up. Cool the burgers a few minutes more, then serve them warm in the buns.

Provolone Stuffed Meatballs

Servings: 4

Cooking Time: 12 Minutes

Ingredients:

- 1 tablespoon olive oil
- 1 small onion, very finely chopped
- 1 to 2 cloves garlic, minced
- ¾ pound ground beef
- ¾ pound ground pork
- ¾ cup breadcrumbs
- ¼ cup grated Parmesan cheese
- ¼ cup finely chopped fresh parsley (or 1 tablespoon dried parsley)
- ½ teaspoon dried oregano
- 1½ teaspoons salt
- freshly ground black pepper
- 2 eggs, lightly beaten
- 5 ounces sharp or aged provolone cheese, cut into 1-inch cubes

Directions:

1. Preheat a skillet over medium-high heat. Add the oil and cook the onion and garlic until tender, but not browned.
2. Transfer the onion and garlic to a large bowl and add the beef, pork, breadcrumbs, Parmesan cheese, parsley, oregano, salt, pepper and eggs. Mix well until all the ingredients are combined. Divide the mixture into 12 evenly sized balls. Make one meatball at a time, by pressing a hole in the meatball mixture with your finger and pushing a piece of provolone cheese into the hole. Mold the meat back into a ball, enclosing the cheese.
3. Preheat the air fryer to 380°F.
4. Working in two batches, transfer six of the meatballs to the air fryer basket and air-fry for 12 minutes, shaking the basket and turning the meatballs a couple of times during the cooking process. Repeat with the remaining six meatballs. You can pop the first batch of meatballs into the air fryer for the last two minutes of cooking to re-heat them. Serve warm.

Chicken Gyros

Servings: 4

Cooking Time: 14 Minutes

Ingredients:

- 4 4- to 5-ounce boneless skinless chicken thighs, trimmed of any fat blobs
- 2 tablespoons Lemon juice
- 2 tablespoons Red wine vinegar
- 2 tablespoons Olive oil
- 2 teaspoons Dried oregano
- 2 teaspoons Minced garlic
- 1 teaspoon Table salt
- 1 teaspoon Ground black pepper
- 4 Pita pockets (gluten-free, if a concern)
- ½ cup Chopped tomatoes
- ½ cup Bottled regular, low-fat, or fat-free ranch dressing (gluten-free, if a concern)

Directions:

1. Mix the thighs, lemon juice, vinegar, oil, oregano, garlic, salt, and pepper in a zip-closed bag. Seal, gently massage the marinade into the meat through the plastic, and refrigerate for at least 2 hours or up to 6 hours. (Longer than that and the meat can turn rubbery.)
2. Set the plastic bag out on the counter (to make the contents a little less frigid). Preheat the air fryer to 375°F .
3. When the machine is at temperature, use kitchen tongs to place the thighs in the basket in one layer. Discard the marinade. Air-fry the chicken thighs undisturbed for 12 minutes, or until browned and an instant-read meat thermometer inserted into the thickest part of one thigh registers 165°F. You may need to air-fry the chicken 2 minutes longer if the machine's temperature is 360°F.
4. Use kitchen tongs to transfer the thighs to a cutting board. Cool for 5 minutes, then set one thigh in each of the pita pockets. Top each with 2 tablespoons chopped tomatoes and 2 tablespoons dressing. Serve warm.

Philly Cheesesteak Sandwiches

Servings: 3
Cooking Time: 9 Minutes

Ingredients:

- ¾ pound Shaved beef
- 1 tablespoon Worcestershire sauce (gluten-free, if a concern)
- ¼ teaspoon Garlic powder
- ¼ teaspoon Mild paprika
- 6 tablespoons (1½ ounces) Frozen bell pepper strips (do not thaw)
- 2 slices, broken into rings Very thin yellow or white medium onion slice(s)
- 6 ounces (6 to 8 slices) Provolone cheese slices
- 3 Long soft rolls such as hero, hoagie, or Italian sub rolls, or hot dog buns (gluten-free, if a concern), split open lengthwise

Directions:

1. Preheat the air fryer to 400°F.
2. When the machine is at temperature, spread the shaved beef in the basket, leaving a ½-inch perimeter around the meat for good air flow. Sprinkle the meat with the Worcestershire sauce, paprika, and garlic powder. Spread the peppers and onions on top of the meat.
3. Air-fry undisturbed for 6 minutes, or until cooked through. Set the cheese on top of the meat. Continue air-frying undisturbed for 3 minutes, or until the cheese has melted.
4. Use kitchen tongs to divide the meat and cheese layers in the basket between the rolls or buns. Serve hot.

Eggplant Parmesan Subs

Servings: 2
Cooking Time: 13 Minutes

Ingredients:

- 4 Peeled eggplant slices (about ½ inch thick and 3 inches in diameter)
- Olive oil spray
- 2 tablespoons plus 2 teaspoons Jarred pizza sauce, any variety except creamy
- ¼ cup (about ⅔ ounce) Finely grated Parmesan cheese
- 2 Small, long soft rolls, such as hero, hoagie, or Italian sub rolls (gluten-free, if a concern), split open lengthwise

Directions:

1. Preheat the air fryer to 350°F .
2. When the machine is at temperature, coat both sides of the eggplant slices with olive oil spray. Set them in the basket in one layer and air-fry undisturbed for 10 minutes, until lightly browned and softened.
3. Increase the machine's temperature to 375°F (or 370°F, if that's the closest setting—unless the machine is already at 360°F, in which case leave it alone). Top each eggplant slice with 2 teaspoons pizza sauce, then 1 tablespoon cheese. Air-fry undisturbed for 2 minutes, or until the cheese has melted.
4. Use a nonstick-safe spatula, and perhaps a flatware fork for balance, to transfer the eggplant slices cheese side up to a cutting board. Set the roll(s) cut side down in the basket in one layer (working in batches as necessary) and air-fry undisturbed for 1 minute, to toast the rolls a bit and warm them up. Set 2 eggplant slices in each warm roll.

Reuben Sandwiches

Servings: 2
Cooking Time: 11 Minutes

Ingredients:

- ½ pound Sliced deli corned beef
- 4 teaspoons Regular or low-fat mayonnaise (not fat-free)
- 4 Rye bread slices
- 2 tablespoons plus 2 teaspoons Russian dressing
- ½ cup Purchased sauerkraut, squeezed by the handful over the sink to get rid of excess moisture
- 2 ounces (2 to 4 slices) Swiss cheese slices (optional)

Directions:

1. Set the corned beef in the basket, slip the basket into the machine, and heat the air fryer to 400°F. Air-fry undisturbed for 3 minutes from the time the basket is put in the machine, just to warm up the meat.

2. Use kitchen tongs to transfer the corned beef to a cutting board. Spread 1 teaspoon mayonnaise on one side of each slice of rye bread, rubbing the mayonnaise into the bread with a small flatware knife.

3. Place the bread slices mayonnaise side down on a cutting board. Spread the Russian dressing over the "dry" side of each slice. For one sandwich, top one slice of bread with the corned beef, sauerkraut, and cheese (if using). For two sandwiches, top two slices of bread each with half of the corned beef, sauerkraut, and cheese (if using). Close the sandwiches with the remaining bread, setting it mayonnaise side up on top.

4. Set the sandwich(es) in the basket and air-fry undisturbed for 8 minutes, or until browned and crunchy.

5. Use a nonstick-safe spatula, and perhaps a flatware fork for balance, to transfer the sandwich(es) to a cutting board. Cool for 2 or 3 minutes before slicing in half and serving.

Inside Out Cheeseburgers

Servings: 2

Cooking Time: 20 Minutes

Ingredients:

- ¾ pound lean ground beef
- 3 tablespoons minced onion
- 4 teaspoons ketchup
- 2 teaspoons yellow mustard
- salt and freshly ground black pepper
- 4 slices of Cheddar cheese, broken into smaller pieces
- 8 hamburger dill pickle chips

Directions:

1. Combine the ground beef, minced onion, ketchup, mustard, salt and pepper in a large bowl. Mix well to thoroughly combine the ingredients. Divide the meat into four equal portions.

2. To make the stuffed burgers, flatten each portion of meat into a thin patty. Place 4 pickle chips and half of the cheese onto the center of two of the patties, leaving a rim around the edge of the patty exposed. Place the remaining two patties on top of the first and press the meat together firmly, sealing the edges tightly. With the burgers on a flat surface, press the sides of the burger with the palm of your hand to create a straight edge. This will help keep the stuffing inside the burger while it cooks.

3. Preheat the air fryer to 370°F.

4. Place the burgers inside the air fryer basket and air-fry for 20 minutes, flipping the burgers over halfway through the cooking time.

5. Serve the cheeseburgers on buns with lettuce and tomato.

Mexican Cheeseburgers

Servings: 4

Cooking Time: 22 Minutes

Ingredients:

- 1¼ pounds ground beef
- ¼ cup finely chopped onion
- ½ cup crushed yellow corn tortilla chips
- 1 (1.25-ounce) packet taco seasoning
- ¼ cup canned diced green chilies
- 1 egg, lightly beaten
- 4 ounces pepper jack cheese, grated
- 4 (12-inch) flour tortillas
- shredded lettuce, sour cream, guacamole, salsa (for topping)

Directions:

1. Combine the ground beef, minced onion, crushed tortilla chips, taco seasoning, green chilies, and egg in a large bowl. Mix thoroughly until combined – your hands are good tools for this. Divide the meat into four equal portions and shape each portion into an oval-shaped burger.

2. Preheat the air fryer to 370°F.

3. Air-fry the burgers for 18 minutes, turning them over halfway through the cooking time. Divide the cheese between the burgers, lower fryer to 340°F and air-fry for an additional 4 minutes to melt the cheese. (This will give you a burger that is medium-well. If you prefer your cheeseburger medium-rare, shorten the cooking

time to about 15 minutes and then add the cheese and proceed with the recipe.)

4. While the burgers are cooking, warm the tortillas wrapped in aluminum foil in a 350°F oven, or in a skillet with a little oil over medium-high heat for a couple of minutes. Keep the tortillas warm until the burgers are ready.

5. To assemble the burgers, spread sour cream over three quarters of the tortillas and top each with some shredded lettuce and salsa. Place the Mexican cheeseburgers on the lettuce and top with guacamole. Fold the tortillas around the burger, starting with the bottom and then folding the sides in over the top. (A little sour cream can help hold the seam of the tortilla together.) Serve immediately.

Fish And Seafood Recipes

Tuna Nuggets In Hoisin Sauce

Servings: 4

Cooking Time: 7 Minutes

Ingredients:

- ½ cup hoisin sauce
- 2 tablespoons rice wine vinegar
- 2 teaspoons sesame oil
- 1 teaspoon garlic powder
- 2 teaspoons dried lemongrass
- ¼ teaspoon red pepper flakes
- ½ small onion, quartered and thinly sliced
- 8 ounces fresh tuna, cut into 1-inch cubes
- cooking spray
- 3 cups cooked jasmine rice

Directions:

1. Mix the hoisin sauce, vinegar, sesame oil, and seasonings together.
2. Stir in the onions and tuna nuggets.
3. Spray air fryer baking pan with nonstick spray and pour in tuna mixture.
4. Cook at 390°F for 3minutes. Stir gently.
5. Cook 2minutes and stir again, checking for doneness. Tuna should be barely cooked through, just beginning to flake and still very moist. If necessary, continue cooking and stirring in 1-minute intervals until done.
6. Serve warm over hot jasmine rice.

Flounder Fillets

Servings: 4

Cooking Time: 8 Minutes

Ingredients:

- 1 egg white
- 1 tablespoon water
- 1 cup panko breadcrumbs
- 2 tablespoons extra-light virgin olive oil
- 4 4-ounce flounder fillets
- salt and pepper
- oil for misting or cooking spray

Directions:

1. Preheat air fryer to 390°F.
2. Beat together egg white and water in shallow dish.
3. In another shallow dish, mix panko crumbs and oil until well combined and crumbly (best done by hand).
4. Season flounder fillets with salt and pepper to taste. Dip each fillet into egg mixture and then roll in panko crumbs, pressing in crumbs so that fish is nicely coated.
5. Spray air fryer basket with nonstick cooking spray and add fillets. Cook at 390°F for 3minutes.
6. Spray fish fillets but do not turn. Cook 5 minutes longer or until golden brown and crispy. Using a spatula, carefully remove fish from basket and serve.

Horseradish-crusted Salmon Fillets

Servings:3

Cooking Time: 8 Minutes

Ingredients:

- ½ cup Fresh bread crumbs (see the headnote)
- 4 tablespoons (¼ cup/½ stick) Butter, melted and cooled
- ¼ cup Jarred prepared white horseradish
- Vegetable oil spray
- 4 6-ounce skin-on salmon fillets (for more information, see here)

Directions:

1. Preheat the air fryer to 400°F.
2. Mix the bread crumbs, butter, and horseradish in a bowl until well combined.
3. Take the basket out of the machine. Generously spray the skin side of each fillet. Pick them up one by one with a nonstick-safe spatula and set them in the basket skin side down with as much air space between them as possible. Divide the bread-crumb mixture between the fillets, coating the top of each fillet with an even layer. Generously coat the bread-crumb mixture with vegetable oil spray.
4. Return the basket to the machine and air-fry undisturbed for 8 minutes, or until the topping has lightly browned and the fish is firm but not hard.
5. Use a nonstick-safe spatula to transfer the salmon fillets to serving plates. Cool for 5 minutes before serving. Because of the butter in the topping, it will stay very hot

for quite a while. Take care, especially if you're serving these fillets to children.

Blackened Red Snapper

Servings: 4

Cooking Time: 8 Minutes

Ingredients:

- 1½ teaspoons black pepper
- ¼ teaspoon thyme
- ¼ teaspoon garlic powder
- ⅛ teaspoon cayenne pepper
- 1 teaspoon olive oil
- 4 4-ounce red snapper fillet portions, skin on
- 4 thin slices lemon
- cooking spray

Directions:

1. Mix the spices and oil together to make a paste. Rub into both sides of the fish.
2. Spray air fryer basket with nonstick cooking spray and lay snapper steaks in basket, skin-side down.
3. Place a lemon slice on each piece of fish.
4. Cook at 390°F for 8 minutes. The fish will not flake when done, but it should be white through the center.

Tilapia Teriyaki

Servings: 3

Cooking Time: 10 Minutes

Ingredients:

- 4 tablespoons teriyaki sauce
- 1 tablespoon pineapple juice
- 1 pound tilapia fillets
- cooking spray
- 6 ounces frozen mixed peppers with onions, thawed and drained
- 2 cups cooked rice

Directions:

1. Mix the teriyaki sauce and pineapple juice together in a small bowl.
2. Split tilapia fillets down the center lengthwise.
3. Brush all sides of fish with the sauce, spray air fryer basket with nonstick cooking spray, and place fish in the basket.
4. Stir the peppers and onions into the remaining sauce and spoon over the fish. Save any leftover sauce for drizzling over the fish when serving.
5. Cook at 360°F for 10 minutes, until fish flakes easily with a fork and is done in center.
6. Divide into 3 or 4 servings and serve each with approximately ½ cup cooked rice.

Shrimp "scampi"

Servings:4

Cooking Time: 5 Minutes

Ingredients:

- 1½ pounds Large shrimp (20–25 per pound), peeled and deveined
- ¼ cup Olive oil
- 2 tablespoons Minced garlic
- 1 teaspoon Dried oregano
- Up to 1 teaspoon Red pepper flakes
- ½ teaspoon Table salt
- 2 tablespoons White balsamic vinegar (see here)

Directions:

1. Preheat the air fryer to 400°F.
2. Stir the shrimp, olive oil, garlic, oregano, red pepper flakes, and salt in a large bowl until the shrimp are well coated.
3. When the machine is at temperature, transfer the shrimp to the basket. They will overlap and even sit on top of each other. Air-fry for 5 minutes, tossing and rearranging the shrimp twice to make sure the covered surfaces are exposed, until pink and firm.
4. Pour the contents of the basket into a serving bowl. Pour the vinegar over the shrimp while hot and toss to coat.

Lobster Tails With Lemon Garlic Butter

Servings: 2

Cooking Time: 5 Minutes

Ingredients:

- 4 ounces unsalted butter
- 1 tablespoon finely chopped lemon zest
- 1 clove garlic, thinly sliced
- 2 (6-ounce) lobster tails
- salt and freshly ground black pepper
- ½ cup white wine
- ½ lemon, sliced
- vegetable oil

Directions:

1. Start by making the lemon garlic butter. Combine the butter, lemon zest and garlic in a small saucepan. Melt and simmer the butter on the stovetop over the lowest possible heat while you prepare the lobster tails.
2. Prepare the lobster tails by cutting down the middle of the top of the shell. Crack the bottom shell by squeezing the sides of the lobster together so that you can access the lobster meat inside. Pull the lobster tail up out of the shell, but leave it attached at the base of the tail. Lay the lobster meat on top of the shell and season with salt and freshly ground black pepper. Pour a little of the lemon garlic butter on top of the lobster meat and transfer the lobster to the refrigerator so that the butter solidifies a little.
3. Pour the white wine into the air fryer drawer and add the lemon slices. Preheat the air fryer to 400°F for 5 minutes.
4. Transfer the lobster tails to the air fryer basket. Air-fry at 370° for 5 minutes, brushing more butter on halfway through cooking. (Add a minute or two if your lobster tail is more than 6-ounces.) Remove and serve with more butter for dipping or drizzling.

Easy Scallops With Lemon Butter

Servings:3

Cooking Time: 4 Minutes

Ingredients:

- 1 tablespoon Olive oil
- 2 teaspoons Minced garlic
- 1 teaspoon Finely grated lemon zest
- ½ teaspoon Red pepper flakes
- ¼ teaspoon Table salt
- 1 pound Sea scallops
- 3 tablespoons Butter, melted
- 1½ tablespoons Lemon juice

Directions:

1. Preheat the air fryer to 400°F.
2. Gently stir the olive oil, garlic, lemon zest, red pepper flakes, and salt in a bowl. Add the scallops and stir very gently until they are evenly and well coated.
3. When the machine is at temperature, arrange the scallops in a single layer in the basket. Some may touch. Air-fry undisturbed for 4 minutes, or until the scallops are opaque and firm.
4. While the scallops cook, stir the melted butter and lemon juice in a serving bowl. When the scallops are ready, pour them from the basket into this bowl. Toss well before serving.

Tuna Patties With Dill Sauce

Servings: 6

Cooking Time: 10 Minutes

Ingredients:

- Two 5-ounce cans albacore tuna, drained
- ½ teaspoon garlic powder
- 2 teaspoons dried dill, divided
- ½ teaspoon black pepper
- ½ teaspoon salt, divided
- ¼ cup minced onion
- 1 large egg
- 7 tablespoons mayonnaise, divided
- ¼ cup panko breadcrumbs
- 1 teaspoon fresh lemon juice
- ¼ teaspoon fresh lemon zest
- 6 pieces butterleaf lettuce
- 1 cup diced tomatoes

Directions:

1. In a large bowl, mix the tuna with the garlic powder, 1 teaspoon of the dried dill, the black pepper, ¼ teaspoon of the salt, and the onion. Make sure to use the back of a fork to really break up the tuna so there are no large chunks.

2. Mix in the egg and 1 tablespoon of the mayonnaise; then fold in the breadcrumbs so the tuna begins to form a thick batter that holds together.
3. Portion the tuna mixture into 6 equal patties and place on a plate lined with parchment paper in the refrigerator for at least 30 minutes. This will help the patties hold together in the air fryer.
4. When ready to cook, preheat the air fryer to 350°F.
5. Liberally spray the metal trivet that sits inside the air fryer basket with olive oil mist and place the patties onto the trivet.
6. Cook for 5 minutes, flip, and cook another 5 minutes.
7. While the patties are cooking, make the dill sauce by combining the remaining 6 tablespoons of mayonnaise with the remaining 1 teaspoon of dill, the lemon juice, the lemon zest, and the remaining ¼ teaspoon of salt. Set aside.
8. Remove the patties from the air fryer.
9. Place 1 slice of lettuce on a plate and top with the tuna patty and a tomato slice. Repeat to form the remaining servings. Drizzle the dill dressing over the top. Serve immediately.

Pecan-orange Crusted Striped Bass

Servings: 2
Cooking Time: 9 Minutes

Ingredients:

- flour, for dredging*
- 2 egg whites, lightly beaten
- 1 cup pecans, chopped
- 1 teaspoon finely chopped orange zest, plus more for garnish
- ½ teaspoon salt
- 2 (6-ounce) fillets striped bass
- salt and freshly ground black pepper
- vegetable or olive oil, in a spray bottle
- Orange Cream Sauce (Optional)
- ½ cup fresh orange juice
- ¼ cup heavy cream
- 1 sprig fresh thyme

Directions:

1. Set up a dredging station with three shallow dishes. Place the flour in one shallow dish. Place the beaten egg whites in a second shallow dish. Finally, combine the chopped pecans, orange zest and salt in a third shallow dish.
2. Coat the fish fillets one at a time. First season with salt and freshly ground black pepper. Then coat each fillet in flour. Shake off any excess flour and then dip the fish into the egg white. Let the excess egg drip off and then immediately press the fish into the pecan-orange mixture. Set the crusted fish fillets aside.
3. Preheat the air fryer to 400°F.
4. Spray the crusted fish with oil and then transfer the fillets to the air fryer basket. Air-fry for 9 minutes at 400°F, flipping the fish over halfway through the cooking time. The nuts on top should be nice and toasty and the fish should feel firm to the touch.
5. If you'd like to make a sauce to go with the fish while it cooks, combine the freshly squeezed orange juice, heavy cream and sprig of thyme in a small saucepan. Simmer on the stovetop for 5 minutes and then set aside.
6. Remove the fish from the air fryer and serve over a bed of salad, like the one below. Then add a sprinkling of orange zest and a spoonful of the orange cream sauce over the top if desired.

Fish Cakes

Servings: 4
Cooking Time: 10 Minutes

Ingredients:

- ¾ cup mashed potatoes (about 1 large russet potato)
- 12 ounces cod or other white fish
- salt and pepper
- oil for misting or cooking spray
- 1 large egg
- ¼ cup potato starch
- ½ cup panko breadcrumbs
- 1 tablespoon fresh chopped chives
- 2 tablespoons minced onion

Directions:

1. Peel potatoes, cut into cubes, and cook on stovetop till soft.

2. Salt and pepper raw fish to taste. Mist with oil or cooking spray, and cook in air fryer at 360°F for 6 to 8minutes, until fish flakes easily. If fish is crowded, rearrange halfway through cooking to ensure all pieces cook evenly.
3. Transfer fish to a plate and break apart to cool.
4. Beat egg in a shallow dish.
5. Place potato starch in another shallow dish, and panko crumbs in a third dish.
6. When potatoes are done, drain in colander and rinse with cold water.
7. In a large bowl, mash the potatoes and stir in the chives and onion. Add salt and pepper to taste, then stir in the fish.
8. If needed, stir in a tablespoon of the beaten egg to help bind the mixture.
9. Shape into 8 small, fat patties. Dust lightly with potato starch, dip in egg, and roll in panko crumbs. Spray both sides with oil or cooking spray.
10. Cook at 360°F for 10 minutes, until golden brown and crispy.

Better Fish Sticks

Servings:3
Cooking Time: 8 Minutes

Ingredients:

- ¾ cup Seasoned Italian-style dried bread crumbs (gluten-free, if a concern)
- 3 tablespoons (about ½ ounce) Finely grated Parmesan cheese
- 10 ounces Skinless cod fillets, cut lengthwise into 1-inch-wide pieces
- 3 tablespoons Regular or low-fat mayonnaise (not fat-free; gluten-free, if a concern)
- Vegetable oil spray

Directions:

1. Preheat the air fryer to 400°F.
2. Mix the bread crumbs and grated Parmesan in a shallow soup bowl or a small pie plate.
3. Smear the fish fillet sticks completely with the mayonnaise, then dip them one by one in the bread-crumb mixture, turning and pressing gently to make an even and thorough coating. Coat each stick on all sides with vegetable oil spray.
4. Set the fish sticks in the basket with at least ¼ inch between them. Air-fry undisturbed for 8 minutes, or until golden brown and crisp.
5. Use a nonstick-safe spatula to gently transfer them from the basket to a wire rack. Cool for only a minute or two before serving.

Sea Bass With Potato Scales And Caper Aïoli

Servings: 2
Cooking Time: 10 Minutes

Ingredients:

- 2 (6- to 8-ounce) fillets of sea bass
- salt and freshly ground black pepper
- ¼ cup mayonnaise
- 2 teaspoons finely chopped lemon zest
- 1 teaspoon chopped fresh thyme
- 2 fingerling potatoes, very thinly sliced into rounds
- olive oil
- ½ clove garlic, crushed into a paste
- 1 tablespoon capers, drained and rinsed
- 1 tablespoon olive oil
- 1 teaspoon lemon juice, to taste

Directions:

1. Preheat the air fryer to 400°F.
2. Season the fish well with salt and freshly ground black pepper. Mix the mayonnaise, lemon zest and thyme together in a small bowl. Spread a thin layer of the mayonnaise mixture on both fillets. Start layering rows of potato slices onto the fish fillets to simulate the fish scales. The second row should overlap the first row slightly. Dabbing a little more mayonnaise along the upper edge of the row of potatoes where the next row overlaps will help the potato slices stick. Press the potatoes onto the fish to secure them well and season again with salt. Brush or spray the potato layer with olive oil.
3. Transfer the fish to the air fryer and air-fry for 8 to 10 minutes, depending on the thickness of your fillets. 1-inch of fish should take 10 minutes at 400°F.

4. While the fish is cooking, add the garlic, capers, olive oil and lemon juice to the remaining mayonnaise mixture to make the caper aïoli.
5. Serve the fish warm with a dollop of the aïoli on top or on the side.

Fried Scallops

Servings:3
Cooking Time: 6 Minutes

Ingredients:

- ½ cup All-purpose flour or tapioca flour
- 1 Large egg(s), well beaten
- 2 cups Corn flake crumbs (gluten-free, if a concern)
- Up to 2 teaspoons Cayenne
- 1 teaspoon Celery seeds
- 1 teaspoon Table salt
- 1 pound Sea scallops
- Vegetable oil spray

Directions:

1. Preheat the air fryer to 400°F.
2. Set up and fill three shallow soup plates or small pie plates on your counter: one for the flour; one for the beaten egg(s); and one for the corn flake crumbs, stirred with the cayenne, celery seeds, and salt until well combined.
3. One by one, dip a scallop in the flour, turning it every way to coat it thoroughly. Gently shake off any excess flour, then dip the scallop in the egg(s), turning it again to coat all sides. Let any excess egg slip back into the rest, then set the scallop in the corn flake mixture. Turn it several times, pressing gently to get an even coating on the scallop all around. Generously coat the scallop with vegetable oil spray, then set it aside on a cutting board. Coat the remaining scallops in the same way.
4. Set the scallops in the basket with as much air space between them as possible. They should not touch. Air-fry undisturbed for 6 minutes, or until lightly browned and firm.
5. Use kitchen tongs to gently transfer the scallops to a wire rack. Cool for only a minute or two before serving.

Shrimp

Servings: 4
Cooking Time: 8 Minutes

Ingredients:

- 1 pound (26–30 count) shrimp, peeled, deveined, and butterflied (last tail section of shell intact)
- Marinade
- 1 5-ounce can evaporated milk
- 2 eggs, beaten
- 2 tablespoons white vinegar
- 1 tablespoon baking powder
- Coating
- 1 cup crushed panko breadcrumbs
- ½ teaspoon paprika
- ½ teaspoon Old Bay Seasoning
- ¼ teaspoon garlic powder
- oil for misting or cooking spray

Directions:

1. Stir together all marinade ingredients until well mixed. Add shrimp and stir to coat. Refrigerate for 1 hour.
2. When ready to cook, preheat air fryer to 390°F.
3. Combine coating ingredients in shallow dish.
4. Remove shrimp from marinade, roll in crumb mixture, and spray with olive oil or cooking spray.
5. Cooking in two batches, place shrimp in air fryer basket in single layer, close but not overlapping. Cook at 390°F for 8 minutes, until light golden brown and crispy.
6. Repeat step 5 to cook remaining shrimp.

Maple-crusted Salmon

Servings: 2
Cooking Time: 8 Minutes

Ingredients:

- 12 ounces salmon filets
- ⅓ cup maple syrup
- 1 teaspoon Worcestershire sauce
- 2 teaspoons Dijon mustard or brown mustard
- ½ cup finely chopped walnuts
- ½ teaspoon sea salt
- ½ lemon
- 1 tablespoon chopped parsley, for garnish

Directions:

1. Place the salmon in a shallow baking dish. Top with maple syrup, Worcestershire sauce, and mustard. Refrigerate for 30 minutes.
2. Preheat the air fryer to 350°F.
3. Remove the salmon from the marinade and discard the marinade.
4. Place the chopped nuts on top of the salmon filets, and sprinkle salt on top of the nuts. Place the salmon, skin side down, in the air fryer basket. Cook for 6 to 8 minutes or until the fish flakes in the center.
5. Remove the salmon and plate on a serving platter. Squeeze fresh lemon over the top of the salmon and top with chopped parsley. Serve immediately.

Black Cod With Grapes, Fennel, Pecans And Kale

Servings: 2

Cooking Time: 15 Minutes

Ingredients:

- 2 (6- to 8-ounce) fillets of black cod (or sablefish)
- salt and freshly ground black pepper
- olive oil
- 1 cup grapes, halved
- 1 small bulb fennel, sliced ¼-inch thick
- ½ cup pecans
- 3 cups shredded kale
- 2 teaspoons white balsamic vinegar or white wine vinegar
- 2 tablespoons extra virgin olive oil

Directions:

1. Preheat the air fryer to 400°F.
2. Season the cod fillets with salt and pepper and drizzle, brush or spray a little olive oil on top. Place the fish, presentation side up (skin side down), into the air fryer basket. Air-fry for 10 minutes.
3. When the fish has finished cooking, remove the fillets to a side plate and loosely tent with foil to rest.
4. Toss the grapes, fennel and pecans in a bowl with a drizzle of olive oil and season with salt and pepper. Add the grapes, fennel and pecans to the air fryer basket and air-fry for 5 minutes at 400°F, shaking the basket once during the cooking time.
5. Transfer the grapes, fennel and pecans to a bowl with the kale. Dress the kale with the balsamic vinegar and olive oil, season to taste with salt and pepper and serve along side the cooked fish.

Spicy Fish Street Tacos With Sriracha Slaw

Servings: 2

Cooking Time: 5 Minutes

Ingredients:

- Sriracha Slaw:
- ½ cup mayonnaise
- 2 tablespoons rice vinegar
- 1 teaspoon sugar
- 2 tablespoons sriracha chili sauce
- 5 cups shredded green cabbage
- ¼ cup shredded carrots
- 2 scallions, chopped
- salt and freshly ground black pepper
- Tacos:
- ½ cup flour
- 1 teaspoon chili powder
- ½ teaspoon ground cumin
- 1 teaspoon salt
- freshly ground black pepper
- ½ teaspoon baking powder
- 1 egg, beaten
- ¼ cup milk
- 1 cup breadcrumbs
- 1 pound mahi-mahi or snapper fillets
- 1 tablespoon canola or vegetable oil
- 6 (6-inch) flour tortillas
- 1 lime, cut into wedges

Directions:

1. Start by making the sriracha slaw. Combine the mayonnaise, rice vinegar, sugar, and sriracha sauce in a large bowl. Mix well and add the green cabbage, carrots, and scallions. Toss until all the vegetables are coated with the dressing and season with salt and pepper. Refrigerate the slaw until you are ready to serve the tacos.

2. Combine the flour, chili powder, cumin, salt, pepper and baking powder in a bowl. Add the egg and milk and mix until the batter is smooth. Place the breadcrumbs in shallow dish.
3. Cut the fish fillets into 1-inch wide sticks, approximately 4-inches long. You should have about 12 fish sticks total. Dip the fish sticks into the batter, coating all sides. Let the excess batter drip off the fish and then roll them in the breadcrumbs, patting the crumbs onto all sides of the fish sticks. Set the coated fish on a plate or baking sheet until all the fish has been coated.
4. Preheat the air fryer to 400°F.
5. Spray the coated fish sticks with oil on all sides. Spray or brush the inside of the air fryer basket with oil and transfer the fish to the basket. Place as many sticks as you can in one layer, leaving a little room around each stick. Place any remaining sticks on top, perpendicular to the first layer.
6. Air-fry the fish for 3 minutes. Turn the fish sticks over and air-fry for an additional 2 minutes.
7. While the fish is air-frying, warm the tortilla shells either in a 350°F oven wrapped in foil or in a skillet with a little oil over medium-high heat for a couple minutes. Fold the tortillas in half and keep them warm until the remaining tortillas and fish are ready.
8. To assemble the tacos, place two pieces of the fish in each tortilla shell and top with the sriracha slaw. Squeeze the lime wedge over top and dig in.

Mahi-mahi "burrito" Fillets

Servings:3

Cooking Time: 10 Minutes

Ingredients:

- 1 Large egg white
- 1½ cups (6 ounces) Crushed corn tortilla chips (gluten-free, if a concern)
- 1 tablespoon Chile powder
- 3 5-ounce skinless mahi-mahi fillets
- 6 tablespoons Canned refried beans
- Vegetable oil spray

Directions:

1. Preheat the air fryer to 400°F.
2. Set up and fill two shallow soup plates or small pie plates on your counter: one with the egg white, beaten until foamy; and one with the crushed tortilla chips.
3. Gently rub ½ teaspoon chile powder on each side of each fillet.
4. Spread (or maybe smear) 1 tablespoon refried beans over both sides and the edges of a fillet. Dip the fillet in the egg white, turning to coat it on both sides. Let any excess egg white slip back into the rest, then set the fillet in the crushed tortilla chips. Turn several times, pressing gently to coat it evenly. Coat the fillet on all sides with the vegetable oil spray, then set it aside. Prepare the remaining fillet(s) in the same way.
5. When the machine is at temperature, set the fillets in the basket with as much air space between them as possible. Air-fry undisturbed for 10 minutes, or until crisp and browned.
6. Use a nonstick-safe spatula to transfer the fillets to a serving platter or plates. Cool for only a minute or so, then serve hot.

Shrimp Patties

Servings: 4

Cooking Time: 10 Minutes

Ingredients:

- ½ pound shelled and deveined raw shrimp
- ¼ cup chopped red bell pepper
- ¼ cup chopped green onion
- ¼ cup chopped celery
- 2 cups cooked sushi rice
- ½ teaspoon garlic powder
- ½ teaspoon Old Bay Seasoning
- ½ teaspoon salt
- 2 teaspoons Worcestershire sauce
- ½ cup plain breadcrumbs
- oil for misting or cooking spray

Directions:

1. Finely chop the shrimp. You can do this in a food processor, but it takes only a few pulses. Be careful not to overprocess into mush.
2. Place shrimp in a large bowl and add all other ingredients except the breadcrumbs and oil. Stir until well combined.

3. Preheat air fryer to 390°F.
4. Shape shrimp mixture into 8 patties, no more than ½-inch thick. Roll patties in breadcrumbs and mist with oil or cooking spray.
5. Place 4 shrimp patties in air fryer basket and cook at 390°F for 10 minutes, until shrimp cooks through and outside is crispy.
6. Repeat step 5 to cook remaining shrimp patties.

Beer-battered Cod

Servings:3
Cooking Time: 12 Minutes

Ingredients:

- 1½ cups All-purpose flour
- 3 tablespoons Old Bay seasoning
- 1 Large egg(s)
- ¼ cup Amber beer, pale ale, or IPA
- 3 4-ounce skinless cod fillets
- Vegetable oil spray

Directions:

1. Preheat the air fryer to 400°F.
2. Set up and fill two shallow soup plates or small pie plates on your counter: one with the flour, whisked with the Old Bay until well combined; and one with the egg(s), whisked with the beer until foamy and uniform.
3. Dip a piece of cod in the flour mixture, turning it to coat on all sides (not just the top and bottom). Gently shake off any excess flour and dip the fish in the egg mixture, turning it to coat. Let any excess egg mixture slip back into the rest, then set the fish back in the flour mixture and coat it again, then back in the egg mixture for a second wash, then back in the flour mixture for a third time. Coat the fish on all sides with vegetable oil spray and set it aside. "Batter" the remaining piece(s) of cod in the same way.
4. Set the coated cod fillets in the basket with as much space between them as possible. They should not touch. Air-fry undisturbed for 12 minutes, or until brown and crisp.
5. Use kitchen tongs to gently transfer the fish to a wire rack. Cool for only a couple of minutes before serving.

Salmon Puttanesca En Papillotte With Zucchini

Servings: 2
Cooking Time: 17 Minutes

Ingredients:

- 1 small zucchini, sliced into ¼-inch thick half moons
- 1 teaspoon olive oil
- salt and freshly ground black pepper
- 2 (5-ounce) salmon fillets
- 1 beefsteak tomato, chopped (about 1 cup)
- 1 tablespoon capers, rinsed
- 10 black olives, pitted and sliced
- 2 tablespoons dry vermouth or white wine 2 tablespoons butter
- ¼ cup chopped fresh basil, chopped

Directions:

1. Preheat the air fryer to 400°F.
2. Toss the zucchini with the olive oil, salt and freshly ground black pepper. Transfer the zucchini into the air fryer basket and air-fry for 5 minutes, shaking the basket once or twice during the cooking process.
3. Cut out 2 large rectangles of parchment paper – about 13-inches by 15-inches each. Divide the air-fried zucchini between the two pieces of parchment paper, placing the vegetables in the center of each rectangle.
4. Place a fillet of salmon on each pile of zucchini. Season the fish very well with salt and pepper. Toss the tomato, capers, olives and vermouth (or white wine) together in a bowl. Divide the tomato mixture between the two fish packages, placing it on top of the fish fillets and pouring any juice out of the bowl onto the fish. Top each fillet with a tablespoon of butter.
5. Fold up each parchment square. Bring two edges together and fold them over a few times, leaving some space above the fish. Twist the open sides together and upwards so they can serve as handles for the packet, but don't let them extend beyond the top of the air fryer basket.
6. Place the two packages into the air fryer and air-fry at 400°F for 12 minutes. The packages should be puffed up and slightly browned when fully cooked. Once cooked, let the fish sit in the parchment for 2 minutes.

7. Serve the fish in the parchment paper, or if desired, remove the parchment paper before serving. Garnish with a little fresh basil.

Coconut-shrimp Po' Boys

Servings: 4
Cooking Time: 5 Minutes

Ingredients:

- ½ cup cornstarch
- 2 eggs
- 2 tablespoons milk
- ¾ cup shredded coconut
- ½ cup panko breadcrumbs
- 1 pound (31–35 count) shrimp, peeled and deveined
- Old Bay Seasoning
- oil for misting or cooking spray
- 2 large hoagie rolls
- honey mustard or light mayonnaise
- 1½ cups shredded lettuce
- 1 large tomato, thinly sliced

Directions:

1. Place cornstarch in a shallow dish or plate.
2. In another shallow dish, beat together eggs and milk.
3. In a third dish mix the coconut and panko crumbs.
4. Sprinkle shrimp with Old Bay Seasoning to taste.
5. Dip shrimp in cornstarch to coat lightly, dip in egg mixture, shake off excess, and roll in coconut mixture to coat well.
6. Spray both sides of coated shrimp with oil or cooking spray.
7. Cook half the shrimp in a single layer at 390°F for 5minutes.
8. Repeat to cook remaining shrimp.
9. To Assemble
10. Split each hoagie lengthwise, leaving one long edge intact.
11. Place in air fryer basket and cook at 390°F for 1 to 2minutes or until heated through.
12. Remove buns, break apart, and place on 4 plates, cut side up.
13. Spread with honey mustard and/or mayonnaise.
14. Top with shredded lettuce, tomato slices, and coconut shrimp.

Butternut Squash–wrapped Halibut Fillets

Servings:3
Cooking Time: 11 Minutes

Ingredients:

- 15 Long spiralized peeled and seeded butternut squash strands
- 3 5- to 6-ounce skinless halibut fillets
- 3 tablespoons Butter, melted
- ¾ teaspoon Mild paprika
- ¾ teaspoon Table salt
- ¾ teaspoon Ground black pepper

Directions:

1. Preheat the air fryer to 375°F .
2. Hold 5 long butternut squash strands together and wrap them around a fillet. Set it aside and wrap any remaining fillet(s).
3. Mix the melted butter, paprika, salt, and pepper in a small bowl. Brush this mixture over the squash-wrapped fillets on all sides.
4. When the machine is at temperature, set the fillets in the basket with as much air space between them as possible. Air-fry undisturbed for 10 minutes, or until the squash strands have browned but not burned. If the machine is at 360°F, you may need to add 1 minute to the cooking time. In any event, watch the fish carefully after the 8-minute mark.
5. Use a nonstick-safe spatula to gently transfer the fillets to a serving platter or plates. Cool for only a minute or so before serving.

Maple Balsamic Glazed Salmon

Servings: 4

Cooking Time: 10 Minutes

Ingredients:

- 4 (6-ounce) fillets of salmon
- salt and freshly ground black pepper
- vegetable oil
- ¼ cup pure maple syrup
- 3 tablespoons balsamic vinegar
- 1 teaspoon Dijon mustard

Directions:

1. Preheat the air fryer to 400°F.
2. Season the salmon well with salt and freshly ground black pepper. Spray or brush the bottom of the air fryer basket with vegetable oil and place the salmon fillets inside. Air-fry the salmon for 5 minutes.
3. While the salmon is air-frying, combine the maple syrup, balsamic vinegar and Dijon mustard in a small saucepan over medium heat and stir to blend well. Let the mixture simmer while the fish is cooking. It should start to thicken slightly, but keep your eye on it so it doesn't burn.
4. Brush the glaze on the salmon fillets and air-fry for an additional 5 minutes. The salmon should feel firm to the touch when finished and the glaze should be nicely browned on top. Brush a little more glaze on top before removing and serving with rice and vegetables, or a nice green salad.

Perfect Soft-shelled Crabs

Servings:2

Cooking Time: 12 Minutes

Ingredients:

- ½ cup All-purpose flour
- 1 tablespoon Old Bay seasoning
- 1 Large egg(s), well beaten
- 1 cup (about 3 ounces) Ground oyster crackers
- 2 2½-ounce cleaned soft-shelled crab(s), about 4 inches across
- Vegetable oil spray

Directions:

1. Preheat the air fryer to 375°F (or 380°F or 390°F, if one of these is the closest setting).
2. Set up and fill three shallow soup plates or small pie plates on your counter: one for the flour, whisked with the Old Bay until well combined; one for the beaten egg(s); and one for the cracker crumbs.
3. Set a soft-shelled crab in the flour mixture and turn to coat evenly and well on all sides, even inside the legs. Dip the crab into the egg(s) and coat well, turning at least once, again getting some of the egg between the legs. Let any excess egg slip back into the rest, then set the crab in the cracker crumbs. Turn several times, pressing very gently to get the crab evenly coated with crumbs, even between the legs. Generously coat the crab on all sides with vegetable oil spray. Set it aside if you're making more than one and coat these in the same way.
4. Set the crab(s) in the basket with as much air space between them as possible. They may overlap slightly, particularly at the ends of their legs, depending on the basket's size. Air-fry undisturbed for 12 minutes, or until very crisp and golden brown. If the machine is at 390°F, the crabs may be done in only 10 minutes.
5. Use kitchen tongs to gently transfer the crab(s) to a wire rack. Cool for a couple of minutes before serving.

Miso-rubbed Salmon Fillets

Servings:3

Cooking Time: 5 Minutes

Ingredients:

- ¼ cup White (shiro) miso paste (usually made from rice and soy beans)
- 1½ tablespoons Mirin or a substitute (see here)
- 2½ teaspoons Unseasoned rice vinegar (see here)
- Vegetable oil spray
- 3 6-ounce skin-on salmon fillets (for more information, see here)

Directions:

1. Preheat the air fryer to 400°F.
2. Mix the miso, mirin, and vinegar in a small bowl until uniform.
3. Remove the basket from the machine. Generously spray the skin side of each fillet. Pick them up one by one with a nonstick-safe spatula and set them in the

basket skin side down with as much air space between them as possible. Coat the top of each fillet with the miso mixture, dividing it evenly between them.

4. Return the basket to the machine. Air-fry undisturbed for 5 minutes, or until lightly browned and firm.

5. Use a nonstick-safe spatula to transfer the fillets to serving plates. Cool for only a minute or so before serving.

Honey Pecan Shrimp

Servings: 4

Cooking Time: 10 Minutes

Ingredients:

- ¼ cup cornstarch
- ¾ teaspoon sea salt, divided
- ¼ teaspoon pepper
- 2 egg whites
- ⅔ cup finely chopped pecans
- 1 pound raw, peeled, and deveined shrimp
- ¼ cup honey
- 2 tablespoons mayonnaise

Directions:

1. In a small bowl, whisk together the cornstarch, ½ teaspoon of the salt, and the pepper.
2. In a second bowl, whisk together the egg whites until soft and foamy. (They don't need to be whipped to peaks or even soft peaks, just frothy.)
3. In a third bowl, mix together the pecans and the remaining ¼ teaspoon of sea salt.
4. Pat the shrimp dry with paper towels. Working in small batches, dip the shrimp into the cornstarch, then into the egg whites, and then into the pecans until all the shrimp are coated with pecans.
5. Preheat the air fryer to 330°F.
6. Place the coated shrimp inside the air fryer basket and spray with cooking spray. Cook for 5 minutes, toss the shrimp, and cook another 5 minutes.
7. Meanwhile, place the honey in a microwave-safe bowl and microwave for 30 seconds. Whisk in the mayonnaise until smooth and creamy. Pour the honey sauce into a serving bowl. Add the cooked shrimp to the serving bowl while hot and toss to coat. Serve immediately.

Sea Scallops

Servings: 4

Cooking Time: 8 Minutes

Ingredients:

- 1½ pounds sea scallops
- salt and pepper
- 2 eggs
- ½ cup flour
- ½ cup plain breadcrumbs
- oil for misting or cooking spray

Directions:

1. Rinse scallops and remove the tough side muscle. Sprinkle to taste with salt and pepper.
2. Beat eggs together in a shallow dish. Place flour in a second shallow dish and breadcrumbs in a third.
3. Preheat air fryer to 390°F.
4. Dip scallops in flour, then eggs, and then roll in breadcrumbs. Mist with oil or cooking spray.
5. Place scallops in air fryer basket in a single layer, leaving some space between. You should be able to cook about a dozen at a time.
6. Cook at 390°F for 8 minutes, watching carefully so as not to overcook. Scallops are done when they turn opaque all the way through. They will feel slightly firm when pressed with tines of a fork.
7. Repeat step 6 to cook remaining scallops.

Shrimp & Grits

Servings: 4

Cooking Time: 5 Minutes

Ingredients:

- 1 pound raw shelled shrimp, deveined (26–30 count or smaller)
- Marinade
- 2 tablespoons lemon juice
- 2 tablespoons Worcestershire sauce
- 1 tablespoon olive oil
- 1 teaspoon Old Bay Seasoning
- ½ teaspoon hot sauce

- Grits
- ¾ cup quick cooking grits (not instant)
- 3 cups water
- ½ teaspoon salt
- 1 tablespoon butter
- ½ cup chopped green bell pepper
- ½ cup chopped celery
- ½ cup chopped onion
- ½ teaspoon oregano
- ¼ teaspoon Old Bay Seasoning
- 2 ounces sharp Cheddar cheese, grated

Directions:

1. Stir together all marinade ingredients. Pour marinade over shrimp and set aside.
2. For grits, heat water and salt to boil in saucepan on stovetop. Stir in grits, lower heat to medium-low, and cook about 5minutes or until thick and done.
3. Place butter, bell pepper, celery, and onion in air fryer baking pan. Cook at 390°F for 2minutes and stir. Cook 6 or 7minutes longer, until crisp tender.
4. Add oregano and 1 teaspoon Old Bay to cooked vegetables. Stir in grits and cheese and cook at 390°F for 1 minute. Stir and cook 1 to 2minutes longer to melt cheese.
5. Remove baking pan from air fryer. Cover with plate to keep warm while shrimp cooks.
6. Drain marinade from shrimp. Place shrimp in air fryer basket and cook at 360°F for 3minutes. Stir or shake basket. Cook 2 more minutes, until done.
7. To serve, spoon grits onto plates and top with shrimp.

Horseradish Crusted Salmon

Servings: 2

Cooking Time: 14 Minutes

Ingredients:

- 2 (5-ounce) salmon fillets
- salt and freshly ground black pepper
- 2 teaspoons Dijon mustard
- ½ cup panko breadcrumbs*
- 2 tablespoons prepared horseradish
- ½ teaspoon finely chopped lemon zest
- 1 tablespoon olive oil
- 1 tablespoon chopped fresh parsley

Directions:

1. Preheat the air fryer to 360°F.
2. Season the salmon with salt and freshly ground black pepper. Then spread the Dijon mustard on the salmon, coating the entire surface.
3. Combine the breadcrumbs, horseradish, lemon zest and olive oil in a small bowl. Spread the mixture over the top of the salmon and press down lightly with your hands, adhering it to the salmon using the mustard as "glue".
4. Transfer the salmon to the air fryer basket and air-fry at 360°F for 14 minutes (depending on how thick your fillet is) or until the fish feels firm to the touch. Sprinkle with the parsley.

Crabmeat-stuffed Flounder

Servings:3

Cooking Time: 12 Minutes

Ingredients:

- 4½ ounces Purchased backfin or claw crabmeat, picked over for bits of shell and cartilage
- 6 Saltine crackers, crushed into fine crumbs
- 2 tablespoons plus 1 teaspoon Regular or low-fat mayonnaise (not fat-free)
- ¾ teaspoon Yellow prepared mustard
- 1½ teaspoons Worcestershire sauce
- ⅛ teaspoon Celery salt
- 3 5- to 6-ounce skinless flounder fillets
- Vegetable oil spray
- Mild paprika

Directions:

1. Preheat the air fryer to 400°F.
2. Gently mix the crabmeat, crushed saltines, mayonnaise, mustard, Worcestershire sauce, and celery salt in a bowl until well combined.
3. Generously coat the flat side of a fillet with vegetable oil spray. Set the fillet sprayed side down on your work surface. Cut the fillet in half widthwise, then cut one of the halves in half lengthwise. Set a scant ⅓ cup of the crabmeat mixture on top of the undivided half of the fish fillet, mounding the mixture to make an oval

that somewhat fits the shape of the fillet with at least a ¼-inch border of fillet beyond the filling all around.

4. Take the two thin divided quarters (that is, the halves of the half) and lay them lengthwise over the filling, overlapping at each end and leaving a little space in the middle where the filling peeks through. Coat the top of the stuffed flounder piece with vegetable oil spray, then sprinkle paprika over the stuffed flounder fillet. Set aside and use the remaining fillet(s) to make more stuffed flounder "packets," repeating steps 3 and

5. Use a nonstick-safe spatula to transfer the stuffed flounder fillets to the basket. Leave as much space between them as possible. Air-fry undisturbed for 12 minutes, or until lightly brown and firm (but not hard).

6. Use that same spatula, plus perhaps another one, to transfer the fillets to a serving platter or plates. Cool for a minute or two, then serve hot.

Lemon-roasted Salmon Fillets

Servings:3

Cooking Time: 7 Minutes

Ingredients:

- 3 6-ounce skin-on salmon fillets
- Olive oil spray
- 9 Very thin lemon slices
- ¾ teaspoon Ground black pepper
- ¼ teaspoon Table salt

Directions:

1. Preheat the air fryer to 400°F.
2. Generously coat the skin of each of the fillets with olive oil spray. Set the fillets skin side down on your work surface. Place three overlapping lemon slices down the length of each salmon fillet. Sprinkle them with the pepper and salt. Coat lightly with olive oil spray.
3. Use a nonstick-safe spatula to transfer the fillets one by one to the basket, leaving as much air space between them as possible. Air-fry undisturbed for 7 minutes, or until cooked through.
4. Use a nonstick-safe spatula to transfer the fillets to serving plates. Cool for only a minute or two before serving.

Fish-in-chips

Servings:4

Cooking Time: 11 Minutes

Ingredients:

- 1 cup All-purpose flour or potato starch
- 2 Large egg(s), well beaten
- 1½ cups (6 ounces) Crushed plain potato chips, preferably thick-cut or ruffled (gluten-free, if a concern)
- 4 4-ounce skinless cod fillets

Directions:

1. Preheat the air fryer to 400°F.
2. Set up and fill three shallow soup plates or small pie plates on your counter: one for the flour, one for the beaten egg(s), and one for the crushed potato chips.
3. Dip a piece of cod in the flour, turning it to coat on all sides, even the ends and sides. Gently shake off any excess flour, then dip it in the beaten egg(s). Gently turn to coat it on all sides, then let any excess egg slip back into the rest. Set the fillet in the crushed potato chips and turn several times and onto all sides, pressing gently to coat the fish. Dip it back in the egg(s), coating all sides but taking care that the coating doesn't slip off; then dip it back in the potato chips for a thick, even coating. Set it aside and coat more fillets in the same way.
4. When the machine is at temperature, set the fillets in the basket with as much air space between them as possible. Air-fry undisturbed for 11 minutes, until golden brown and firm but not hard.
5. Use kitchen tongs to transfer the fillets to a wire rack. Cool for just a minute or two before serving.

Crunchy And Buttery Cod With Ritz® Cracker Crust

Servings: 2

Cooking Time: 10 Minutes

Ingredients:

- 4 tablespoons butter, melted
- 8 to 10 RITZ® crackers, crushed into crumbs
- 2 (6-ounce) cod fillets
- salt and freshly ground black pepper
- 1 lemon

Directions:

1. Preheat the air fryer to 380°F.
2. Melt the butter in a small saucepan on the stovetop or in a microwavable dish in the microwave, and then transfer the butter to a shallow dish. Place the crushed RITZ® crackers into a second shallow dish.
3. Season the fish fillets with salt and freshly ground black pepper. Dip them into the butter and then coat both sides with the RITZ® crackers.
4. Place the fish into the air fryer basket and air-fry at 380°F for 10 minutes, flipping the fish over halfway through the cooking time.
5. Serve with a wedge of lemon to squeeze over the top.

Fried Shrimp

Servings:3

Cooking Time: 7 Minutes

Ingredients:

- 1 Large egg white
- 2 tablespoons Water
- 1 cup Plain dried bread crumbs (gluten-free, if a concern)
- ¼ cup All-purpose flour or almond flour
- ¼ cup Yellow cornmeal
- 1 teaspoon Celery salt
- 1 teaspoon Mild paprika
- Up to ½ teaspoon Cayenne (optional)
- ¾ pound Large shrimp (20–25 per pound), peeled and deveined
- Vegetable oil spray

Directions:

1. Preheat the air fryer to 400°F.
2. Set two medium or large bowls on your counter. In the first, whisk the egg white and water until foamy. In the second, stir the bread crumbs, flour, cornmeal, celery salt, paprika, and cayenne (if using) until well combined.
3. Pour all the shrimp into the egg white mixture and stir gently until all the shrimp are coated. Use kitchen tongs to pick them up one by one and transfer them to the bread-crumb mixture. Turn each in the bread-crumb mixture to coat it evenly and thoroughly on all sides before setting it on a cutting board. When you're done coating the shrimp, coat them all on both sides with the vegetable oil spray.
4. Set the shrimp in as close to one layer in the basket as you can. Some may overlap. Air-fry for 7 minutes, gently rearranging the shrimp at the 4-minute mark to get covered surfaces exposed, until golden brown and firm but not hard.
5. Use kitchen tongs to gently transfer the shrimp to a wire rack. Cool for only a minute or two before serving.

Salmon

Servings: 4

Cooking Time: 8 Minutes

Ingredients:

- Marinade
- 3 tablespoons low-sodium soy sauce
- 3 tablespoons rice vinegar
- 3 tablespoons ketchup
- 3 tablespoons olive oil
- 3 tablespoons brown sugar
- 1 teaspoon garlic powder
- ½ teaspoon ground ginger
- 4 salmon fillets (½-inch thick, 3 to 4 ounces each)
- cooking spray

Directions:

1. Mix all marinade ingredients until well blended.
2. Place salmon in sealable plastic bag or shallow container with lid. Pour marinade over fish and turn to coat well. Refrigerate for 30minutes.
3. Drain marinade, and spray air fryer basket with cooking spray.
4. Place salmon in basket, skin-side down.
5. Cook at 360°F for 10 minutes, watching closely to avoid overcooking. Salmon is done when just beginning to flake and still very moist.

Potato-wrapped Salmon Fillets

Servings:3

Cooking Time: 8 Minutes

Ingredients:

- 1 Large 1-pound elongated yellow potato(es), peeled
- 3 6-ounce, 1½-inch-wide, quite thick skinless salmon fillets
- Olive oil spray
- ¼ teaspoon Table salt
- ¼ teaspoon Ground black pepper

Directions:

1. Preheat the air fryer to 400°F.
2. Use a vegetable peeler or mandoline to make long strips from the potato(es). You'll need anywhere from 8 to 12 strips per fillet, depending on the shape of the potato and of the salmon fillet.
3. Drape potato strips over a salmon fillet, overlapping the strips to create an even "crust." Tuck the potato strips under the fillet, overlapping the strips underneath to create as smooth a bottom as you can. Wrap the remaining fillet(s) in the same way.
4. Gently turn the fillets over. Generously coat the bottoms with olive oil spray. Turn them back seam side down and generously coat the tops with the oil spray. Sprinkle the salt and pepper over the wrapped fillets.
5. Use a nonstick-safe spatula to gently transfer the fillets seam side down to the basket. It helps to remove the basket from the machine and set it on your work surface (keeping in mind that the basket's hot). Leave as much air space as possible between the fillets. Air-fry undisturbed for 8 minutes, or until golden brown and crisp.
6. Use a nonstick-safe spatula to gently transfer the fillets to serving plates. Cool for a couple of minutes before serving.

Crab Stuffed Salmon Roast

Servings: 4

Cooking Time: 20 Minutes

Ingredients:

- 1 (1½-pound) salmon fillet
- salt and freshly ground black pepper
- 6 ounces crabmeat
- 1 teaspoon finely chopped lemon zest
- 1 teaspoon Dijon mustard
- 1 tablespoon chopped fresh parsley, plus more for garnish
- 1 scallion, chopped
- ¼ teaspoon salt
- olive oil

Directions:

1. Prepare the salmon fillet by butterflying it. Slice into the thickest side of the salmon, parallel to the countertop and along the length of the fillet. Don't slice all the way through to the other side – stop about an inch from the edge. Open the salmon up like a book. Season the salmon with salt and freshly ground black pepper.
2. Make the crab filling by combining the crabmeat, lemon zest, mustard, parsley, scallion, salt and freshly ground black pepper in a bowl. Spread this filling in the center of the salmon. Fold one side of the salmon over the filling. Then fold the other side over on top.
3. Transfer the rolled salmon to the center of a piece of parchment paper that is roughly 6- to 7-inches wide and about 12-inches long. The parchment paper will act as a sling, making it easier to put the salmon into the air fryer. Preheat the air fryer to 370°F. Use the parchment paper to transfer the salmon roast to the air fryer basket and tuck the ends of the paper down beside the salmon. Drizzle a little olive oil on top and season with salt and pepper.
4. Air-fry the salmon at 370°F for 20 minutes.
5. Remove the roast from the air fryer and let it rest for a few minutes. Then, slice it, sprinkle some more lemon zest and parsley (or fresh chives) on top and serve.

Crunchy Clam Strips

Servings:3

Cooking Time: 8 Minutes

Ingredients:

- ½ pound Clam strips, drained
- 1 Large egg, well beaten
- ½ cup All-purpose flour
- ½ cup Yellow cornmeal
- 1½ teaspoons Table salt

- 1½ teaspoons Ground black pepper
- Up to ¾ teaspoon Cayenne
- Vegetable oil spray

Directions:

1. Preheat the air fryer to 400°F.
2. Toss the clam strips and beaten egg in a bowl until the clams are well coated.
3. Mix the flour, cornmeal, salt, pepper, and cayenne in a large zip-closed plastic bag until well combined. Using a flatware fork or small kitchen tongs, lift the clam strips one by one out of the egg, letting any excess egg slip back into the rest. Put the strips in the bag with the flour mixture. Once all the strips are in the bag, seal it and shake gently until the strips are well coated.
4. Use kitchen tongs to pick out the clam strips and lay them on a cutting board (leaving any extra flour mixture in the bag to be discarded). Coat the strips on both sides with vegetable oil spray.
5. When the machine is at temperature, spread the clam strips in the basket in one layer. They may touch in places, but try to leave as much air space as possible around them. Air-fry undisturbed for 8 minutes, or until brown and crunchy.
6. Gently dump the contents of the basket onto a serving platter. Cool for just a minute or two before serving hot.

Italian Tuna Roast

Servings: 8

Cooking Time: 21 Minutes

Ingredients:

- cooking spray
- 1 tablespoon Italian seasoning
- ⅛ teaspoon ground black pepper
- 1 tablespoon extra-light olive oil
- 1 teaspoon lemon juice
- 1 tuna loin (approximately 2 pounds, 3 to 4 inches thick, large enough to fill a 6 x 6-inch baking dish)

Directions:

1. Spray baking dish with cooking spray and place in air fryer basket. Preheat air fryer to 390°F.
2. Mix together the Italian seasoning, pepper, oil, and lemon juice.
3. Using a dull table knife or butter knife, pierce top of tuna about every half inch: Insert knife into top of tuna roast and pierce almost all the way to the bottom.
4. Spoon oil mixture into each of the holes and use the knife to push seasonings into the tuna as deeply as possible.
5. Spread any remaining oil mixture on all outer surfaces of tuna.
6. Place tuna roast in baking dish and cook at 390°F for 20 minutes. Check temperature with a meat thermometer. Cook for an additional 1 minutes or until temperature reaches 145°F.
7. Remove basket from fryer and let tuna sit in basket for 10minutes.

Bacon-wrapped Scallops

Servings: 4

Cooking Time: 8 Minutes

Ingredients:

- 16 large scallops
- 8 bacon strips
- ½ teaspoon black pepper
- ¼ teaspoon smoked paprika

Directions:

1. Pat the scallops dry with a paper towel. Slice each of the bacon strips in half. Wrap 1 bacon strip around 1 scallop and secure with a toothpick. Repeat with the remaining scallops. Season the scallops with pepper and paprika.
2. Preheat the air fryer to 350°F.
3. Place the bacon-wrapped scallops in the air fryer basket and cook for 4 minutes, shake the basket, cook another 3 minutes, shake the basket, and cook another 1 to 3 to minutes. When the bacon is crispy, the scallops should be cooked through and slightly firm, but not rubbery. Serve immediately.

Firecracker Popcorn Shrimp

Servings: 6
Cooking Time: 8 Minutes

Ingredients:

- ½ cup all-purpose flour
- 2 teaspoons ground paprika
- 1 teaspoon garlic powder
- ½ teaspoon black pepper
- ¼ teaspoon salt
- 2 eggs, whisked
- 1½ cups panko breadcrumbs
- 1 pound small shrimp, peeled and deveined

Directions:

1. Preheat the air fryer to 360°F.
2. In a medium bowl, place the flour and mix in the paprika, garlic powder, pepper, and salt.
3. In a shallow dish, place the eggs.
4. In a third dish, place the breadcrumbs.
5. Assemble the shrimp by covering them in the flour, then dipping them into the egg, and then coating them with the breadcrumbs. Repeat until all the shrimp are covered in the breading.
6. Liberally spray the metal trivet that fits in the air fryer basket with olive oil mist. Place the shrimp onto the trivet, leaving space between the shrimp to flip. Cook for 4 minutes, flip the shrimp, and cook another 4 minutes. Repeat until all the shrimp are cooked.
7. Serve warm with desired dipping sauce.

Coconut Shrimp

Servings: 4
Cooking Time: 12 Minutes

Ingredients:

- 1 pound large shrimp (about 16 to 20), peeled and de-veined
- ½ cup flour
- salt and freshly ground black pepper
- 2 egg whites
- ½ cup fine breadcrumbs
- ½ cup shredded unsweetened coconut
- zest of one lime
- ½ teaspoon salt
- ⅛ to ¼ teaspoon ground cayenne pepper
- vegetable or canola oil
- sweet chili sauce or duck sauce (for serving)

Directions:

1. Set up a dredging station. Place the flour in a shallow dish and season well with salt and freshly ground black pepper. Whisk the egg whites in a second shallow dish. In a third shallow dish, combine the breadcrumbs, coconut, lime zest, salt and cayenne pepper.
2. Preheat the air fryer to 400°F.
3. Dredge each shrimp first in the flour, then dip it in the egg mixture, and finally press it into the breadcrumb-coconut mixture to coat all sides. Place the breaded shrimp on a plate or baking sheet and spray both sides with vegetable oil.
4. Air-fry the shrimp in two batches, being sure not to over-crowd the basket. Air-fry for 5 minutes, turning the shrimp over for the last minute or two. Repeat with the second batch of shrimp.
5. Lower the temperature of the air fryer to 340°F. Return the first batch of shrimp to the air fryer basket with the second batch and air-fry for an additional 2 minutes, just to re-heat everything.
6. Serve with sweet chili sauce, duck sauce or just eat them plain!

Lightened-up Breaded Fish Filets

Servings: 4
Cooking Time: 10 Minutes

Ingredients:

- ½ cup all-purpose flour
- ½ teaspoon cayenne pepper
- 1 teaspoon garlic powder
- ½ teaspoon black pepper
- ¼ teaspoon salt
- 2 eggs, whisked
- 1½ cups panko breadcrumbs
- 1 pound boneless white fish filets
- 1 cup tartar sauce
- 1 lemon, sliced into wedges

Directions:

1. In a medium bowl, mix the flour, cayenne pepper, garlic powder, pepper, and salt.

2. In a shallow dish, place the eggs.
3. In a third dish, place the breadcrumbs.
4. Cover the fish in the flour, dip them in the egg, and coat them with panko. Repeat until all fish are covered in the breading.
5. Liberally spray the metal trivet that fits inside the air fryer basket with olive oil mist. Place the fish onto the trivet, leaving space between the filets to flip. Cook for 5 minutes, flip the fish, and cook another 5 minutes. Repeat until all the fish is cooked.
6. Serve warm with tartar sauce and lemon wedges.

Curried Sweet-and-spicy Scallops

Servings:3

Cooking Time: 5 Minutes

Ingredients:

- 6 tablespoons Thai sweet chili sauce
- 2 cups (from about 5 cups cereal) Crushed Rice Krispies or other rice-puff cereal
- 2 teaspoons Yellow curry powder, purchased or homemade (see here)
- 1 pound Sea scallops
- Vegetable oil spray

Directions:

1. Preheat the air fryer to 400°F.
2. Set up and fill two shallow soup plates or small pie plates on your counter: one for the chili sauce and one for crumbs, mixed with the curry powder.
3. Dip a scallop into the chili sauce, coating it on all sides. Set it in the cereal mixture and turn several times to coat evenly. Gently shake off any excess and set the scallop on a cutting board. Continue dipping and coating the remaining scallops. Coat them all on all sides with the vegetable oil spray.
4. Set the scallops in the basket with as much air space between them as possible. Air-fry undisturbed for 5 minutes, or until lightly browned and crunchy.
5. Remove the basket. Set aside for 2 minutes to let the coating set up. Then gently pour the contents of the basket onto a platter and serve at once.

Fish And “chips”

Servings: 2

Cooking Time: 10 Minutes

Ingredients:

- ½ cup flour
- ½ teaspoon paprika
- ¼ teaspoon ground white pepper (or freshly ground black pepper)
- 1 egg
- ¼ cup mayonnaise
- 2 cups salt & vinegar kettle cooked potato chips, coarsely crushed
- 12 ounces cod
- tartar sauce
- lemon wedges

Directions:

1. Set up a dredging station. Combine the flour, paprika and pepper in a shallow dish. Combine the egg and mayonnaise in a second shallow dish. Place the crushed potato chips in a third shallow dish.
2. Cut the cod into 6 pieces. Dredge each piece of fish in the flour, then dip it into the egg mixture and then place it into the crushed potato chips. Make sure all sides of the fish are covered and pat the chips gently onto the fish so they stick well.
3. Preheat the air fryer to 370°F.
4. Place the coated fish fillets into the air fry basket. (It is ok if a couple of pieces slightly overlap or rest on top of other fillets in order to fit everything in the basket.)
5. Air-fry for 10 minutes, gently turning the fish over halfway through the cooking time.
6. Transfer the fish to a platter and serve with tartar sauce and lemon wedges.

Shrimp Po’boy With Remoulade Sauce

Servings: 6

Cooking Time: 8 Minutes

Ingredients:

- ½ cup all-purpose flour
- ½ teaspoon paprika
- 1 teaspoon garlic powder
- ½ teaspoon black pepper

- ¼ teaspoon salt
- 2 eggs, whisked
- 1½ cups panko breadcrumbs
- 1 pound small shrimp, peeled and deveined
- Six 6-inch French rolls
- 2 cups shredded lettuce
- 12 ⅛-inch tomato slices
- ¾ cup Remoulade Sauce (see the following recipe)

Directions:

1. Preheat the air fryer to 360°F.
2. In a medium bowl, mix the flour, paprika, garlic powder, pepper, and salt.
3. In a shallow dish, place the eggs.
4. In a third dish, place the panko breadcrumbs.
5. Covering the shrimp in the flour, dip them into the egg, and coat them with the breadcrumbs. Repeat until all shrimp are covered in the breading.
6. Liberally spray the metal trivet that fits inside the air fryer basket with olive oil spray. Place the shrimp onto the trivet, leaving space between the shrimp to flip. Cook for 4 minutes, flip the shrimp, and cook another 4 minutes. Repeat until all the shrimp are cooked.
7. Slice the rolls in half. Stuff each roll with shredded lettuce, tomato slices, breaded shrimp, and remoulade sauce. Serve immediately.

Coconut Jerk Shrimp

Servings:3

Cooking Time: 8 Minutes

Ingredients:

- 1 Large egg white(s)
- 1 teaspoon Purchased or homemade jerk dried seasoning blend (see the headnote)
- ¾ cup Plain panko bread crumbs (gluten-free, if a concern)
- ¾ cup Unsweetened shredded coconut
- 12 Large shrimp (20–25 per pound), peeled and deveined
- Coconut oil spray

Directions:

1. Preheat the air fryer to 375°F .
2. Whisk the egg white(s) and seasoning blend in a bowl until foamy. Add the shrimp and toss well to coat evenly.
3. Mix the bread crumbs and coconut on a dinner plate until well combined. Use kitchen tongs to pick up a shrimp, letting the excess egg white mixture slip back into the rest. Set the shrimp in the bread-crumb mixture. Turn several times to coat evenly and thoroughly. Set on a cutting board and continue coating the remainder of the shrimp.
4. Lightly coat all the shrimp on both sides with the coconut oil spray. Set them in the basket in one layer with as much space between them as possible. (You can even stand some up along the basket's wall in some models.) Air-fry undisturbed for 6 minutes, or until the coating is lightly browned. If the air fryer is at 360°F, you may need to add 2 minutes to the cooking time.
5. Use clean kitchen tongs to transfer the shrimp to a wire rack. Cool for only a minute or two before serving.

Crispy Smelts

Servings:3

Cooking Time: 20 Minutes

Ingredients:

- 1 pound Cleaned smelts
- 3 tablespoons Tapioca flour
- Vegetable oil spray
- To taste Coarse sea salt or kosher salt

Directions:

1. Preheat the air fryer to 400°F.
2. Toss the smelts and tapioca flour in a large bowl until the little fish are evenly coated.
3. Lay the smelts out on a large cutting board. Lightly coat both sides of each fish with vegetable oil spray.
4. When the machine is at temperature, set the smelts close together in the basket, with a few even overlapping on top. Air-fry undisturbed for 20 minutes, until lightly browned and crisp.
5. Remove the basket from the machine and turn out the fish onto a wire rack. The smelts will most likely come out as one large block, or maybe in a couple of large pieces. Cool for a minute or two, then sprinkle the smelts with salt and break the block(s) into much smaller sections or individual fish to serve.

Sweet Potato–wrapped Shrimp

Servings:3

Cooking Time: 6 Minutes

Ingredients:

- 24 Long spiralized sweet potato strands
- Olive oil spray
- ¼ teaspoon Garlic powder
- ¼ teaspoon Table salt
- Up to a ⅛ teaspoon Cayenne
- 12 Large shrimp (20–25 per pound), peeled and deveined

Directions:

1. Preheat the air fryer to 400°F.
2. Lay the spiralized sweet potato strands on a large swath of paper towels and straighten out the strands to long ropes. Coat them with olive oil spray, then sprinkle them with the garlic powder, salt, and cayenne.
3. Pick up 2 strands and wrap them around the center of a shrimp, with the ends tucked under what now becomes the bottom side of the shrimp. Continue wrapping the remainder of the shrimp.
4. Set the shrimp bottom side down in the basket with as much air space between them as possible. Air-fry undisturbed for 6 minutes, or until the sweet potato strands are crisp and the shrimp are pink and firm.
5. Use kitchen tongs to transfer the shrimp to a wire rack. Cool for only a minute or two before serving.

Super Crunchy Flounder Fillets

Servings:2

Cooking Time: 6 Minutes

Ingredients:

- ½ cup All-purpose flour or tapioca flour
- 1 Large egg white(s)
- 1 tablespoon Water
- ¾ teaspoon Table salt
- 1 cup Plain panko bread crumbs (gluten-free, if a concern)
- 2 4-ounce skinless flounder fillet(s)
- Vegetable oil spray

Directions:

1. Preheat the air fryer to 400°F.
2. Set up and fill three shallow soup plates or small pie plates on your counter: one for the flour; one for the egg white(s), beaten with the water and salt until foamy; and one for the bread crumbs.
3. Dip one fillet in the flour, turning it to coat both sides. Gently shake off any excess flour, then dip the fillet in the egg white mixture, turning it to coat. Let any excess egg white mixture slip back into the rest, then set the fish in the bread crumbs. Turn it several times, gently pressing it into the crumbs to create an even crust. Generously coat both sides of the fillet with vegetable oil spray. If necessary, set it aside and continue coating the remaining fillet(s) in the same way.
4. Set the fillet(s) in the basket. If working with more than one fillet, they should not touch, although they may be quite close together, depending on the basket's size. Air-fry undisturbed for 6 minutes, or until lightly browned and crunchy.
5. Use a nonstick-safe spatula to transfer the fillet(s) to a wire rack. Cool for only a minute or two before serving.

Blackened Catfish

Servings: 4

Cooking Time: 8 Minutes

Ingredients:

- 1 teaspoon paprika
- 1 teaspoon garlic powder
- 1 teaspoon onion powder
- 1 teaspoon ground dried thyme
- ½ teaspoon ground black pepper
- ⅛ teaspoon cayenne pepper
- ½ teaspoon dried oregano
- ⅛ teaspoon crushed red pepper flakes
- 1 pound catfish filets
- ½ teaspoon sea salt
- 2 tablespoons butter, melted

- 1 tablespoon extra-virgin olive oil
- 2 tablespoons chopped parsley
- 1 lemon, cut into wedges

Directions:

1. In a small bowl, stir together the paprika, garlic powder, onion powder, thyme, black pepper, cayenne pepper, oregano, and crushed red pepper flakes.
2. Pat the fish dry with paper towels. Season the filets with sea salt and then coat with the blackening seasoning.
3. In a small bowl, mix together the butter and olive oil and drizzle over the fish filets, flipping them to coat them fully.
4. Preheat the air fryer to 350°F.
5. Place the fish in the air fryer basket and cook for 8 minutes, checking the fish for doneness after 4 minutes. The fish will flake easily when cooked.
6. Remove the fish from the air fryer. Top with chopped parsley and serve with lemon wedges.

Recipe Index

I

J

K

L

M

N

O

P

Q

R

S

T